Clinical Approach to Jaundice

Clinical Approach to Jaundice

Edited by

RAKESH TANDON

S.K. ACHARYA

On behalf of

The Indian College of Physicians

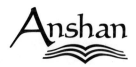

© Rakesh Tandon, S.K. Acharya, 2004

First published in 2004 by Byword Viva Publishers Private Limited
New Delhi, India. e-mail: bywordviva@yahoo.co.uk

and co-published by

ANSHAN LIMITED
6 Newlands Road, Tunbridge Wells, Kent. TN4 9AT. UK
Tel/Fax: +44(o)1892 557767
e-mail: info@anshan.co.uk
Web site: www.anshan.co.uk

Every effort has been made to check drug dosages in this book,
however it is still possible that errors have occurred. Also dosage
schedules are constantly being revised and new side-effects
recognized. For these reasons the reader is urged to consult drug
manufacturers' printed instructions, particularly the recommended
dose, advice on administration and adverse reactions before
administering any of the drugs recommended in this book.

British Library Cataloguing in Publication Data
A catalogue record for this book is available from the British Library

Not for sale in India, Pakistan, Nepal, Sri Lanka and Bangladesh

ISBN 1-904798-09-8

Project Editor: Swati Sharma
Copy Editior: Nimrat D. Khandpur
Illustrator and Typesetter: Harjeet Kaur Chhatwal
Cover Design: Terence Griffiths

Printed in India by Sanat Printers Private Limited

Foreword

The past couple of years have witnessed spectacular advances in the field of jaundice, both in terms of enhanced understanding and the availability of a rich panoply of therapeutic options. The access to superb, non-invasive techniques of investigation, such as ultrasonography, computerized tomography (CT), magnetic resonance imaging (MRI), etc. coupled with invasive investigations in selected cases, has enabled gastroenterologists and physicians to evaluate patients with jaundice with great precision.

This monograph on jaundice will be of immense help not only for gastroenterologists and physicians but also specialists from other medical disciplines such as radiologists, surgeons, obstetricians, paediatricians, oncologists, pathologists and nutritionists.

The efforts of the editors Drs Rakesh Tandon and S.K. Acharya in unifying diverse aspects of jaundice in a concise monograph are laudable. I am sure this book will find a permanent place on the desks of gastroenterologists, physicians and other members of the medical fraternity.

P.C. MANORIA
Dean
Indian College of Physicians

Bhopal
May 2004

Preface

Jaundice is a common symptom that occurs in a variety of hepatobiliary and haematological disorders. In addition, a wide spectrum of pathophysiological processes may cause hyperbilirubinaemia, which presents with only jaundice without any other associated clinical manifestation, and often poses a diagnostic dilemma. A comprehensive, rational and clinical approach to jaundice is thus a necessity for most physicians. Unfortunately, however, no book or compendium presenting such a clinical approach was available till date. It is to fill this lacuna that the Indian College of Physicians decided to produce a monograph on the *Clinical Approach to Jaundice* and we were assigned the job. In this monograph, we have attempted to present a format that would help physicians to adopt logical diagnostic and management alogrithms in their clinical practice.

The book starts with a step-by-step diagnostic approach to the evaluation of jaundice. Hepatitis, biliary tract diseases, systemic infections, haematological diseases, drugs, liver tumours have all been discussed in this monograph with a 'new look', considering jaundice as the dominant clinical manifestation. The book also contains a chapter on various diagnostic and 'state-of-the-art' treatment schedules in each of these disease states.

Histopathology of the liver and nutritional management in jaundice are unique features of this book. These chapters highlight the common principles of diagnosis and management of apparently dissimilar conditions in a cohesive manner.

Eminent gastroenterologists and hepatologists have contributed to this book by providing their insights into individual conditions associated with jaundice. They are experts with years of experience in clinical problem-solving and research in the respective areas on which they have contributed to this book.

We, the editors and the Indian College of Physicians, would feel satisfied if this book does indeed assist physicians to help the numerous patients presenting to them with jaundice.

RAKESH TANDON
S.K. ACHARYA

New Delhi
May 2004

Contents

Contributors

S.K. ACHARYA
Department of Gastroenterology
and Human Nutrition
All India Institute of
Medical Sciences
New Delhi

N. AGARWAL
Department of Gastroenterology
SMS Hospital and Medical College
Jaipur

A.C. ANAND
Department of Gastroenterology
Army Hospital R&R and
Base Hospital, Armed Forces
Medical Services
New Delhi

ANIL ARORA
Department of Gastroenterology
Sir Ganga Ram Hospital
New Delhi

RUPA BANERJEE
Department of Gastroenterology
Asian Institute of Gastroenterology
Hyderabad

JAYA BENJAMIN
Department of Gastroenterology
and Human Nutrition
All India Institute of
Medical Sciences
New Delhi

Y.K. CHAWLA
Department of Gastroenterology
Postgraduate Institute of Medical
Education and Research
Chandigarh

GOURDAS CHOUDHURI
Department of Gastroenterology
Sanjay Gandhi Postgraduate
Institute of Medical Sciences
Lucknow

S. DATTA GUPTA
Department of Pathology
All India Institute of
Medical Sciences
New Delhi

USHA DUTTA
Department of Gastroenterology
Postgraduate Institute of Medical
Education and Research
Chandigarh

MANISHA DWIVEDI
Department of Gastroenterology
Moti Lal Nehru Medical College
Allahabad

PRAMOD KUMAR GARG
Department of Gastroenterology
All India Institute of
Medical Sciences
New Delhi

DEEPAK GOVIL
Department of GI Surgery
Pushpawati Singhania Research
Institute for Liver, Renal and
Digestive Diseases
New Delhi

MANPREET S. GULATI
Department of Radiodiagnosis
All India Institute of
Medical Sciences
New Delhi

ANIL JAIN
Department of Medicine
Maulana Azad Medical College
New Delhi

SANJAY JAIN
Department of Gastroenterology
Sir Ganga Ram Hospital
New Delhi

Y.K. JOSHI
Department of Gastroenterology
and Human Nutrition
All India Institute of
Medical Sciences
New Delhi

P. KAR
Department of Medicine
Maulana Azad Medical College
New Delhi

MANDHIR KUMAR
Department of Gastroenterology
Sir Ganga Ram Hospital
New Delhi

MANOJ KUMAR
Department of Gastroenterology
GB Pant Hospital
New Delhi

ARUN KUNDRA
Department of Medicine
Maulana Azad Medical College
New Delhi

K. MADAN
Department of Gastroenterology
and Human Nutrition
All India Institute of
Medical Sciences
New Delhi

SRI PRAKASH MISRA
Department of Gastroenterology
Moti Lal Nehru Medical College
Allahabad

S. MUKHOPADHYAY
Department of Pathology
All India Institute of
Medical Sciences
New Delhi

S. NIJHAWAN
Department of Gastroenterology
SMS Hospital and Medical College
Jaipur

SHASHI B. PAUL
Department of Radiodiagnosis
All India Institute of
Medical Sciences
New Delhi

RAJESH PURI
Department of Gastroenterology
Sir Ganga Ram Hospital
New Delhi

P. PURI
Department of Gastroenterology
Army Hospital R&R and
Base Hospital
Armed Forces Medical Services
New Delhi

R.R. RAI
Department of Gastroenterology
SMS Hospital and Medical College
Jaipur

S.K. SARIN
Department of Gastroenterology
GB Pant Hospital
New Delhi

SANJEEV SACHDEVA
Department of Gastroenterology
Sanjay Gandhi Postgraduate
Institute of Medical Sciences
Lucknow

VIVEK A. SARASWAT
Department of Gastroenterology
Sanjay Gandhi Postgraduate
Institute of Medical Sciences
Lucknow

MALATHI SATHIYASEKARAN
Department of Gastroenterology
KKCTH and SMF Hospitals
Chennai

M.P. SHARMA
Department of Gastroenterology
and Human Nutrition
All India Institute of
Medical Sciences
New Delhi

DINESH KUMAR SINGAL
Department of Gastroenterology
Pushpawati Singhania Research
Institute for Liver, Renal and
Digestive Diseases
New Delhi

S.S. SIDDHU
Division of Gastroenterology
Department of Medicine
Dayanand Medical College
and Hospital
Ludhiana

RANDHIR SUD
Department of Gastroenterology
Sir Ganga Ram Hospital
New Delhi

RAKESH TANDON
Department of Gastroenterology
Pushpawati Singhania Research
Institute for Liver, Renal and
Digestive Diseases
New Delhi

Abbreviations

3D CTC min IP	Three-dimensional computerized tomographic cholangiography with minimum intensity projection	BSP	bromosulphthalein
		BUN	blood urea nitrogen
		CAVH	continuous arteriovenous haemodialysis
5' NT	5'-nucleotidase	CBC	complete blood counts
AAA	aromatic amino acids	CBD	common bile duct
ADH	alcohol dehydrogenase	CCA	cholangiocarcinoma
AE	alveolar echinococcosis	CDS	clinical diagnostic scale
AFP	alpha-fetoprotein	CE	cystic echinococcosis
AHF	acute hepatic failure	CEA	carcinoembryonic antigen
AIDS	acquired immune deficiency syndrome	CECT	contrast-enhanced computed tomography
AIH	autoimmune hepatitis	CLD	chronic liver disease
ALA	amoebic liver abscess	cMOAT	canalicular multispecific anion transporter
ALD	alcoholic liver disease		
ALDH	aldehyde dehydrogenase	CMV	cytomegalovirus
ALF	acute liver failure	COPD	chronic obstructive pulmonary disease
ALP	alkaline phosphatase		
ALS	artificial liver support	CSF	cerebrospinal fluid
ALT	alanine aminotransferase	CT	computerized tomography
AMA	antimitochondrial antibodies	CTC	computerized tomographic cholangiography
ANA	antinuclear antibodies		
APTT	activated partial thromboplastin time	CTL	cytotoxic T lymphocytes
		CTP	Child–Turcotte–Pugh
ARDS	adult respiratory distress syndrome	CUC	chronic ulcerative colitis
		CVH	chronic viral hepatitis
ARF	acute renal failure	CVP	central venous pressure
ASGPR	asialoglycoprotein receptor	CVS	cardiovascular system
ASMA	anti-smooth muscle antibodies	CVVH	continuous venovenous haemodialysis
AST	aspartate aminotransferase	CYP2E1	cytochrome P450 2E1
ATP	adenosine triphosphate	DD	death domain
AVH	acute viral hepatitis	DIC	disseminated intravascular coagulation
BA	biliary atresia		
BCAA	branched-chain amino acids	DILD	drug-induced liver disease
BCG	bacillus Calmette–Guérin	DPG	diphosphoglycerate
BDG	bilirubin diglucuronide	ds	double-stranded
BMG	bilirubin monoglucuronide	EAA	essential amino acids
BMI	body mass index	EASLD	European Association for the Study of Liver Diseases
BSEP	bile salt export pump		

EBV	Epstein–Barr virus	HEV	hepatitis E virus
EHBA	extrahepatic biliary atresia	HGV	hepatitis G virus
EHPVO	extrahepatic portal vein obstruction	HIDA	hepatobiliary scan with an iminodiacetic acid
EIA	enzyme-linked immunoassay	HIV	human immunodeficiency virus
ELISA	enzyme-linked immunosorbent assay	HLA	human leucocyte antigen
ERC	endoscopic retrograde cholangiography	HPA	hepatobiliary and pancreatic ascariasis
ERCP	endoscopic retrograde cholangiopancreaticography	HRP	histidine-rich protein
		HRS	hepatorenal syndrome
ESPEN	European Association for Parenteral and Enteral Nutrition	HSV	herpes simplex virus
		HV	hepatic vein
		HVOTO	hepatic venous outflow tract obstruction
ESR	erythrocyte sedimentation rate	HVPG	hepatic vein pressure gradient
EUS	endoscopic ultrasound		
FAD	flavin adenine dinucleotide	IASL	International Association for the Study of the Liver
FFP	fresh frozen plasma		
FHF	fulminant hepatic failure	ICP	intracranial pressure
FNAC	fine-needle aspiration cytology	ICU	intensive care unit
		IDA	iminodiacetic acid
FNH	focal nodular hyperplasia	IFN	interferon
FSE	fast-spin echocardiography	IHA	indirect haemagglutination
GBV	GB virus	Ig	immunoglobulin
G6PD	glucose-6-phosphate dehydrogenase	IHBR	intrahepatic biliary radicle
		IL	interleukin
GABA	gamma amino butyric acid	IMD	inherited metabolic disorders
GGT	gamma-glutamyl transpeptidase		
		INH	idiopathic neonatal hepatitis
GI	gastrointestinal	INR	international normalized ratio
GVHD	graft-versus-host disease	IOUS	intraoperative ultrasonography
H&E	haematoxylin and eosin		
HAART	highly active antiretroviral therapy	IUGR	intrauterine growth retardation
HAI	histological activity index	KF	Kayser–Fleischer
HASTE	half-Fourier turbo-spin echocardiography	LCHAD	long chain 3-hydroxyl CoA dehydrogenase
HAV	hepatitis A virus	LDH	lactose dehydrogenase
HBcAg	hepatitis B c antigen	LFT	liver function tests
HBeAg	hepatitis B e antigen	LKM	liver kidney microsome
HBIG	hepatitis B immune globulin	LOHF	late-onset hepatic failure
HBsAg	hepatitis B s antigen	LP	liver–pancreas
HBV	hepatitis B virus	MARS	molecular adsorbents recirculating system
HCC	hepatocellular carcinoma		
HCV	hepatitis C virus	MCT	medium-chain triglycerides
HD	Hodgkin disease	MM	multiple myeloma
HDL	high-density lipoprotein	MRC	magnetic resonance cholangiography
HDV	hepatitis D virus		
HE	hepatic encephalopathy	MRCP	magnetic resonance cholangiopancreaticography
HELLP	haemolysis, elevated liver enzymes and low platelets		

MRI	magnetic resonance imaging	RBF	renal blood flow
MRP	multidrug resistance-associated protein	RFA	radiofrequency ablation
		RIA	radioimmunoassay
MTBE	methyl-tert-butyl-ether	RIBA	recombinant immunoblot assay
NAD	nicotinamide dinucleotide		
NAFLD	non-alcoholic fatty liver disease	RPC	recurrent pyogenic cholangitis
NANE	non-A, non-E	RT	reverse transcription
NASH	non-alcoholic steatohepatitis	SAM-e	S-adenosyl methionine
NCS	neonatal cholestasis syndrome	SEN-V	SEN virus
		SENSE	sensitivity encoding
NF	nuclear factor	SHF	subacute hepatic failure
NF-κB	nuclear factor kappa B	SMA	smooth muscle antibodies
NHL	non-Hodgkin lymphoma	SMASH	simultaneous acquisition of spatial harmonics
NK	natural killer		
NNH	neonatal hapatitis	SOLs	space-occupying lesions
NTCP	sodium taurocholate co-transporter	SPECT	single-photon emission computed tomography
NSAIDs	non-steroidal anti-inflammatory drugs	ss	single-stranded
		TGF	transforming growth factor
OATP	organic anion-transporting polypeptide	TLC	total leucocyte count
		TNF	tumour necrosis factor
OLT	orthotopic liver transplantation	TORCH	toxoplasma, rubella, cytomegalovirus, herpesvirus
OPD	outpatient department	TPN	total parenteral nutrition
ORF	open reading frames	TSS	toxic shock syndrome
OT	oxaloacetic transaminase	TTV	TT virus
PAS	periodic acid Schiff	TyPICAL	Tolerance, Physical dependence, Impaired Control or craving for ALcohol
PBC	primary biliary cirrhosis		
PBD	percutaneous biliary drainage		
PC	percutaneous cholecystostomy	UCB	unconjugated bilirubin
		UDCA	ursodeoxycholic acid
PCA	patient-controlled analgesia	UDP	uridine diphosphate
PCR	polymerase chain reaction	UDPG	uridine diphosphoglucuronyl transferase
PCT	porphyria cutanea tarda		
PFIC	progressive familial intrahepatic cholestasis	UGI	upper gastrointestinal
		UGT	uridine glucuronyl transferase
PIBD	paucity of the intrahepatic bile ducts	ULN	upper limit of normal
		USG	ultrasonography
PPN	partial parenteral nutrition	UTI	urinary tract infection
PSC	primary sclerosing cholangitis	VBDS	vanishing bile duct syndrome
PT	prothrombin time	VOD	veno-occlusive disease
PTBD	percutaneous transhepatic biliary drainage	VZV	Varicella zoster
		WBC	white blood cell
PTC	percutaneous transhepatic cholangiography	WM	Waldenström macroglobulinaemia
PTT	partial thromboplastin time	YMDD	tyrosine–methionine–aspartate–aspartate
RAI	rejection activity index		
RBC	red blood cell		

CHAPTER 1

Introduction to jaundice

RAKESH TANDON, S.K. ACHARYA

Jaundice (icterus) is the most important and visible symptom of hepatobiliary disorders. The term jaundice indicates yellow discoloration of the sclera, mucous membranes, skin and nail beds. Such yellow discoloration of various body tissues is due to hyperbilirubinaemia, which has innumerable causes and its optimal management has been a challenge for clinicians since centuries.

During the past few decades, the elucidation and understanding of bilirubin metabolism, and easy access to various biochemical and imaging techniques have made it possible to identify the underlying pathogenetic process causing jaundice. On the other hand, sophisticated and powerful investigative techniques, unless used judiciously, may expose a patient to unnecessary discomfort, risk and cost. Therefore, a rational approach to a patient with jaundice requires optimal selection of diagnostic and therapeutic techniques based on meticulous clinical assessment of the probable pathogenetic process causing jaundice. This would provide a definitive diagnosis of the cause of jaundice in most patients.

BILIRUBIN METABOLISM

Bilirubin is a tetrapyrrole end-product of haem degradation. Approximately 4 mg/kg of bilirubin is produced daily, 70% of which is derived from haemoglobin degradation in senescent erythrocytes and newly formed erythrocytes in the bone narrow or circulation (ineffective erythropoiesis). The remaining bilirubin is derived from the breakdown of non-haemoglobin haemoproteins in the liver such as catalase and cytochrome oxidases.

The degradation of haem to bilirubin is a two-step process. Initially, the haem is broken down to biliverdin by the microsomal enzyme haem oxygenase and subsequently biliverdin is converted to bilirubin by a cytosolic enzyme biliverdin reductase. This catabolism of haemoglobin to bilirubin occurs in macrophages in the spleen, liver and bone marrow. Bilirubin then gets converted

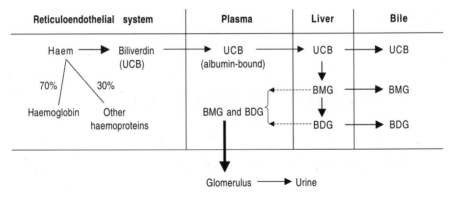

Fig. 1. Bilirubin metabolism
UCB: unconjugated bilirubin; BMG: bilirubin monoglucuronide; BDG: bilirubin diglucuronide

to water-soluble conjugates in the liver and is secreted in the bile. Bilirubin metabolism and elimination is a multi-step process. An inherited or acquired disorder interfering at any step of the bilirubin metabolism may cause hyper-bilirubinaemia and jaundice. Figure 1 shows the details of bilirubin metabolism.

Bilirubin from the blood is transferred to the hepatocyte across its basolateral (sinusoidal) surface by a carrier protein, organic anion transport polypeptide-2 (OATP-2). Inside the cytosol of the hepatocyte, cytosolic binding proteins (e.g. ligands, fatty acid binding proteins) direct the bilirubin to the endoplasmic reticulum where it is converted to bilirubin mono- and diglucuronides (BMG, BDG) with the help of an enzyme uridine diphosphoglucuronyl transferase (UDPG). BMG and BDG are water-soluble substances that get excreted through the apical (canalicular) membrane of the hepatocytes into the bile canaliculus by an adenosine triphosphate (ATP)-dependent pump which is a peptide and is known as multidrug resistance-associated protein 2 (MRP2), which also transports many other organic anions such as bromosulphthalein (BSP). Approximately 80% of the bilirubin gets excreted as BDG and a small amount gets excreted as BMG and unconjugated bilirubin. Reabsorption of bile through the gallbladder and intestine is negligible. However, bilirubin is deconjugated by bacterial enzymes in the terminal ileum and colon, and gets converted to colourless tetrapyrrols such as urobilinogens. About 20% of urobilinogens are absorbed and excreted in the urine.

The normal bilirubin concentration in the serum of an adult is <1.5 mg/dl, and <5% of circulating bilirubin is present in the conjugated form. Jaundice becomes evident when the level of serum bilirubin is >3 mg/dl. Usually, estimation of serum bilirubin is expressed as direct (conjugated), indirect (unconjugated) and total bilirubin.

DIFFERENTIAL DIAGNOSIS OF JAUNDICE

Jaundice occurs either due to increase in bilirubin formation or decrease in hepatic clearance. Causes of jaundice can be broadly categorized into three:

1. Isolated disorders of bilirubin metabolism
2. Liver diseases
3. Obstruction of the intra- or extrahepatic bile ducts.

Isolated disorders of bilirubin metabolism include various inherited or acquired conditions leading to unconjugated or conjugated hyperbilirubinaemia. Table I shows the causes, pathogenetic processes and interpretation of various investigations for unconjugated hyperbilirubinaemia and Table II gives the causes, mechanisms and investigations for conjugated hyperbilirubinaemia.

A general alogrithm for evaluating a patient with jaundice is given in Chapter 2. However, the sequential approach essentially involves the following three steps:

1. Clinical evaluation and screening laboratory tests (LFT, haemogram and USG) to differentiate between various categories of jaundice as described earlier;
2. Formulation of a working differential diagnosis under each category of hyperbilirubinaemia. The specific tests used in such patients include various serological tests for hepatitis viruses, autoantibodies, copper and iron metabolism, liver histology, imaging techniques such as MRI/CT scan, cholangiography, etc.;
3. Consideration of intervention strategies.

Table I. Causes, mechanisms and investigations in unconjugated hyperbilirubinaemia

Causes	Mechanisms	Investigations

Increased bilirubin production	• Haemolytic anaemias
	• Ineffective erythropoiesis
	  — Vitamin B_{12}/folate deficiency
	  — Sideroblastic anaemia
	  — Massive transfusion
	  — Polycythaemia vera
	• Large haematoma
		• Serum bilirubin <5 mg/dl
		• Normal AST/ALT/serum ALP
		• Low haemoglobin
		• Characteristic clinical picture
		• Normal urine colour
		• ↑Urobilinogin in urine

Decreased bilirubin uptake and conjugation	• Drugs
	  Rifampicin—competitive inhibition of bilirubin uptake
	• Gilbert syndrome
	  Relative deficiency in UDPG (UGT-1 gene mutation)
	• Crigler–Najjar syndromes types I and II
	  UGT-1 activity absent (UDPG very low or absent)
	• Physiological jaundice of the newborn
	  Delayed UGT-1 gene expression (UDPG production delayed)
		• Serum bilirubin <5 mg/dl (marked rise in the Crigler–Najjar syndrome type II and physiological jaundice)
		• AST:ALT normal
		• Haemoglobin normal

UDPG: uridine diphosphoglucuronyl transferase; UGT: uridine glucuronyl transferase

Table II. Causes, mechanisms and investigations in conjugated hyperbilirubinaemia

Causes	Mechanisms	Investigations
Inherited disorders	• Dubin–Johnson syndrome (DJS) and Rotor syndrome —Absence of multidrug resistance-associated protein 2 (MRP2) peptide on canalicular membrane	• Serum bilirubin: 5–15 mg/dl • ALT/AST/serum ALP normal • BSP excretion decreased in DJS • Liver biopsy—centrizonal lipofuscin pigments
Liver disease	• Acute viral hepatitis (A–E) • Drug/toxin-induced liver injury • Alcoholic hepatitis • Hepatic venous outflow tract obstruction (HVOTO) • Ischaemic liver injury • Interited disorders such as Wilson disease	• Serum bilirubin >5 mg/dl • Abnormal hepatic enzymes • Specific tests for hepatitis virus/Wilson disease/HVOTO are diagnostic

Cholestatic disease	• Obstructive jaundice
	  —Due to mechanical obstruction of the bile ducts (e.g. choledocholithiasis, carcinoma of the pancreas, carcinoma of the gallbladder, ampullary cancer, biliary strictures)
	• Intrahepatic cholestasis
	  —Hepatitis virus
	  —Drugs
	  —Bile duct diseases such as primary biliary cirrhosis, primary sclerosing cholangitis, vanishing bile duct syndrome
	  —Cholestasis of pregnancy
	  —Benign recurrent intrahepatic cholestasis
	  —Total parenteral nutrition
		• Serum bilirubin >10 mg/dl
		• Serum ALP ↑↑
		• Characteristic imaging and histology
		• Characteristic serology

A thorough clinical examination, LFT and USG usually provide definitive diagnosis in two-thirds of jaundiced patients. More sophisticated and specialized investigations may be needed in the remaining. The following chapters discuss the specific situations and necessary diagnostic approaches for jaundice.

CHAPTER 2

Diagnostic approach to jaundice

A.C. ANAND, P. PURI

Jaundice is a common feature of both acute and chronic liver diseases as well as disorders of a non-hepatic origin. The word 'jaundice' comes from the French word *jaune,* which means yellow. Jaundice is characterized by yellow discoloration of the skin, sclera and mucous membranes due to elevated serum bilirubin levels. Jaundice can be recognized clinically at serum bilirubin levels of 3 mg/dl or more. Besides a rise in the bilirubin level, yellowness of the skin can be due to carotenoderma, use of the drug quinacrine and excessive exposure to phenols. Carotenoderma is due to the overingestion of carotene; in this condition, the pigment is deposited mainly on the palms, soles and nasolabial folds with sparing of the sclera.[1,2]

Jaundice can occur in four different ways. First, there may be an increased bilirubin load as in haemolysis. Second, there may be a disturbance in the hepatic uptake and transport of bilirubin within the hepatocytes. Third, there may be defects in conjugation and, finally, there may be defects in the excretion of conjugated bilirubin across the canalicular cell membrane or an obstruction of the large biliary channels. Table I gives the differential diagnosis of jaundice.

HISTORY

A detailed history and clinical examination provide vital clues towards the aetiology of jaundice. The onset of jaundice in viral hepatitis is associated with a prodrome of anorexia, nausea, vomiting, malaise and myalgia. The onset of cholestasis, on the other hand, is insidious. A history of acute viral hepatitis (AVH) in the family, intravenous drug use or transfusion of blood products suggest the possibility of AVH. A history of fever with chills and rigors, or right upper abdominal pain or a past history of biliary surgery would suggest cholangitis. Cholestasis is associated with pruritus and clay-coloured stools. On the other hand, dark urine and pale stools exclude the possibility of haemolytic jaundice. A history of multiple sex partners, travel, ethanol intake,

Table I. Differential diagnosis of jaundice

Mechanism	Type of jaundice	Cause of jaundice
Isolated elevation of serum bilirubin	Unconjugated hyperbilirubinaemia	• Increased bilirubin production (e.g. haemolysis), ineffective erythropoiesis, resorption of haematomas • Decreased hepatocellular uptake (e.g. rifampicin) • Decreased conjugation (e.g. Gilbert syndrome, Crigler–Najjar syndrome)
	Conjugated hyperbilirubinaemia	• Dubin–Johnson syndrome • Rotor syndrome
Hepatocellular jaundice	Acute or subacute hepatocellular injury	Viral hepatitis, alcohol, drugs, ischaemic hepatitis, Wilson disease, acute fatty liver of pregnancy
	Chronic hepato-cellular disease	Viral hepatitis, alcoholic liver disease, autoimmune hepatitis, haemochromatosis, Wilson disease, non-alcoholic steatohepatitis, α_1-antitrypsin deficiency
	Hepatic disorders with prominent cholestasis	• Diffuse infiltrative disorders (e.g. granulomatous diseases such as mycobacterial infections, sarcoidosis, lymphoma, drugs), amyloidosis, malignancy • Inflammation of the intrahepatic bile ductules and/or portal tracts (e.g. primary biliary cirrhosis), graft-versus-host disease, drugs (e.g. chlorpromazine) • Miscellaneous, such as benign recurrent intrahepatic cholestasis, use of oestrogens and steroids, total parenteral nutrition, bacterial infections, paraneoplastic syndromes, intrahepatic cholestasis of pregnancy, postoperative cholestasis
Obstruction of the bile ducts	Benign	Choledocholithiasis, primary sclerosing cholangitis, AIDS cholangiopathy, postsurgical strictures, pancreatitis
	Malignant	Carcinoma gallbladder, periampullary carcinoma, cholangiocarcinoma, carcinoma of the head of the pancreas

drugs, blood transfusion, needlestick exposure and tattooing is also important. Previous biliary surgery with subsequent jaundice may suggest strictures, residual stones or hepatitis. A family history of jaundice or liver disease suggests the possibility of hereditary hyperbilirubinaemia or a genetic disorder such as Wilson disease. Table II outlines the important points to be considered while taking the history of a patient with jaundice.

PHYSICAL EXAMINATION

Stigmata of chronic liver disease, ascites and encephalopathy suggest that the jaundice is hepatocellular in origin. High fever and right upper abdominal tenderness suggest a diagnosis of cholangitis and choledocholithiasis, while a palpable abdominal mass suggests a malignant obstructive jaundice. A right upper abdominal scar or palpable gallbladder suggests obstructive jaundice. Certain physical findings may suggest a particular liver disease, such as the hyperpigmentation of haemochromatosis, xanthomas of primary biliary cirrhosis and Kayser–Fleischer (KF) rings of Wilson disease. A systemic illness should be excluded, e.g. distended jugular veins in constrictive pericarditis or right

Table II. Important points to be considered while taking the history of a patient with jaundice

Duration of jaundice

Previous attacks of jaundice

Weight loss

Colour of urine and stool

History of unconjugated hyperbilirubinaemia/haemolysis
- Normal coloured urine/cola colour in haemolysis
- Recurrent episodes
- Recurrent anaemia
- No prodrome/cholestatic features

History suggestive of viral hepatitis/drug-induced hepatitis
- Contact with other jaundiced patients
- History of injections or blood transfusions
- Exposure to drugs
- Prodrome of anorexia, nausea, vomiting

History suggestive of cholestasis
- Pruritius
- Clay-coloured stools

History suggestive of bile duct stones/cholangitis/obstructive jaundice
- Pain
- Chills, fever, systemic symptoms
- Biliary surgery

---

heart failure in a patient with hepatomegaly and ascites. A hard nodular liver may be due to primary or secondary malignancy. Diffuse lymphadenopathy may suggest infectious mononucleosis or lymphoma as the aetiology.

LABORATORY, RADIOLOGICAL AND HISTOLOGICAL EVALUATION

The liver is a complex organ with numerous metabolic and excretory functions, and no single test can assess the overall hepatic function. Thus, a number of laboratory tests are usually combined to detect liver dysfunction, assess its severity and determine the aetiology. In most cases, the aetiology can be established by simple non-invasive tests, but many patients require referral to a specialist for management of the disease.[3] Radiological imaging techniques and liver biopsy often provide essential diagnostic information; however, their use should be tailored to the specific clinical circumstances.

SERUM BIOCHEMICAL TESTS

Bilirubin

In adults, the normal serum bilirubin concentration is <1.5 mg/dl,[4] of which <5% is in the conjugated form. The serum bilirubin level is measured by the van den Bergh reaction. While the conjugated bilirubin reacts quickly, the unconjugated fraction requires the addition of ethanol or urea as an 'accelerator' to allow its reaction with the diazo reagent.[5] In haemolysis or genetic disorders such as Gilbert syndrome, there is unconjugated hyperbilirubinaemia (over 90% of circulating bilirubin is unconjugated), while in hepatocellular or obstructive jaundice, the bilirubin is conjugated (over 50% of circulating bilirubin is conjugated). The degree of elevation of serum bilirubin often correlates poorly with clinical severity. Unconjugated bilirubin is not excreted in the urine and thus in unconjugated hyperbilirubinaemia, bilirubin is absent in the urine.

Serum enzymes

Enzymes raised in hepatocellular injury

Aminotransferases include alanine aminotransferase (ALT), located primarily in liver cytosol, and aspartate aminotransferase (AST), which is also a mitochondrial enzyme. ALT is found mainly in the liver while AST is also found in other tissues such as skeletal and cardiac muscle. ALT is more specific than AST in detecting liver disease. AST and ALT are released following hepatocyte injury/necrosis. A marked rise in serum transaminases, with levels >1000 U/L, is seen in AVH, ischaemic hepatitis and drug-induced liver disease. On the other hand, in alcoholic liver disease, the enzyme levels are rarely >200–300 U/L, with an AST:ALT ratio >2:1.[3]

Enzymes raised in cholestasis

These include alkaline phosphatase (ALP), gamma-glutamyl transpeptidase (GGT) and 5'-nucleotidase (5' NT). ALP isoenzymes are also present in the bone and placenta. If the source of an isolated increase in ALP is not clinically clear, a concomitant elevation of GGT or 5' NT indicates a hepatobiliary origin. GGT levels are often disproportionately elevated in alcoholic liver disease.

Proteins

Albumin

Albumin is synthesized by the liver and has a half-life of 15–20 days. Decreased levels of albumin are seen in advanced cirrhosis and signify severe hepatic dysfunction. The serum albumin level usually remains normal in acute hepatitis; falling values in this setting imply an unusually severe course.

Globulins

Non-specific diffuse elevation is common in chronic liver disease. There is a disproportionate elevation of IgG in autoimmune hepatitis, IgM in primary biliary cirrhosis and IgA in alcoholic liver disease.

International normalized ratio and prothrombin time

The international normalized ratio (INR)/PT is a valuable index of the ability of the liver to synthesize vitamin K-dependent clotting factors. An increasing INR/PT implies relatively severe hepatocellular dysfunction. The INR/PT may be deranged in cholestasis as well, but this is due to the malabsorption of vitamin K and is rapidly corrected by the parenteral administration of vitamin K.

Other tests

Other tests include the serological/replicative markers appropriate for the specific diagnosis of acute or chronic viral hepatitis: antimitochondrial antibody for primary biliary cirrhosis; antinuclear factor, anti-smooth muscle antibody and anti-liver kidney microsome (LKM) antibody seen in autoimmune hepatitis; alpha-fetoprotein, which is raised in hepatocellular carcinoma; and serum caeruloplasmin for Wilson disease.

IMAGING PROCEDURES

The preferred order for imaging tests cannot be fixed and varies not only with the setting of an individual patient but also with the facilities and practices of the institution. In general, radiological imaging (in some cases radiology-guided fine-needle aspiration cytology [FNAC]) is important for the diagnosis of a focal liver mass or biliary disease.[6] However, imaging plays little role in the evaluation of diffuse hepatocellular disease such as hepatitis.

Ultrasonography

USG is the most widely used imaging procedure. It is a valuable but operator-dependent investigation. It has a sensitivity of 55%–91% and a specificity of 82%–95% to detect biliary obstruction. Although USG may not detect stones in the extrahepatic bile duct, which may be obscured by overlying gas, it reliably establishes the presence of a dilated biliary tree, thereby implying mechanical obstruction. Besides its value in differentiating intrahepatic from extrahepatic cholestasis, USG can also pick up evidence of associated abnormalities such as portal hypertension, focal lesions and fatty liver.

Computerized tomography

CT has a sensitivity of 63%–96% and a specificity of 93%–100% to detect biliary obstruction. Non-calcified cholesterol gall stones can be easily missed on CT scan because they may be isodense with bile.

Endoscopic retrograde cholangiopancreaticography

ERCP not only permits direct visualization of the biliary tree but also allows therapeutic intervention, e.g. removal of common bile duct stones or biliary stenting. It is the gold standard test for the evaluation of extrahepatic biliary diseases causing jaundice.

Percutaneous transhepatic cholangiography

In PTC, direct contrast visualization of the biliary tree is obtained via a percutaneous needle puncture of the liver. This is done less often than ERCP, but is especially useful if there is high biliary obstruction, e.g. a tumour at the bifurcation of the hepatic ducts. It also permits therapeutic intervention such as stent insertion to bypass a ductal malignancy.

Magnetic resonance cholangiopancreaticography

MRCP is an expensive but valuable imaging technique. MRCP is superior to USG and CT in detecting biliary obstruction. It has a sensitivity of 82%–100% and a specificity of 92%–98% to detect biliary obstruction.

LIVER BIOPSY

Percutaneous liver biopsy provides important diagnostic information at a relatively low risk, but is needed in only a minority of cases with hepatic dysfunction. Major indications include chronic hepatitis, cirrhosis, unexplained liver enzyme abnormalities, hepatosplenomegaly of unknown aetiology, suspected infiltrative disorder, suspected granulomatous disease, etc. Relative contraindications include a tendency for clinical bleeding, INR >1.5 or PT >3 s above the control value, severe thrombocytopenia and marked ascites. The risk of fatal haemorrhage in patients undergoing percutaneous liver biopsy is 0.4% if they have a malignancy and 0.04% if they have non-malignant disease.[7]

APPROACH TO A CASE OF JAUNDICE

The rational selection of these tests is based on a detailed history and physical examination to arrive at an initial differential diagnosis, which would decide the sequence of further evaluation. Basic laboratory tests either confirm the clinical diagnosis or provide additional information. The next step involves the use of various imaging techniques, which further narrow the possibilities. In a small number of cases, liver biopsy may be necessary.

The clinical assessment and basic biochemical parameters lead to three broad subgroups of patients:

1. *Isolated elevation of serum bilirubin*: when the AST, ALT and ALP levels are normal;
2. *Hepatocellular jaundice*: when the AST and ALT levels are elevated out of proportion to the ALP level;

3. *Cholestatic jaundice*: when the ALP level is elevated out of proportion to the AST and ALT levels.

Assessment of the patient should address the following questions:

1. Is the jaundice caused by haemolysis, an isolated disorder of bilirubin metabolism, hepatocellular dysfunction or biliary obstruction?
2. If hepatobiliary disease is present, is the condition acute or chronic?
3. If cholestasis is present, is it intrahepatic or extrahepatic in origin?
4. Is the jaundice due to a primary liver disorder or a systemic disorder involving the liver?
5. What is the aetiology: viral infection, alcohol or drug intake, etc.?

When the liver enzymes are normal, the possible aetiologies are limited, and include haemolysis and genetic disorders of bilirubin uptake, conjugation or excretion. When the liver enzymes are elevated, the key to the appropriate and timely evaluation of jaundice is the distinction between hepatocellular and obstructive jaundice. The differentiating features between these two are given in Table III.

Further evaluation is then directed towards which of these three broad subgroups are suggested by the clinical examination and basic biochemical parameters. Figure 1 is an algorithm for the evaluation of patients with jaundice.

Table III. Distinguishing features of obstructive and hepatocellular jaundice

		Obstructive jaundice	Hepatocellular jaundice
History	Abdominal pain	+	+/−
	Fever, rigors	+	Fever only in prodrome
	Prior biliary surgery	+	
	Prodrome		+
	Family history of jaundice		+
	Known infectious exposure/exposure to hepatotoxin/receipt of blood products, use of intravenous drugs		+
Physical examination	High fever	+	
	Palpable gallbladder	+	
	Palpable abdominal mass	+	
	Abdominal scar	+	
	Ascites	±	+
	Stigmata of liver disease		+
	Hepatic encephalopathy		+
Laboratory investigations	AST, ALT, ALP	ALP > AST, ALT	ALP < AST, ALT
	Deranged PT normalizes with injection of vitamin K	Yes	No

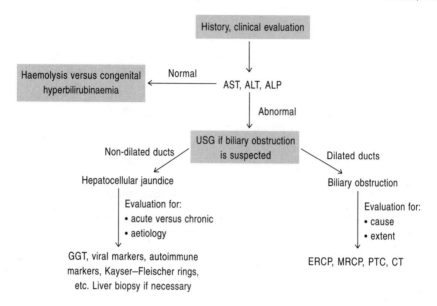

Fig. 1. Evaluation of a patient with jaundice

Isolated elevation of serum bilirubin

Isolated elevation of serum bilirubin could indicate either unconjugated or conjugated hyperbilirubinaemia.

Unconjugated hyperbilirubinaemia

In patients with this condition, the main aim of evaluation is to differentiate between haemolysis and disorders of uptake/conjugation of bilirubin. Haemolysis is confirmed by the presence of anaemia along with a raised reticulocyte count, urobilinogen in the urine, estimation of plasma and urine haemoglobin, and evidence of haemolysis in the peripheral blood smear. On confirmation of haemolysis, further tests are directed to determine its aetiology.

In the absence of haemolysis, the intake of drugs such as rifampicin must be excluded as these interfere with the uptake of hepatic bilirubin.[8] Genetic disorders associated with unconjugated hyperbilirubinaemia include the Gilbert syndrome and Crigler–Najjar syndrome types I and II.[9-11] In Crigler–Najjar syndrome type I, there is complete absence of uridine diphosphate (UDP) glucuronyl transferase; these children develop kernicterus and often die. Patients with Crigler–Najjar syndrome type II have bilirubin levels between 6 and 25 mg/dl. Patients with Gilbert syndrome have mild unconjugated hyperbilirubinaemia. A fasting test with 400 cal for 72 hours may show a rise in serum bilirubin, and administration of phenobarbitone results in a fall in bilirubin levels. In the absence of haemolysis, a mild rise in the bilirubin levels may be attributed to the Gilbert syndrome and no further evaluation is warranted.

Conjugated hyperbilirubinaemia

Elevation of conjugated bilirubin may be due to Dubin–Johnson or Rotor syndromes. In the Dubin–Johnson syndrome, black pigmentation is seen on liver biopsy. However, both are benign and differentiating tests are unnecessary.

HEPATOCELLULAR JAUNDICE

Hepatocellular jaundice may be caused by acute or chronic liver disease such as viral hepatitis, alcohol/drug toxicity, Wilson disease, haemochromatosis and autoimmune hepatitis. Investigations for a viral aetiology should be carried out, which include tests for HBsAg, IgM HBc, IgM anti-HAV and IgM anti-HEV. Clinical examination and basic biochemical screening may suggest other aetiologies. In such a situation or if the viral markers are negative, tests for other aetiologies may be carried out, such as KF rings and serum caeruloplasmin for Wilson disease; and antinuclear factor, antismooth muscle antibody and anti-LKM antibody for autoimmune hepatitis.

CHOLESTATIC JAUNDICE

When clinical evaluation and LFT suggest cholestasis, it is imperative to differentiate between intrahepatic and extrahepatic cholestasis (Table IV). The presence of dilated intrahepatic biliary radicles on USG differentiates the two conditions. However, the biliary radicles may not be dilated on USG in the presence of extrahepatic cholestasis in some situations such as early/partial obstruction or when the ducts are unable to dilate due to fibrosis, e.g. primary sclerosing cholangitis or cirrhosis.

In intrahepatic cholestasis, further evaluation includes appropriate serological tests and liver biopsy, while in extrahepatic cholestasis, the next step would be to determine the site and cause of the obstruction. CT scan further delineates a focal/mass lesion, and imaging-guided FNAC can provide a tissue diagnosis. The biliary

Table IV. Causes of cholestasis

Intrahepatic cholestasis	Extrahepatic cholestasis
Cholestatic phase of acute viral hepatitis	*Benign*
Alcoholic hepatitis	Choledocholithiasis
Drug-induced liver disease	Primary sclerosing cholangitis
Primary biliary cirrhosis	Chronic pancreatitis
Primary sclerosing cholangitis	AIDS cholangiopathy
Total parenteral nutrition	Postsurgical biliary strictures
Graft-versus-host disease	*Malignant*
Cholestasis of pregnancy	Carcinoma of the head of the pancreas
Sepsis	Carcinoma gallbladder
Benign postoperative cholestasis	Cholangiocarcinoma
Fibrosing cholestatic hepatitis	Periampullary carcinoma
	Obstruction of the common bile duct due to metastatic nodes

anatomy would be better delineated using non-invasive MRCP or minimally invasive ERCP (which can be combined with a therapeutic procedure).

JAUNDICE IN SPECIAL SITUATIONS

In special situations, the approach to a patient with jaundice will vary as the causes will be different.

Jaundice in newborns

Jaundice becomes clinically apparent when a baby has a serum bilirubin level >5 mg/dl, and is first seen on the face and later spreads to the trunk. The commonest cause is physiological hyperbilirubinaemia, which peaks at 48–72 hours in full-term infants and 4–5 days in premature ones. The serum bilirubin level does not exceed 13 mg/dl in full-term infants and 15 mg/dl in preterm infants. The direct bilirubin fraction is generally <2 mg/dl in physiological neonatal jaundice. This type of jaundice disappears by 1 week in full-term and by 2 weeks in premature infants. If the unconjugated bilirubin levels do not conform to the above, one should consider either increased production of bilirubin (haemolysis or haematoma) or delayed excretion of bilirubin due to inherited disorders (Crigler–Najjar syndrome, Dubin–Johnson syndrome, Rotor syndrome), hypothyroidism and prematurity.

Breast-milk jaundice is seen exclusively in neonates. The usual causes of conjugated hyperbilirubinaemia (>15% of the total bilirubin in normal conditions) are infections (sepsis, perinatally acquired viral infections including hepatitis, and intrauterine viral infections such as hepatitis B or TORCH), metabolic abnormalities (Rotor and Dubin–Johnson syndromes, α_1-antitrypsin deficiency, galactosaemia, tyrosinosis, cystic fibrosis, hereditary fructose deficiency) and anatomical abnormalities (biliary atresia, Alagille syndrome [ductopenia] and obstructions as with a choledochal cyst).[12] Drug-induced cholestasis is also a possibility in hospitalized patients.

Jaundice in pregnancy

This can be due to the usual causes but one should look for disorders peculiar to pregnancy. These include obstetric cholestasis, acute fatty liver of pregnancy, toxaemias of pregnancy, and the HELLP (haemolysis, elevated liver enzymes, low platelets) syndrome.[13]

Postoperative jaundice

This condition can have multiple causes such as increased bilirubin load (blood transfusions, haemolysis, haematoma formation), hepatocellular damage (related to pre-existing hepatic disease or fresh viral hepatitis, sepsis, ischaemic hepatopathy caused by hypotension or hypoxaemia during surgery, drug-induced hepatitis, congestive cardiac failure and general anaesthetic-induced hepatic damage) or less often due to extrahepatic biliary obstruction by gall stones, ascending cholangitis, pancreatitis or bile duct injury.[14] Similarly, jaundice in immunosuppressed patients, such as those who are recipients of allografts or immunosuppressive therapy or those with malignancy receiving anticancer chemotherapy, may be related to drug toxicity, viral hepatitis (especially fibrosing cholestatic hepatitis), sepsis or biliary complications. Malignancy such as lymphoma can *per se* cause jaundice.[15]

CONCLUSION

A variety of disorders can cause jaundice and the ideal approach remains a challenge. Clinical evaluation alone can suggest the correct diagnosis in over two-thirds of cases. There is a wide array of diagnostic, biochemical and imaging techniques for the evaluation of a patient with jaundice. However, over-reliance on laboratory data without adequate clinical assessment often results in unnecessary expense, delay in diagnosis and unwarranted risks.

REFERENCES

1. Christopher R, Rangaswamy GR, Santhoshkumar N, Shetty KT. Carotenoderma in metabolic carotenemia. *Indian Pediatr* 1997;**34**:1032–4.
2. Lascari AD. Carotenemia. A review. *Clin Pediatr* 1981;**20**:25–9.
3. Beckingham IJ, Ryder SD. Investigation of liver and biliary disease. *BMJ* 2001;**322**:33–6.
4. Berk PD. Bilirubin metabolism and the hereditary hyperbilirubinemias. *Semin Liver Dis* 1994;**14**:321–2.
5. Lidofsky SD. Jaundice. In: Feldman M, Friedman LS, Sleisenger MH (eds). *Sleisenger and Fordtran's gastrointestinal and liver disease. Vol. 1.* 7th ed. Philadelphia: WB Saunders; 2002:249–62.
6. Reddy SI, Grace ND. Liver imaging. A hepatologist's perspective. *Clin Liver Dis* 2002; **6**:297–310.
7. McGill DB, Rakela J, Zinsmeister AR, Ott BJ. A 21-year experience with major hemorrhage after percutaneous liver biopsy. *Gastroenterology* 1990;**99**:1396–400.
8. LaPerche Y, Graillot C, Arondel J, Berthelot P. Uptake of rifampicin by isolated liver cells: Interaction with sulfobromophthalein uptake and evidence for separate carriers. *Biochem Pharmacol* 1979;**28**:2065–9.
9. Berk PD, Noyer C. Hereditary hyperbilirubinaemias. In: Haubrich WA, Schaffner F, Berk JE (eds). *Bockus gastroenterology. Vol. 3.* 5th ed. Philadelphia: WB Saunders; 1995:1906–30.
10. Seppen J, Bosma PJ, Goldhoorn BG, *et al.* Discrimination between Crigler–Najjar types I and II by expression of mutant bilirubin uridine diphosphate-glucuronosyl-transferase. *J Clin Invest* 1994;**94**:2385–91.
11. Borlak J, Thum T, Landt O, *et al.* Molecular diagnosis of a familial nonhemolytic hyperbilirubinemia (Gilbert's syndrome) in healthy subjects. *Hepatology* 2000;**32**:792–5.
12. Dennery PA, Seidman DS, Stevenson DK. Neonatal hyperbilirubinaemia. *N Engl J Med* 2001;**344**:581–90.
13. Knox TA, Olans LB. Liver disease in pregnancy. *N Engl J Med* 1996;**335**:569–75.
14. Molina EG, Reddy KR. Postoperative jaundice. *Clin Liver Dis* 1999;**3**:477–88.
15. Ravindra KV, Stringer MD, Prasad KR, Kinsey SE, Lodge JP. Non-Hodgkin lymphoma presenting with obstructive jaundice. *Br J Surg* 2003;**90**:845–9.

CHAPTER 3

Radiological management of the jaundiced patient

MANPREET S. GULATI, SHASHI B. PAUL

Non-surgical intervention in the biliary tract including percutaneous transhepatic biliary drainage (PTBD) was introduced in the early 1970s. Though percutaneous transhepatic cholangiography (PTC) was performed for several years before the development of PTBD, therapeutic biliary interventions had remained outside the domain of radiologists. During the past 30 years, improved diagnostic imaging techniques and interventional hardware, developments in endoscopy, and the experience gained through clinical trials have revolutionized and clearly defined the role of percutaneous biliary interventions.

The practice of PTC has progressively diminished in the face of non-invasive imaging techniques such as ultrasonography (USG), magnetic resonance cholangiography (MRC), 3-D intravenous computerized tomographic cholangiography (3-D CTC) and the recently available 3-D CTC with minimum intensity projection (3-D CTC min IP). The diagnostic role of endoscopic retrograde cholangiography (ERC) has further reduced in recent years. PTC is now reserved only for problematic cases and for evaluation immediately before percutaneous intervention.

Percutaneous transhepatic biliary drainage, which was initially proposed as a routine preoperative measure for patients with severe obstructive jaundice, is now more of a palliative procedure in patients with an inoperable malignant obstruction. This has been made possible by improved preoperative patient preparation, good antibiotic therapy, improved surgical techniques and easy availability of expertise in endoscopic biliary drainage. One of the most important recent advances has been the introduction of self-expanding metallic stents for use in malignant obstructions. The use of covered metallic stents, removable metallic stents and the biodegradable stents currently being developed might be good strategies for the management of benign strictures. PTBD also continues to play a very important role in the management of suppurative cholangitis, postoperative obstructions and select patients with cholelithiasis. Percutaneous access to the biliary system is also possible via a T-tube tract in a postoperative (cholecystectomy) situation, providing an opportunity for performing percutaneous stone extraction from the biliary tract.

This chapter discusses all the aforementioned percutaneous interventional radiological techniques, indications for their use and other relevant issues.

PALLIATIVE BILIARY DRAINAGE FOR MALIGNANT STRICTURES

Malignant biliary obstruction is a not uncommonly encountered clinical problem in routine gastrointestinal medical and surgical practice. It is particularly common in India because of the high incidence of carcinoma of the gallbladder,[1] which frequently involves the bile ducts at the hepatic hilum. Carcinoma of the head of the pancreas and ampulla, cholangiocarcinoma, and metastatic hilar and peripancreatic adenopathy are other important causes of malignant biliary obstruction.

Biliary obstruction is potentially fatal because of the adverse pathological effects including depressed immunity, impaired phagocytic activity, reduced Kupffer cell function and paucity of bile salts reaching the gut, with consequent endotoxaemia, septicaemia and renal failure.[2] There is, therefore, a need to decompress the biliary system. The majority of malignant hepatic tumours, such as carcinoma of the gallbladder and pancreas, and cholangiocarcinoma, are unresectable.[3,4] Only 20%–30% of these tumours are resectable at the time of diagnosis.[3,5] Palliation of the malignant obstruction relieves the patient of itching and jaundice, reduces the risk of infection and septicaemia, and generally improves the quality of life. Surgical, endoscopic and interventional radiological percutaneous techniques are available for palliation. Non-surgical techniques are preferred because these are associated with lower morbidity and mortality.

Endoscopic stenting, in general, is preferred over percutaneous techniques because of a higher success rate, shorter hospital stay, lower complication rate and a lower 30-day mortality,[6] and also the fact that this is a tool that provides direct access to the treating gastroenterologist. The percutaneous approach is required only in situations in which endoscopic drainage has failed or is not possible, such as a previous Billroth II surgery, duodenal obstruction by a tumour, high hilar obstruction not negotiable by the transpapillary route, periampullary diverticulum and a large, papillary, fungating growth that makes cannulation difficult.[2] Hilar malignant strictures are particularly difficult to traverse via the endoscopic approach. In India, since carcinoma of the gallbladder commonly invades the hilar strictures and is the commonest cause of malignant biliary obstruction,[3] percutaneous drainage is a very important palliative option that has not been fully utilized. In clinical practice, a cohesive team comprising a gastroenterologist, a surgeon and a radiologist should adopt a multidisciplinary approach to the management of the patient before treatment is initiated.

The role of imaging before palliative biliary drainage

Since the management of malignant biliary obstruction depends on the resectability of the underlying tumour, patients should undergo accurate staging following diagnosis. One of the important goals of preoperative imaging is to identify vascular invasion by the tumour at the hepatic hilum. Hitherto, angiography was used to identify the vascular anatomy prior to surgery in carcinoma of the gallbladder[7] and hilar cholangiocarcinoma.[8-10] Recently, dual-phase helical CT has been used to evaluate vascular invasion in hilar tumours.[11,12] As a single modality, it can not only detect the malignancy, but also has the potential of comprehensively evaluating each patient for criteria of unresectability.[3] In a study by Kumaran et al.,[3] vascular invasion was diagnosed whenever the mass was in close contact with the artery/vein and there was loss of the intervening fat plane. The presence of irregularity of the luminal outline, narrowing of the calibre of the blood vessel in serial images and the presence of a tumour on both sides of the vessel were considered definite evidence of invasion.

High-quality 3-D reconstruction images made possible by helical CT are uniquely suitable for the depiction of the complex anatomy of the biliary tract. Van Beers et al.[13] evaluated 3-D CTC done by 3-D reconstructions following slow intravenous infusion of the cholangiographic agent iodipamide. Kwon et al.[14] utilized combined oral and intravenous cholangiographic agents prior to helical CT. Zeman et al.[15] devised a protocol extending the application of 3-D CT to preoperative planning for patients with obstructive pancreatic or biliary neoplasms in whom oral and intravenous cholangiographic agents have limited efficacy due to impaired biliary excretion. 3-D reconstructions can be successfully produced by taking advantage of the negative contrast effect of low-attenuation bile in the dilated ducts relative to the adjacent enhanced liver. 3-D CTC min IP can determine the level and cause of biliary obstruction. It can be obtained from regular thin-section helical CT data and may be a strong competitor against MRC because of the additional information on adjacent soft tissues such as contiguous organ involvement, regional metastasis, vascular invasion and ductal involvement itself. In a study by Park et al.,[16] the diagnostic potential of 3-D CTC min IP was considered in 9 patients, with PTC as the gold standard. 3-D CTC min IP demonstrated dilated intrahepatic ducts up to the tertiary branches and correctly diagnosed the level of biliary obstruction in all the patients. We have been using this modality for the past two years in all hilar malignant lesions. Not only is the resectability of the tumour better defined,[3] but the identification of variant ductal anatomy is also possible. Additionally, it helps in choosing a duct appropriate for drainage.

MRI as well as CT are performed for detecting direct spread of the tumour to the liver and hepatic metastases. Visualization of the intrahepatic bile ducts on MRI depends on the size of the ducts, concentration of bile, pulse sequence used, motion artifact and periportal high signal. CT and USG are more sensitive than MRI for detecting intrahepatic bile duct dilatation. The advent of MRC, wherein solid organs and moving fluid appear as low-intensity signals against stationary fluid (bile), which appears as a high-intensity signal, has been a very useful development for the imaging of biliary disease. Either gradient echocardiographic or fast-spin echocardiographic (FSE) sequences are obtained, and 3-D maximum intensity projection is used to reconstruct the projectional images. MRC can thus combine the advantages of projectional and sectional imaging methods. The half-Fourier turbo spin echo (HASTE) sequence is currently favoured and some newer sequences such as simultaneous acquisition of spatial harmonics (SMASH) and sensitivity encoding (SENSE) are also on the horizon.[5] MRC has the advantages of being non-invasive and free from complications.[17] Ductal dilatation, strictures and anatomical variation are well depicted by this technique, which makes this modality well suited for planning the optimal therapeutic approach for patients with biliary obstruction.

Invasive PTC is thus indicated only when: (i) the above-mentioned imaging modalities are not available; and (ii) as a first step in therapeutic percutaneous biliary intervention.

PERCUTANEOUS INTERVENTION IN MALIGNANT BILIARY OBSTRUCTION

All patients with potentially resectable tumours should undergo surgery. Biliary drainage is required in the preoperative stage in patients with high serum bilirubin levels or cholangitis and a potentially resectable tumour. In patients with an unresectable tumour, palliative drainage can be offered as the only definitive treatment.

Preoperative PTBD

Although the practice of PTBD prior to surgery is controversial,[2] it is advocated by many surgeons before curative resection to correct the metabolic derangement produced by biliary obstruction and decrease the complications of biliary surgery in the jaundiced patient. Either internal or external biliary drainage catheters or, more preferably, plastic stents are inserted 2–6 weeks prior to elective surgery. Many surgeons advise preoperative PTBD because biliary catheters are easy to locate at surgery, particularly during difficult dissection of lesions at the hepatic hilum.[18]

Palliation of malignant biliary obstruction using PTBD

PTBD is now the standard management for patients with incurable malignant biliary obstruction, particularly in certain specific situations.

The indications for PTBD are as follows:

- to treat cholangitis secondary to obstruction;
- to treat symptomatic obstructive jaundice when an endoscopic retrograde approach fails or is not possible (as discussed earlier);
- to gain access to the biliary system to perform transhepatic brachytherapy for cholangiocarcinoma; and
- preoperative decompression and stent placement to assist in surgical manipulation (controversial).

The relative contraindications for PTBD are as follows:

- an incorrectable bleeding diathesis;
- a large volume of ascites (the procedure may be difficult with a potential for bile peritonitis. A left-sided approach should be considered in such cases);
- segmental isolated intrahepatic obstructions that do not cause marked symptoms should not be drained. Bacterial contamination usually occurs when an isolated ductal system is accessed. As a consequence of this contamination, it is often impossible to withdraw drainage even if it is not required clinically. Thus, a patient could be left with a permanent, unwanted and potentially problematic drainage catheter; and
- a totally uncooperative patient (may require general anaesthesia or heavy conscious sedation).

Preparation for PTBD

Blood tests

Coagulation profile: The international normalized ratio (INR) should be less than 1.5. Vitamin K, fresh frozen plasma and platelets (as needed) should be administered to correct any coagulopathy.

Liver function tests: Serum bilirubin and ALP levels should be checked (an elevated ALP level, even in the setting of a near-normal bilirubin level, indicates a low-grade obstruction).

Baseline renal function: Blood urea and creatinine should be checked, especially before administering pre-procedure nephrotoxic antibiotics.

Informed consent

The procedure should be explained completely to the patient, outlining the risks with specific attention to sepsis and bleeding.

Prophylactic antibiotics

Appropriate antibiotics are administered 1–2 hours before the procedure to avoid biliary sepsis. The spectrum of antibiotic coverage must include both Gram-positive and -negative organisms. In our set-up, a combination of third-generation cephalosporins, amikacin and metronidazole is administered in appropriate dosages. The antibiotics should be continued for 24–72 hours following the procedure. A regular appraisal should be done to identify the prevalent infectious organisms and their drug resistance pattern in the local setting.

Sedation/analgesia

The patient should be given a clear liquid diet several hours before the procedure (for conscious sedation) with a well-functioning intravenous line and adequate hydration. Pre-procedural sedation is helpful but not mandatory. It is performed under conscious sedation (midazolam and fentanyl) with a liberal infiltration of local anaesthetic at the site and capsule of the liver.

It is best to prepare a wide area which will permit access to the biliary system from both the left and right sides, as needed.

Procedure

Technical approach: entry from the right or left side

We use the Bismuth–Corlette classification[19] to initially categorize the biliary obstruction. According to this classification system: (i) type 1 obstruction occurs distal to the confluence of the right and left hepatic ducts (primary confluence); (ii) type 2 obstruction involves the primary but not the secondary confluence; (iii) type 3 involves the primary confluence and, additionally, either the right (type 3a) or left (type 3b) secondary confluence; and (iv) type 4 involves the secondary confluence of both the right and left hepatic ducts. Whether to use a right- or left-sided approach must be decided on a case-by-case basis. Extensive right-sided disease with sparing of the left side makes the decision easy (left-sided approach), as does a patient with an atrophic left lobe (right-sided approach).

It is worth mentioning some broad guidelines that we use in our set-up. In the case of a type 1 lesion, there are two advantages in approaching from the right side (especially right anterior): the angle of approach to the point of obstruction is 90° or greater, making for easy catheter insertion; and the radiologist's hands are well away from the primary X-ray beam. The advantage of using the left-sided approach is that USG can be utilized for the initial puncture, accidental breach of the pleural space is avoided, and the patient has less catheter-related discomfort (the right intercostal approach being more painful). This left-sided approach is also preferable when there is ascites.

When the obstruction is at the confluence, the situation is more complex. It is important to be aware of the anatomy of the right and left hepatic ducts. The right hepatic duct is short, unlike the left which is 2–3 cm long until its bifurcation into the segmental ducts. Thus, a catheter placed in the right system initially drains a greater part of the liver because of the size difference between the lobes. However, once the tumour grows, the situation reverses because the catheter placed in the right side now drains only one segment, whereas the left-sided catheter drains the entire left lobe. Thus, for type 2 lesions, either the right anterior system or the left system is chosen (the left is chosen if the left lobe of the liver is of good size). For type 3a lesions, if there is extensive involvement of the right secondary confluence, we do either a single left-sided drainage or ideally combine it with right anterior or posterior drainage (keeping in mind the cost of the procedure, life expectancy and subjective assessment of the amount of liver to be drained as seen on CT). It has been shown that drainage of 25% of the liver volume using a single catheter/endoprosthesis may be sufficient.[20] For type 3b lesions, the approach is similar. For type 4 lesions, at least two drains should be used. Lobes and segments which are atrophic are excluded from the proposed drainage plan. A duct suspected to be already infected or contaminated due to the procedure is always drained.

Technique

After opacification of the ducts by PTC, the study is reviewed to select the best bile duct to puncture. The duct should be punctured at a peripheral location to gain a sufficient length of duct above the obstructing lesion, avoid injury to the large portal venous and arterial structures present at the hilum of the liver and reduce the length of the transhepatic tract. The left ducts are catheterized via an anterior subxiphoid approach. USG guidance can often be helpful for dilated left ducts. For the right lateral approach, the point of skin entry should be intercostal and lower than the costophrenic angle. The entry point should be chosen so as to allow the shortest path to the target duct. A well-chosen path will facilitate subsequent manoeuvres by minimizing any sharp angles along its course.

In some cases, the duct punctured at the time of the original diagnostic PTC provides a suitable site for cannulation, in which case a conversion system (described below) can be used. However, it is important to resist the temptation to convert a suboptimal PTC entry site. One should keep switching between the anteroposterior and lateral views to observe the progress of the needle towards the target duct. Intermediate oblique views are also of great help. A variety of needle systems can be successfully used to gain access to the bile ducts. These systems are of two main types: (i) those using a fine 21 or 22 gauge needle for the initial puncture followed by the insertion of a 0.018" wire (Seldinger technique) and subsequent conversion using a Neff, Cope or similar set; and (ii) those in which the puncture is performed using an 18–19 gauge needle covered by a flexible 4.8 F sheath. Once the needle is removed, the sheath will accept a 0.038" guidewire; the sheath can then be advanced over the guidewire into the bile duct. Once the duct is catheterized, the next step is to cross the lesion/obstruction and gain access to the duodenum (Fig. 1). This often requires the use of an angiographic or biliary manipulation catheter, and a hydrophilic guidewire (such as Terumo). In the case of a difficult-to-traverse obstruction, finer guidewires and microcatheters can be used. Additionally, it may be necessary to establish peripheral drainage for a short time and then bring the patient back for a subsequent, or very rarely, a third attempt. With the obstruction crossed, the angiographic catheter should be advanced over the hydrophilic guidewire into the bowel. The guidewire is then removed and a stiff wire such as the Amplatz super stiff, Ultrastiff or Lunderquist is used. With the stiff wire in place, the transhepatic tract can be dilated using serial dilators to accommodate the large-bore drainage catheter. A variety of drainage catheters are available with different characteristics suited for specific clinical situations.

Biliary drainage can be established in three ways:

1. *External biliary drainage:* The percutaneous catheter is positioned within the biliary tree and is attached to a collection bag outside the body to allow external drainage of bile. As an initial step, this allows the patient to recover

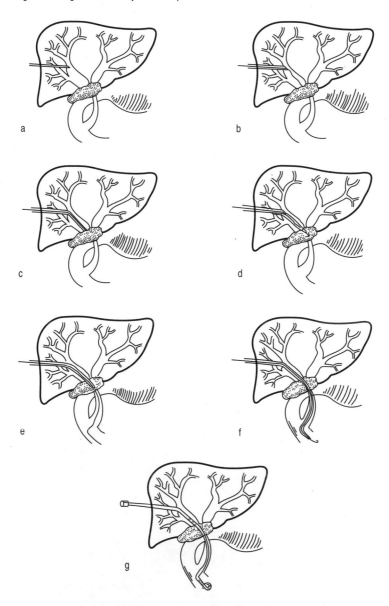

Fig. 1. The technique of placing a ring biliary catheter. (a) A needle is placed under ultrasound or fluoroscopic control (following PTC). The duct to be punctured is carefully chosen. Bile is aspirated and contrast injected to confirm correct positioning. (b) An extra-stiff guidewire is passed through the needle into the system. While keeping the guidewire steady, the needle is withdrawn over the guidewire and replaced by a 4–5 F angiographic or biliary manipulation catheter. (c) The stiff guidewire is replaced by a hydrophilic guidewire and the catheter guidewire assembly is brought close to the tumour. (d) The guidewire is slightly withdrawn so that it comes to lie within the catheter, and the catheter is 'dug' into the tumour. (e) The guidewire is again pushed, and will usually cross the obstruction into the distal duct and duodenum. Repetitive forward and backward movement of the guidewire may be required. (f) The catheter is moved over the wire into the duodenum. The hydrophilic guidewire is again exchanged for an extra-stiff guidewire. The transhepatic tract and obstruction are dilated by serial dilators. (g) A ring biliary catheter is finally pushed over the guidewire, with its end lying in the duodenum, facilitating internal and external drainage because of the multiple side-holes in its distal part.

from an acute septic state due to cholangitis. Indeed, an attempt to traverse the obstruction should not be made in such situations to avoid any extra manipulation as it can lead to cholangiovenous reflux into the blood stream and cause septicaemia/toxaemia, which can develop very rapidly. External drainage also allows time for clots or debris to clear and the percutaneous tract to mature, but is not suitable in the long term because of large fluid and electrolyte losses. The diversion of bile salts from the gut adversely affects the general state of well-being. The patient may be advised to regularly drink the drained-out bile. The bile can be mixed with an aerated drink for this purpose or given through a nasogastric tube. Sepsis and pericatheter leakage are other problems. The catheter is also a grim reminder to the patient of his malignancy.

2. *Internal–external drainage:* This involves positioning the PTBD catheter across the obstruction and into the duodenum (Fig. 2). There are multiple side-holes in the distal part of the catheter shaft (ring biliary drainage catheter available from Cook, Bard, etc.). If a standard catheter is not available, several side-holes can be punched into an ordinary drainage catheter over a distance of 10–12 cm in the distal part of the catheter, which can satisfactorily function as a ring biliary drainage catheter. Because of the multiple side-holes, which come to lie both above and below the obstruction, the catheter not only drains the bile out into the bag connected externally but, when capped outside, serves to drain the bile internally across the obstruction. Although it is preferable to replace this tube with an endoprosthesis or stent within

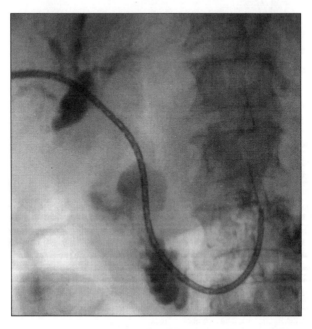

Fig. 2. A ring biliary catheter inserted percutaneously from the right side with the proximal part in the right ducts and the distal part in the duodenum. Note the side-holes present in the entire distal length of the catheter.

48–72 hours, cost and other considerations may dictate that long-term drainage be allowed to continue via such a catheter. The advantages of internal–external drainage are that fluid loss is eliminated and the bile drains into the bowel. Such catheters are easily exchanged over a guidewire on an outpatient basis so that the problem of catheter obstruction can be managed. Pain, infection and bile leakage at the skin-entry site may be the problems encountered with this technique.

3. *Implanted endoprosthesis:* This provides all the advantages of internal drainage without the problems associated with the percutaneous catheter exiting from the skin. In most situations, stenting is done in the second sitting (especially for plastic stents), after having placed an external or preferably a ring biliary catheter which has been draining for 24–72 hours. This is to avoid the discomfort of dilatation of the transhepatic tract up to 10–12 F in one session.

Initially, a careful cholangiogram should be performed to delineate the exact extent of obstruction and determine where the stent is to be positioned. Malignant obstructions should be overstented, with the stent extending well past the borders of the stricture to maintain patency as the tumour enlarges. After a stiff wire is placed across the stricture, a vascular introducer sheath of an appropriate size (usually 8 or 9 F) is placed. In most situations, it is advantageous to balloon-dilate the stricture (using a balloon 8–10 mm in diameter) prior to stent placement, particularly for self-expanding metallic stents, to facilitate rapid expansion of the device. This leads to more efficient bile drainage, and minimizes the chances of cholangitis and bile leakage.

A variety of plastic and metallic biliary endoprostheses are available. The more commonly used plastic endoprostheses, which are far cheaper than the metallic ones, include the Carey Coons Percuflex (Meditech), Ring Kerlan, Lunderquist Owman Teflon (Cook), Lammer polyurethane (Cook) stents, etc. We have also used pieces of catheters cut to the desired length after creating multiple side-holes, or even the distal part of the ring biliary catheter with the proximal part serving as the pusher. The Carey Coons stent is a 19 cm long tube, 12 F or 14 F with multiple side-holes and a gradual 90° bend in its most distal part. A 3-0 nylon suture is attached to the proximal shaft, extending to a silastic button, which acts as a subcutaneous anchor preventing distal migration of the stent. The Ring Kerlan stent is 12 F in diameter. It is made from Percuflex, with its length varying from 8 cm to 10 cm and is perforated throughout its shaft. A Mallecot mushroom tip is present at the trailing end for stabilization. A loop suture for repositioning is present proximal to the Mallecot. The Lunderquist Owman Teflon catheter is available in various sizes from 8 F to 12 F and is tapered at both ends.

We normally place a loop of suture around the proximal side-hole emerging from the proximal end-hole while pushing the stent, so that the stent can be pulled back in case it gets pushed further inside than necessary. We have occasionally had to use a vascular snare to reposition a distally migrated stent at the time of deployment (Fig. 3). These, and other routinely used endoscopic stents (even those with flaps), can be easily pushed through a large 10–12 F

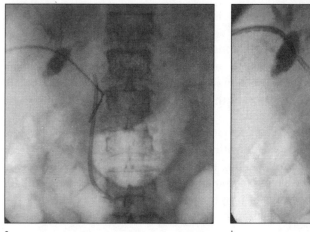
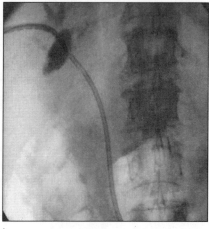

a   b

Fig. 3. (a) A percutaneously inserted plastic stent, which had migrated distal to the obstruction, being repositioned using a vascular snare. (b) The stent has been repositioned and an access catheter is placed proximal to it in the right duct, to reintervene if required.

sheath (after placing it across the obstruction) using any appropriate blunt head catheter to serve as a pusher. Once the stent is accurately in place, the suture can be removed, followed by withdrawal of the sheath over the stent till it is just proximal to the stent. The guidewire is then withdrawn from within the stent, finally releasing it. During the three steps, the pusher is kept steady with its head firm against the proximal end of the stent. The pusher is then removed over the guidewire. An external drainage catheter can be left inside with its tip just proximal to the stent (Fig. 3b), which can be used to flush the system for 24–48 hours, when it can be removed after a check cholangiogram.

Metallic stents of various types are used with the intent of achieving a higher patency rate and better bile flow.[21] These are positioned in a compressed state (7–12 F) but expand to achieve a diameter of 8–12 mm. This offers the advantage of placing a stent of a large diameter with minimal trauma. The newer stents with a 7 F delivery system can be positioned in a single sitting because the tract has to be dilated only up to 8 F and hence avoids the morbidity of multiple procedures. Metallic stents include the balloon-expandable stents (Palmaz, Johnson & Johnson and Tantalum Strecker, Boston Scientific Corp.). These stents are positioned over a balloon angioplasty catheter and deployed by inflating the balloon. Metallic stents are not preferred because of their poor radial force and inflexibility.

Self-expanding stents with very good radial force, such as the Gianturco Rosch Z stents (Cook), Wallstents (Cook), Nitinol Strecker (Boston Scientific Corp.), Memotherm (Bard) and Zilver stents (Cook), are available. The Z stent is made of stainless steel wire (0.016–0.018″ diameter) and has 6 zigzag bends. It is available in various lengths (1.5–9 cm) and diameters (6–12 mm), and is deployed through a 10–12 F introducer/sheath system, with a method of delivery very similar to that used for the plastic stent. The problem with Z stents is that of tumour ingrowth through the relatively wide mesh holes. The most widely used Wallstent endoprosthesis is deployed via a 7–8 F delivery catheter, which is very flexible and allows for easy, sheath-free passage through hard malignancies. It can vary from a length of 20 mm to 94 mm and is available in predetermined diameters of 8 mm, 10 mm and 12 mm. Its chief disadvantage is longitudinal shortening (up to 40%), which has to be taken into account for precise positioning.

The newer nitinol stents, such as the Memotherm and Zilver, have virtually no shortening when compared to the Wallstent, and these are also relatively more flexible and very kink-resistant. For deployment, the delivery system is introduced over an extra-stiff guidewire and the stent positioned across the obstruction. The stent is then released by retraction of the outer membrane covering it, which lies in a constrained state (Fig. 4).

It is generally advisable to have the distal end of the stent project through the ampulla into the duodenum.[18] This is because the rigid nature of the stent can sometimes cause kinking of the lower part of the common bile duct (CBD), which may cause obstruction (with the newer flexible nitinol stents, this may be unnecessary). Additionally, it is easier to cannulate them endoscopically for clearance or for additional endoprosthesis insertion. If the stent projects too far into the duodenum, it can cause erosion of the opposite wall. The proximal end should be well above the obstruction to minimize tumour overgrowth, while avoiding placement of the proximal end in the liver track. Side branches covered by the stent during placement are not associated with branch occlusion.[22]

Once the stent is in position, a cholangiogram is done through the side arm of the introducer sheath to determine if contrast flows freely across the obstruction (Fig. 4e). If the system is being adequately drained, a drainage catheter replaces the introducer sheath, its tip positioned proximal to the stent, to facilitate 4–6 hourly flushing of the system and perform a cholangiogram 24–48 hours later, as well as to assess stent patency. If all is well, the drainage catheter can be removed.

Stenting of hilar strictures

This presents the most challenging problem for biliary interventionists. Hilar strictures can be treated by using a single stent if there is free communication between the right and left duct systems. If no opacification of the left-sided system is seen at PTC and there is adequate opacification of the right-sided system, then again a single stent may be used on the right side. The same is true of the left side provided the left lobe is hypertrophied and will provide adequate biliary drainage. If, however, there is opacification of the system of the opposite side, and the drainage will be inadequate with a single stent, then double stenting should be done through a unilateral or bilateral transhepatic route. In the unilateral route, two stents are placed from a single track, one passing from the right to the left hepatic duct and the second from the right hepatic duct to the CBD, or an equivalent arrangement from the left side in a Y-shaped configuration

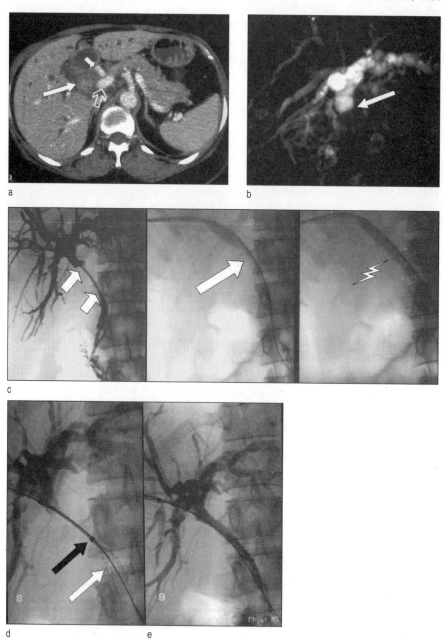

Fig. 4. Metallic stent placement in a patient with unresectable carcinoma of the gallbladder.
(a) Contrast-enhanced axial CT image showing a mass (large arrow) arising from the gallbladder and
encasing the main portal vein (open arrow) and hepatic artery (small arrow). The intrahepatic biliary ducts
are also dilated. (b) MRC frontal projection showing a block of the common hepatic duct 2 cm beyond the
confluence (arrow). (c) A ring biliary drainage catheter has been placed and the cholangiogram shows the
extent of the stricture (small arrows). This was dilated using a balloon catheter which initially shows a waist
(large arrow) at the site of the stricture and later disappears (wavy arrow), indicating adequate dilatation. (d)
A nitinol stent (Memotherm) is being deployed at the site of the stricture. A partially open stent mesh (white
arrow) is seen being released by the withdrawal of the covering membrane (black arrow). (e) Following
deployment, a cholangiogram done from the access catheter shows good patency of the stent.

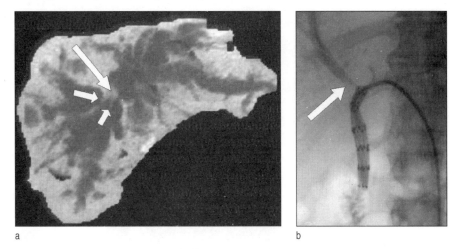

a   b

Fig. 5. Malignant hilar biliary obstruction. Hilar reconstruction. (a) CT cholangiogram axial minimum intensity projection (as seen from below) shows a blocked primary confluence (large arrow) and right secondary confluence (small arrows). (b) Hilar reconstruction done from the left transhepatic access. An indigenous plastic stent (arrow) has been placed connecting the right and left ducts, and a metallic Z stent has been placed between the left and common ducts.

(Fig. 5). The duct expands to accommodate both stents without any problem. In the bilateral route, one stent each is placed from the right and left side tracts, with the distal ends of both stents placed in the CBD in X-shaped configuration.

Combined transhepatic endoscopic approach (Rendezvous procedure)

Transhepatic placement of a catheter of small diameter across the obstructed duct and into the duodenum offers a second chance for the endoscopist. This arrangement is very useful when the endoscopist has initially failed to negotiate the obstruction in an earlier attempt and it is not advisable to create a large transhepatic track because of the risk of bile leakage into the peritoneum, or in patients with coagulopathy. With a transhepatically inserted 4 or 5 F catheter negotiated across the obstruction into the duodenum, a 450 cm exchange guidewire such as Zebra (Microvasive) is inserted into the catheter. The patient is placed in the prone oblique position for insertion of the endoscope. The endoscopist grasps the lower end of the guidewire with a snare or biopsy forceps and brings it out of the proximal end of the endoscope biopsy channel, while the radiologist keeps feeding the wire at the skin-entry site. The transhepatic catheter is now withdrawn so that its tip lies in the intrahepatic portion of the biliary tree above the malignant stricture. The endoscopist proceeds with the placement of a large-bore biliary endoprosthesis in the standard fashion, while the guidewire is held taut between the endoscopic and percutaneous ends (Fig. 6). When the endoprosthesis is in position and free egress of bile is noticed, the transhepatic catheter can be removed. However, if the position of endoprosthesis or adequacy of decompression is doubtful, the transhepatic catheter may be retained for observation and reintervention, if required.

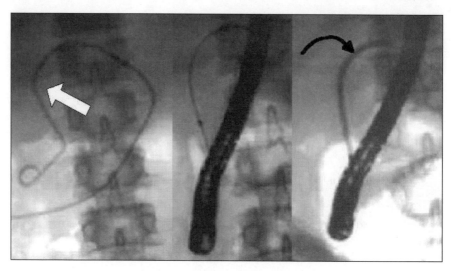

Fig. 6. The Rendezvous procedure. An 8 F ring biliary catheter (straight arrow) was placed earlier using the left-sided transhepatic route in a patient who had a hilar stricture. The patient had developed ascites and a plastic stent placement was planned. A 450 cm Zebra guidewire was introduced through the catheter, which was snared by an endoscope placed in the duodenum, and was brought out through the endoscope.
By keeping the guidewire taut at the cutaneous entry site and the proximal end of the endoscope, a 10 F plastic stent (curved arrow) was deployed via the endoscope.

Post-procedure management following biliary drainage

- Patients should be hospitalized for at least 24 hours following biliary drainage, and monitored for sepsis and vital signs.
- An appropriate combination of antibiotics should be continued after drainage is established.
- The internal–external biliary drainage catheter should be used for external drainage for the first 12–24 hours. If the catheter permits drainage of bile into the bowel, then the drainage catheter can be capped to allow internal drainage. If the patient is able to tolerate internal drainage for 8–12 hours, then he/she can be discharged. If internal drainage is not possible, then external bag drainage must be maintained. The bile output can range from 400 to 800 ml/day. With external drainage, dehydration can occur, unless adequate steps are taken to replace the lost fluids.
- Biliary drainage catheters should be forward flushed with normal saline every 48 hours. This helps prevent debris from accumulating in the catheter and causing it to occlude.
- The dressing around the drainage catheter should be changed at least every 48 hours and bathing avoided. Also, the biliary drainage catheters should be changed every 3–4 months.
- Pericatheter leakage is the result of catheter occlusion or displacement. Fluoroscopic evaluation is essential for determining and correcting this problem. Serum bilirubin values may be followed as an indicator of adequate drainage. Depending on the size and type of drain, it takes 10–15 days on an

average for the bilirubin levels to drop by 50%. If the bilirubin level starts rising, catheter occlusion should be suspected.

- After adequate drainage, biliary sepsis should be relieved. If sepsis remains a problem, then additional studies should be performed to determine the cause, which can either be catheter occlusion or undrained biliary ducts. A thorough cholangiogram with special attention to the ductal anatomy can sometimes identify a missing ductal segment, indicating an isolated undrained system. Alternatively, an MRC or CT cholangiogram can be performed.
- Late sepsis manifesting as fever, several days or weeks after the patient has been adequately drained, is usually indicative of obstruction of the drainage catheter. If the patient has a capped biliary catheter, the tube should be uncapped to allow the bile to drain externally. If externalizing the drainage catheter resolves the infection, then fluoroscopic evaluation of the catheter can be performed electively. However, if fever persists after externalization, then an emergency catheter evaluation should be performed. If catheter obstruction is not the source of sepsis, then the patient should be evaluated for undrained ductal segments.

Complications

Complications of percutaneous biliary interventions can be divided into early, that is, procedural complications and late complications.[18] Most procedural complications are related to the initial biliary drainage with mortality ranging from 0% to 2.8%;[23,24] major complications occur in 3.5%–9.5%.[25,26] Also, a larger number of procedure-related deaths have been reported for malignant (3%) compared to benign disease (0%).[27,28] This is also true of procedure-related complications (7% v. 2%). Minor complications such as mild, self-limiting haemobilia, fever and transient bacteraemia, occur in up to 66% of patients.[29]

Immediate complications

These may be:

1. *Sedation:* Problems may occur if care is not taken to constantly monitor patients during and after the procedure for complications of cardiorespiratory depression. Pulse oximetry should be used for monitoring all patients undergoing procedures involving conscious sedation.
2. *Haemorrhage:* Mild haemobilia is common, occurring in up to 16% of cases.[24] More severe bleeding requiring transfusion occurs in approximately 3% of patients.[30] Haemorrhage is minimized by the correction of coagulation defects and avoidance of percutaneous intervention in patients with severe incorrectable coagulopathies. It is usually self-limiting and seldom requires treatment. If the bleeding is mild and venous in origin, repositioning the catheter so that the trailing side-holes are located within the biliary tree and not within the hepatic

parenchyma, and upsizing the catheter to tamponade the bleeding point usually suffice. The catheter should be regularly irrigated with saline to maintain its patency and clear any thrombus from the bile ducts. If haemobilia does not resolve with these measures or is severe, vascular embolization should be performed through the transhepatic track or by hepatic arteriography.[18]

3. *Sepsis:* Manipulation of catheters and guidewires within an infected biliary tract can produce rapid bacteraemia, which may progress to septicaemic shock if antibiotic coverage is not administered prior to the procedure. Intravenous antibiotics should be continued following biliary drainage until the catheter is removed.

4. Pericatheter leak may occur in approximately 15% of patients.[31]

5. Pancreatitis occurs in 0%–4% of patients.[31]

6. Pneumothorax, haemothorax, bilothorax are rare complications (<1%).[32,33]

7. Contrast reaction is seen in <2% of patients.[31]

Delayed complications

These include the following:

1. Cholangitis: Approximately 50% of bile cultures will be positive when obtained at initial puncture.[27] When an internal–external drainage is performed with an 8 F catheter, recurrent cholangitis secondary to inadequate drainage is possible. The rate of sepsis will decrease if this is replaced by a 10–12 F drain.[34]

2. Catheter dislodgement occurs in approximately 15%–20% of patients.[24,35]

3. Peritonitis is seen in 1%–3%.[31]

4. Hypersecretion of bile (0%–5%):[28] This can cause considerable fluid and electrolyte imbalance and is usually seen within several days of drainage.

5. A biliopleural fistula[32] may occur.

6. In some patients, there may be skin infection or irritation.

7. An intrahepatic/perihepatic abscess may form.

8. Metastatic seeding of the serosa or tract with cholangiocarcinoma[28] and pancreatic carcinoma[24,36] has been reported.

Some routine precautions that help in markedly reducing the incidence of complications are given in Table I.[37]

Plastic versus metallic stent placement

Short-term complications are similar to those related to PTBD, such as cholangitis, haemorrhage and bile leakage. Metallic stent placement is associated with a lower incidence of cholangitis than with plastic stents.[38] Stents are prone to obstruction, but over the long term, expandable metallic stents have a better patency rate than plastic stents: 272 *v.* 96 days in a randomized trial by Lammer.[21] Obstruction of the plastic stent is caused by bile decomposition, deposition and encrustation, usually following bacterial contamination. This would require replacement either by

Table I. Methods to reduce the frequency of complications of percutaneous biliary interventions

---

Sepsis
    Antibiotic prophylaxis
    Minimal manipulation
    Restrict volume of contrast injected and aspirate bile prior to contrast injection
Haemorrhage
    Normalize coagulation factors
    Fine-needle coaxial technique
    Peripheral duct puncture
    Careful positioning of side-holes to avoid communication with an intrahepatic vessel
    Avoid puncture of extrahepatic ducts
    Single puncture site in liver capsule
Bile leak
    Careful positioning of side-holes
    Ensure adequate drainage by careful positioning of side-holes
Cholangitis
    Irrigation of catheter with sterile saline
    Large diameter catheters (12 F) for long drainage
    Routine tube exchange every 2–3 months
Catheter dislodgement
    Safety stitch method
    Self-retaining (pigtail) catheter

---

endoscopic or percutaneous means. Metallic stents, on the other hand, get obstructed due to tumour overgrowth and/or impaction of food debris. Unblocking metallic stents involves a repeat intervention, such as the introduction of a plastic or metallic stent within the obstructed lumen of the stent. In our set-up, since carcinoma of the gallbladder is the commonest cause of biliary obstruction and patients have a relatively shorter life span after diagnosis, reintervention is very rarely required. Plastic stents are prone to migration (early or late), which occurs in 3%–6% of cases.[18,21,39] Although metallic stents may get dislodged by balloon dilatation immediately after deployment, long-term spontaneous migration is very unusual.[40,41]

Patients should be followed up by clinical criteria, liver function tests and USG to detect early signs of stent occlusion.

Clinical results

PTBD

The results of various series are given in Table II.[35,42–47] In general, the technical success rate varies from 86% to 100% with successful drainage rates of 81%–96%. The reported 30-day mortality rate is 1%–49% and complication rate 6%–58%. This marked variation in results is probably due to differences in the criteria for patient selection, the experience and expertise of different operators, and the criteria used to define success and complications.

Plastic and metallic stenting

The evaluation of patency rates for stents in malignant biliary obstruction is

Table II. Results of percutaneous transhepatic biliary drainage in malignant obstruction

Authors	Number of patients	Technical success (%)	Success of drainage (%)	30-day mortality (%)	Complication rate (%)
Pereiras et al.[42]	12	100	83	–	58
Vorgeli et al.[43]	76	97	92	27	20
Joseph et al.[44]	39	90	–	49	53
Lammer and Neumayer[45]	162	100	96	15	9
Schild et al.[46]	220	–	92	1	22
Gazzaniga et al.[35]	362	97	81	–	15
Murai et al.[47]	92	86	–	–	–

Table III. Obstruction rate of plastic and metallic stents in malignant biliary obstruction

Authors	Number of patients	Obstruction rate (%)		Median duration of patency (days)	
		Plastic stents	Metallic stents	Plastic stents	Metallic stents
Davids et al. [38]	105	54	33	126	273
Knyrim et al. [48]	62	43	22	–	–
Lammer et al.[49]	101	27	19	96	272

difficult because some patients may die with patent stents while others may die with occult stent occlusion, making data collection and analysis difficult. Additionally, because stents occlude over time, patient groups with short mean survival times have improved stent patency rates compared to those with longer mean survival times. Therefore, retrospective analysis of stent patency is difficult and not so useful. Only well-designed, prospective, randomized controlled trials with stent occlusion as a measurable end-point can provide the necessary information (Table III).[18] The most recent of these by Lammer et al.,[49] which compared the transhepatic placement of metallic and plastic stents, showed that the occlusion rates for metallic stents were significantly lower than those for plastic stents (19% v. 27%), the median duration of patency of metallic stents was longer (272 v. 96 days) and the 30-day mortality was significantly lower for metallic stents (10% v. 24%). Finally, placement of a metallic stent was associated with a significantly shorter hospital stay (10 v. 21 days) and lower overall costs per patient.

Rationalizing biliary drainage and stenting in malignant obstruction

PTBD should be done only in those patients with malignant obstruction who are clearly symptomatic, such as those with intense pruritus and acute cholangitis, to improve the quality of life if curative resection is not possible. In patients with unresectable disease who do not have any of these indications, one should consciously decide not to undertake the procedure to avoid complications. The decision to provide PTBD should be taken after close consultation and discussion among the physician, surgeon and radiologist, as emphasized earlier.

In India, cost considerations largely dictate the materials used for PTBD and stenting. The number of catheters or stents used (just enough to provide satisfactory drainage), reuse of introducing materials, innovations such as in-house conversion of external drainage catheters to external–internal catheters by punching multiple side-holes, and using pieces of catheters as plastic stents by creating side-holes and flaps are some of the measures that we frequently adopt. Since the patency of plastic and metallic stents is similar during the first 3 months after stent insertion, only patients with a life expectancy of more than 3 months should be offered expandable metallic stents.[50] Plastic stents can also be easily exchanged by endoscopic or percutaneous means. If plastic stents occlude rapidly and repeatedly, metallic stents should be used. Patients who are in good health with a life expectancy of more than 3 months, and those from remote areas with no facility for stent exchange, are good candidates for metallic stents.

As expertise increases in the deployment technique of metallic stents, there is a great need to indigenously develop cheap, truly biocompatible metallic stents of good quality, which can be introduced via a small opening, are easily available, and have a reusable delivery system. This has the potential to substantially bring down costs. Currently, a good-quality metallic stent (including the delivery system) costs between Rs 26 000 and Rs 50 000. A plastic stent, with and without a delivery system, costs Rs 5000 and Rs 1500, respectively. Rationalizing the procedure by careful selection of patients, the nature of the procedure and cost-effective materials can go a long way in giving the maximum benefit to the maximum number of patients with malignant biliary obstruction.

Other interventions in malignant biliary obstruction

Biliary cytology and biopsy procedures

In suspected malignant biliary obstruction, the percutaneous tract can be used for cytological or histological confirmation. Bile collected from the external drainage bag is more likely to yield positive cytology than the fluid obtained at PTC alone.[51] Cytological study is positive in about 50% of patients with cholangiocarcinoma, although the reported sensitivity varies widely.[51,52] The positive cytology rate is lower for primary pancreatic tumours.[54]

If cytology is negative, percutaneous biopsy can be done under cholangio-graphic or USG guidance. Alternatively, the cholangiographic tract can also be used to obtain brushings or for biopsy using a pair of forceps, bioptome or myocardial biopsy needle; a needle biopsy can also be performed through a transhepatic sheath.

Endoluminal irradiation

Inoperable malignant biliary obstructive lesions can be subjected to endoluminal radiotherapy after the insertion of catheters and stents through the obstructive lesion. This method is particularly useful in patients with cholangiocarcinomas because some of these patients may live for years, and the combination of stenting and radiotherapy provides a much better and longer-lasting palliation than stenting alone.[54] Very high doses of local radiation can be administered by means of iridium-192 (^{192}Ir) seeds with little exposure to the liver beyond the tumour. Unfortunately, patients treated with endoluminal radiotherapy are subject to episodes of severe cholangitis, periductal abscess and haemobilia.[55]

PERCUTANEOUS INTERVENTION IN BENIGN BILIARY OBSTRUCTION

The majority of benign strictures are a result of upper abdominal surgery, particularly cholecystectomy. Bile ductal injuries are seen in 0%–4% of open cholecystectomies and 0%–2% of open procedures.[56,57] The other most common cause of iatrogenic stricture is anastomotic stricture following biliary–enteric anastomosis. Most anastomotic strictures are extrahepatic and can present several years following surgery. Multiple intrahepatic strictures are usually a manifestation of sclerosing cholangitis or bile duct ischaemia. The latter can occur due to hepatic artery occlusion following liver transplantation, cholecystectomy or hepatic chemoembolization. Multiple intrahepatic benign strictures are the most difficult to treat.

Patients with benign strictures present with recurrent jaundice, cholangitis and pain. Intrahepatic calculi are commonly found above benign strictures. These also contribute to intermittent obstruction. If the underlying cause is not treated, chronic biliary sepsis and obstruction may result in chronic liver insufficiency and may progress to biliary cirrhosis.

Assessment by imaging

The principles of non-invasive radiological evaluation remain the same as those for malignant obstruction. For more direct evaluation, ERC is usually employed to define the exact location, length and character of the biliary stricture. However, for patients with very tight and hilar strictures, PTC is usually required due to insufficient opacification of the proximal ducts by ERC. Additionally, PTBD can be performed immediately following PTC.

Management options

Benign strictures have a tendency to restenose following treatment and hence are difficult to treat. The main treatment options available are surgery and radiological dilatation.

Surgery

This treatment essentially involves resection of the strictured segment and primary anastomosis of the duct, or the formation of biliary–enteric anastomosis (hepatico- and choledochoduodenostomy or -jejunostomy). Surgery involving strictures close to the liver hilum is challenging, especially in patients with involvement of the hepatic ducts. For multiple intrahepatic strictures, liver transplantation is the only surgical option. The reported recurrence rate of strictures following surgical treatment is 7%–30%.[56,57] The surgical treatment of recurrent strictures is even more difficult, with a re-recurrence rate of 22% and mortality rate of 10%.[57] Concurrent hepatobiliary disease, portal hypertension and scarring of the liver hilum from previous surgery increase the duration of surgery, morbidity and mortality.[58]

Radiological balloon stricturoplasty

This method involves securing an access to the biliary system in the same manner as described for PTBD. Since benign strictures require repeat treatment because of frequent restenosis, surgeons should actively consider creating access jejunal loops, which may be placed at the time of formation of the bilioenteric anastomosis as a prelude to balloon dilatation. The access point of this loop is fixed to the anterior abdominal wall and is identified by a radio-opaque marker, such as a ring of metallic sutures or surgical staples (Fig. 7). It is usually easy to puncture the access loop and then gain retrograde access to the anastomosis for repeat interventions without the need for PTBD.

Once access to the anastomosis is gained via the biliary tract or access loop, the stricture is crossed with a wire and a catheter. A balloon catheter is then placed across the stricture and inflated to dilate the stricture (Fig. 7b). There are no clear guidelines available in the literature as to the length of time for which the balloon is to be kept in the inflated state. In our centre, we usually dilate the stricture for 10 min and look for recoil or 'waist' formation in the balloon on repeat inflation to consider a longer period of inflation at a higher pressure. A catheter of a large diameter is left across the anastomosis to prevent restenosis during the initial period of healing by fibrosis and to provide ready access to the system.

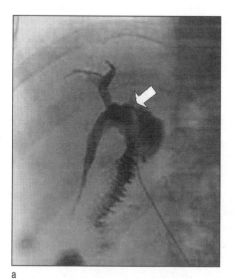 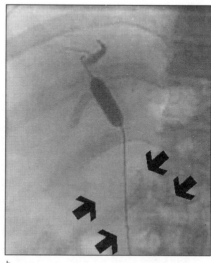

a   b

Fig. 7. A patient operated for cholecystectomy also underwent biliary–enteric anastomosis and presented with repeated attacks of cholangitis. (a) A cholangiogram done by placing a catheter in the intrahepatic biliary ducts via the access loop (multiple black arrows) shows an anastomotic stricture (white arrow). (b) A balloon catheter has been used to dilate the stricture.

This catheter is removed 6 weeks later after ensuring a satisfactory cholangiogram and asymptomatic clinical status of the patient.

The complications are similar to those seen with PTBD. Success rates range from 70% to 93%.[59-61] Balloon dilatation for sclerosing cholangitis has a much lower success rate of 42%–59%.[59] However, this subgroup of patients are poor surgical candidates and balloon stricturoplasty is a good temporizing measure in patients scheduled for liver transplantation.

Radiological endoprosthesis placement

Most patients with benign biliary strictures are relatively young and are expected to lead near-normal lives once the obstruction is relieved. Therefore, the treatment provided should be durable and without major long-term complications. There is no role for plastic endoprostheses placement in the management of benign biliary strictures, mainly due to their early occlusion. Metallic endoprostheses should be placed only as a last resort in these patients (patients unfit or unsuitable for surgery, failed repeated balloon dilatations) because of stent-related problems, such as recurrent cholangitis, stent occlusion and stone formation. Three-year patency rates for benign strictures following insertion of Gianturco stents are 68.7%.[62] Biodegradable and drug-eluting (which prevent obstruction) stents are experimental at present, and might be useful options in the future.

Percutaneous cholecystostomy

Catheterization of the gallbladder can provide temporizing or even definite therapy for various gallbladder diseases such as acute cholecystitis, hydrops and empyema. Often, these conditions could be associated with distal ductal obstruction due to calculi and can present with jaundice. Percutaneous cholecystostomy (PC) can not only temporize the acute episode by providing good gallbladder drainage but can also provide drainage for the biliary system, especially in patients with non-dilated ducts and distal obstruction. The drawback of PC in such patients is that cannulation of the cystic duct is difficult and, therefore, further therapeutic procedures, such as balloon dilatation, endoprostheses insertion and stone removal, are difficult, though not impossible.

Technique

The technique of PC is simple and may be a bedside procedure, using mobile USG, in intensive care units (Figs 8a and b). CT may be used as the method for guidance as well. The gallbladder is punctured through the liver with a needle (18–22 G). The transhepatic approach is adopted on the premise that by entering the gallbladder through the bare area of the liver, the chances of bile leakage would be less and any leak would get tamponaded against the adjacent adherent liver surface. It has been reported that the transperitoneal approach is as effective with a similar rate of bile leakage.[63] The transperitoneal approach should, however, be adopted only if there are problems with the transhepatic approach, such as adjacent liver metastasis.[64] A sample of the bile should be sent for

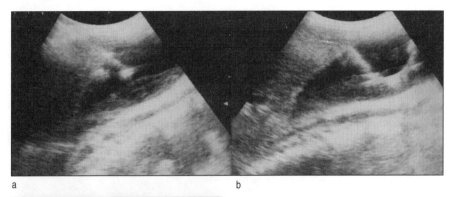

a   b

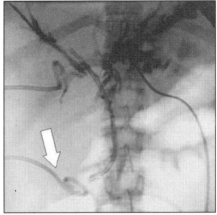

Fig. 8. Percutaneous cholecystostomy in a case of empyema of the gallbladder with cholangiocarcinoma. (a) A needle has been advanced transhepatically into the gallbladder lumen under USG guidance. (b) A metallic guidewire has been introduced through the needle, allowing it to coil within the lumen. (c) Multiple catheters are seen, placed earlier into the blocked and isolated biliary ducts. A catheter (arrow) is seen in the gallbladder.

c

bacteriological studies. The Cope catheter is introduced for drainage using the standard Seldinger technique, which has the advantage of forming a suture-activated, distal, self-retaining loop. This prevents accidental displacement of the tube and, in the transperitoneal approach, can be used to draw the gallbladder up against the anterior abdominal wall to prevent bile leakage.[64] The cholecystostomy catheter should remain inside for about 8–10 days. Cholecystography should be performed to demonstrate the patency of the cystic and bile ducts (Fig. 8c).

Complications

The complications that can occur are bile peritonitis, vasovagal reactions, malposition of the catheter and haemorrhage, which can, at times, be fatal. The reported incidence of complications is, however, low if proper precautions are taken.

Percutaneous stone removal

Percutaneous treatment is seldom necessary for CBD stones as endoscopic removal is feasible in most cases. In a few instances, when endoscopy is not possible (local anatomical variation, previous surgery with biliary–enteric anastomosis), percutaneous management is useful. The advantages of this route are: the possibility of performing associated choledochoscopy, intraluminal lithotripsy or lithotomy and the absence of permanent sphincterotomy.[63] Different techniques can be used to remove the stones. Balloon dilatation of the sphincter will allow the stones to be pushed and flushed through the papilla (Fig. 9). In a series of 31 patients, the success rate was 87%,[65] with a mean treatment time of 16 days. Dormia baskets help to retrieve the stones, as long as the stones are large enough to be strongly crushed in them. Mechanical or laser lithotripsy can be undertaken to break large stones into smaller fragments and has a high success rate.[63]

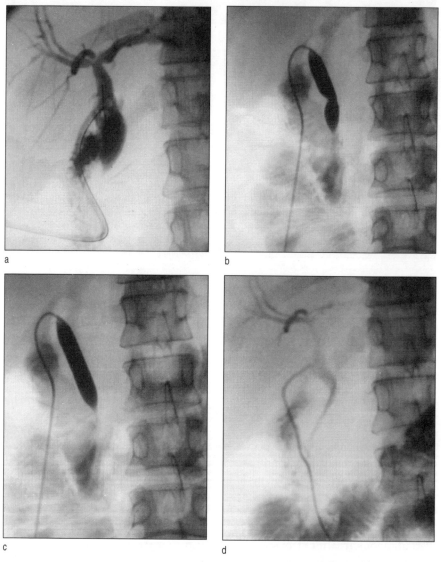

a

b

c

d

Fig. 9. Post-cholecystectomy percutaneous removal of stones via a T-tube tract. (a) A T-tube cholangiogram showing retained stones (seen as filling defects) in the common bile duct. (b) A balloon sphincterotomy showing a 'waist' at the site of the sphincter. (c) An inflated balloon being used to chase the stones across the sphincterotomy. (d) A cholangiogram done following the clearance of stones shows no filling defects.

Percutaneous dissolution

Percutaneous dissolution of gall stones can be done with agents such as methyl-tert-butyl-ether (MTBE) or mono-octanoin. These agents are administered into the gallbladder via PC. Instillation is performed manually with continuous infusion and 4–6 aspirations per minute. The average treatment time is 5 hours per day for 1–3 days. The disadvantages of MTBE infusion are the necessity of manual infusion and aspiration of fluid over such a protracted period, sedation due to systemic absorption, and the risk of duodenitis and intravascular haemolysis. The efficacy of MTBE may be enhanced with stone fragmentation, which increases the surface area–volume ratio.[66] The effectiveness has been reported to be between 84% and 90% in various series.[67] This technique, however, cannot be used in the presence of acute cholecystitis, cholangitis, pancreatitis or in the presence of heavily calcified stones. At present, the technique is reserved for patients who are at high risk for general anaesthesia.

T-tube manipulations

Retained ductal stones (or stones that form years after cholecystectomy) are generally first approached by endoscopic sphincterotomy. However, a T-tube already in place facilitates percutaneous extraction (Figs 9 and 10). For this technique, it is important to allow the tract to mature for at least 5 weeks after surgery. Following cholangiography, the T-tube is removed over an extra-stiff guidewire, and a large sheath introduced. With the sheath in place, stones can be removed in the manner elaborated in the section on percutaneous stone removal. With experience, successful stone extraction using a T-tube can be achieved in 95% of cases with complications arising in only 4%.[68]

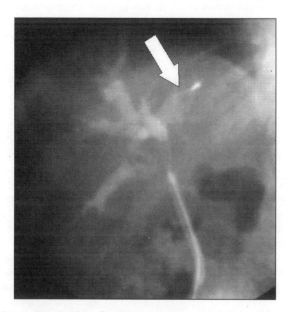

Fig. 10. A trapped stone (arrow) within a Dormia basket being removed via the T-tube tract

ACKNOWLEDGEMENT

We wish to thank Professor S.K. Acharya, Editor, *Tropical Gastroenterology*, for kindly consenting to the reproduction of the text and figures from the authors' review article in the same journal.[69]

REFERENCES

1. Das DK, Tripathy RP, Bhambham S, Chachra KL, Sodhani P, Malhotra V. Ultrasound guided fine-needle aspiration cytology diagnosis of gallbladder lesion. *Diagn Cytopathol* 1998; **18:**258–64.

2. Garg PK, Tandon RK. Nonsurgical drainage for biliary obstruction. *Indian J Gastroenterol* 1994;**13:**118–27.

3. Kumaran V, Gulati MS, Paul SB, Pande GK, Sahni P, Chattopadhyay TK. The role of dual phase helical CT in assessing resectability of carcinoma of the gallbladder. *Eur Radiol* 2002;**12:**1993–9.

4. Blumgart LH. Cholangiocarcinoma. In: Blumgart LH (ed). *Surgery of the liver and biliary tract.* Edinburgh: Churchill Livingstone; 1998:721–53.

5. Pillai VAK, Shreekumar KP, Prabhu NK, Moorthy S. Utility of MR cholangiography in planning transhepatic biliary interventions in malignant hilar obstructions. *Indian J Radiol Imag* 2002;**12:**37–42.

6. Speer AG, Russel CG, Hatfield ARW. Randomised trial of endoscopic versus percutaneous stent insertion in malignant obstructive jaundice. *Lancet* 1987;**11:**57–62.

7. Kersjes W, Koster O, Heuer M, Schneider B. [A comparison of imaging procedures in the diagnosis of gallbladder and bile duct carcinomas.] *Rofo Fortschr Geb Rontgenstr Neuen Bildgeb Verfahr* 1990;**153:**174–80.

8. Gulliver DJ, Baker ME, Cheng CA, Meyers WC, Papas TN. Malignant biliary obstruction: Efficacy of thin section dynamic CT in determining resectability. *AJR Am J Roentgenol* 1992;**159:**503–7.

9. Choi BI, Lee JH, Han MC, Kim SH, Yi JG, Kim CW. Hilar cholangiocarcinoma: Comparative study with sonography and CT. *Radiology* 1989;**172:**689–92.

10. de Aretxabala X, Roa I, Burgos L, *et al.* Gallbladder cancer in Chile. A report on 54 potentially resectable tumours. *Cancer* 1992;**69:**60–5.

11. Cha JH, Han JK, Kim TK, *et al.* Preoperative evaluation of Klatskin tumour: Accuracy of spiral CT in determining vascular invasion as a sign of unresectability. *Abdom Imaging* 2000;**25:**500–7.

12. Feydy A, Vilgrain V, Denys A, *et al.* Helical CT assessment in hilar cholangiocarcinoma: Correlation with surgical and pathologic findings. *AJR Am J Roentgenol* 1999;**172:**73–7.

13. Van Beers BE, Lacrosse M, Trigaux JP, de Canniere L, De Ronde T, Pringot J. Non invasive imaging of the biliary tree before or after laparoscopic cholecystectomy: Use of three dimensional spiral CT cholangiography. *AJR Am J Roentgenol* 1994;**162:**1331–5.

14. Kwon AH, Uetsuji S, Yamada O, Inoue T, Kamiyama Y, Boku T. Three dimensional reconstruction of the biliary tract using spiral computed tomography. *Br J Surg* 1995;**82:**260–3.

15. Zeman RK, Berman PM, Silverman PM, *et al.* Biliary tract: Three dimensional helical CT without cholangiographic contrast material. *Radiology* 1995;**196:**865–7.

16. Park SJ, Han JK, Kim TK, Choi BI. Three-dimensional spiral CT cholangiography with minimum intensity projection in patients with suspected obstructive biliary disease: Comparison with percutaneous transhepatic cholangiography. *Abdom Imaging* 2001;**26:**281–6.

17. Adamck HE, Albert J, Lietz M, Breer H, Schilling D, Riemann JF. A prospective evaluation of magnetic resonance cholangiography in patients with suspected bile duct obstruction. *Gut* 1998;**43:**680–3.

18. Morgan RA, Adam A. Percutaneous management of biliary obstruction. In: Gazelle GS, Saini S, Mueller PR (eds). *Hepatobiliary and pancreatic radiology imaging and intervention.* Stuttgart: Thieme; 1998:677–709.

19. Bismuth H, Corlette MB. Intrahepatic cholangioenteric anastomosis in carcinoma of the hilus of the liver. *Surg Gynecol Obstetr* 1975;**140:**170–8.

20. Polydorou AA, Chisholm EM, Romanos AA, *et al.* A comparison of right versus left hepatic duct endoprosthesis insertion in malignant hilar biliary obstruction. *Endoscopy* 1989; **21:**266–71.

21. Lammer JL. Biliary endoprostheses: Plastic versus metal stents. *Radiol Clin North Am* 1990;**28:**1211–22.

22. Nicholson DA, Cheety N, Jackson J. Patency of side branches after peripheral placement of metallic biliary endoprosthesis. *J Vasc Interv Radiol* 1992;**3:**127–30.

23. Ferrucci JT Jr, Mueller PR, Harbim WP. Percutaneous transhepatic biliary drainage: Technique, results and applications. *Radiology* 1980;**135:**1–13.

24. Hamlin JA, Friedman M, Stein MG, Bray JF. Percutaneous biliary drainage: Complications of 118 consecutive catheterizations. *Radiology* 1986;**158:**199–202.

25. Lamaris JS, Stoker J, Dees J, Nix GA, Van Blankenstein M, Jeekel J. Nonsurgical palliative treatment of patients with malignant biliary obstruction—the place of endoscopic and percutaneous drainage. *Clin Radiol* 1987;**38:**603–8.

26. Clark RA, Mitchell SE, Colley DP, Alexander E. Percutaneous catheter biliary decompression. *AJR Am J Roentgenol* 1981;**137:**503–9.

27. Yee AC, Ho CS. Complications of transhepatic biliary drainage: Benign vs malignant diseases. *AJR Am J Roentgenol* 1987;**148:**1207–9.

28. Carrasco CH, Zornoza J, Bechtel WJ. Malignant biliary obstruction: Complications of percutaneous biliary drainage. *Radiology* 1984;**152:**343–6.

29. Berquist TH, May GR, Johnson CM, Adson MA, Thistle JL. Percutaneous biliary decompression: Internal and external drainage in 50 patients. *AJR Am J Roentgenol* 1981;**136:**901–6.

30. Mueller PR, van Sonnenberg E, Ferrucci JT Jr. Percutaneous biliary drainage: Technical and catheter-related problems in 200 procedures. *AJR Am J Roentgenol* 1982;**138:**17–23.

31. Rosenblatt M, Aruny JE, Kandarpa K. Transhepatic cholangiography, biliary decompression, endobiliary stenting, and cholecystostomy. In: Kandarpa K, Aruny JE (eds). *Handbook of interventional radiology procedures.* Philadelphia: Lippincott Williams & Wilkins; 2002:302–31.

32. Strange C, Allen ML, Freedland PN, Cunningham J, Sahn SA. Biliopleural fistula as a complication of percutaneous biliary drainage: Experimental evidence for pleural inflammation. *Am Rev Respir Dis* 1988;**137:**959–61.

33. Dawson SL, Neff CC, Mueller PR, Ferrucci JT Jr. Fatal hemothorax after inadvertent transpleural biliary drainage. *AJR Am J Roentgenol* 1983;**141:**33–4.

34. Denning DA, Ellison EC, Carey LC. Preoperative percutaneous transhepatic biliary decompression lowers operative morbidity in patients with obstructive jaundice. *Am J Surg* 1991;**141:**61–5.

35. Gazzaniga GM, Faggioni A, Bondanza G, *et al.* Percutaneous transhepatic biliary drainage—twelve years' experience. *Hepatogastroenterology* 1991;**38:**154–9.

36. Cutherell L, Wanebo HJ, Tegtmeyer CJ. Catheter tract seeding after percutaneous biliary drainage for pancreatic cancer. *Cancer* 1986;**57:**2057–60.

37. Wittich GR, van Sonnenberg E, Simeone JF. Results and complications of percutaneous drainage. *Semin Interv Radiol* 1985;**2:**39–49.

38. Davids PH, Groen AK, Rauws EA, Tytgat GN, Huibregtse K. Randomised trial of self expanding metallic stents versus polyethylene stents for distal malignant biliary obstruction. *Lancet* 1992;**340:**1488–92.

39. Mueller PR, Ferrucci JT Jr, Teplick SK, *et al.* Biliary stent endoprosthesis: Analysis of complications in 113 patients. *Radiology* 1985;**156:**637–9.

40. Asch MR, Jaffer NM, Baron DL. Migration of a biliary Wallstent into the duodenum. *J Vasc Interv Radiol* 1993;**4:**381–3.

41. Abramson AF, Javit DJ, Mitty HA, Train JS, Dan SJ. Wallstent migration following deployment in right and left hepatic ducts. *J Vasc Interv Radiol* 1992;**3:**463–5.

42. Pereiras RV Jr, Rheingold OJ, Huston D, *et al.* Relief of malignant obstructive jaundice by percutaneous insertion of a permanent prosthesis in the biliary tree. *Ann Intern Med* 1978;**89:**589–93.

43. Vorgeli DR, Gummy AB, Weese JL. Percutaneous transhepatic cholangiography, drainage and biopsy in patients with malignant biliary obstruction. An alternate to surgery. *Am J Surg* 1985;**150:**243–7.

44. Joseph PK, Bizer LS, Sprayregan SS, Gliedman ML. Percutaneous transhepatic biliary drainage. Results and complications in 81 patients. *JAMA* 1986;**255:**2763–7.

45. Lammer J, Neumayer K. Biliary drainage endoprosthesis: Experience with 201 patients. *Radiology* 1986;**159:**625–9.

46. Schild H, Klose KJ, Staritz M, *et al.* [The results and complications of 616 percutaneous transhepatic biliary drainages.] *Rofo Fortschr Geb Rontgenstr Neuen Bildgeb Verfahr* 1989;**151:**289–93.

47. Murai R, Hashiguchi F, Kusuyama A, *et al.* Percutaneous stenting for malignant biliary stenosis. *Surg Endosc* 1991;**5:**140–2.

48. Knyrim K, Wagner HJ, Pausch J, Vakil N. A prospective, randomized, controlled trial of metal stents for malignant obstruction of the common bile duct. *Endoscopy* 1993;**25:**207–12.

49. Lammer J, Hausegger KA, Fluckiger F, *et al.* Common bile duct obstruction due to malignancy: Treatment with plastic versus metal stents. *Radiology* 1996;**201:**167–72.

50. Dhil V, Huibregtse K. Endoscopic placement of expandable biliary stents: Current applicability. *Indian J Gastroenterol* 1996;**15:**142–6.

51. Okuda K, Ohto M, Tsuhiya Y. The role of ultrasound, percutaneous transhepatic cholangiography, computed tomographic scanning and magnetic resonance imaging in the preoperative assessment of bile duct cancer. *World J Surg* 1988;**12:**18–26.

52. Harell GS, Anderson MF, Berry PF. Cytologic bile examination in the diagnosis of biliary duct neoplastic strictures. *AJR Am J Roentgenol* 1981;**137:**1123–6.

53. Gunther RW, Schild H, Thelen M. Percutaneous transhepatic biliary drainage: Experience with 311 procedures. *Cardiovasc Intervent Radiol* 1988;**11:**65–71.

54. Ede RJ, Williams SJ, Hatfield ARW, McIntyre S, Mair G. Endoscopic management of inoperable cholangiocarcinoma using iridium-192. *Br J Surg* 1988;**76:**867–9.

55. Meyers WC, Jones RS. Internal radiation for the bile duct cancer. *World J Surg* 1988;**35:**213–14.

56. Bismuth H. Postoperative strictures of the bile duct. In: Blumgart LH (ed). *The biliary tract: Clinical surgery international.* 5th ed. Edinburgh: Churchill Livingstone; 1982:209–18.

57. Pellagrini CA, Thomas MJ, Way LW. Recurrent biliary stricture: Pattern of recurrence and outcome of surgical therapy. *Am J Surg* 1984;**14:**175–80.

58. Pitt HA, Miyamoto T, Parapatis SK. Factors influencing outcome in patients with post-operative biliary strictures. *Am J Surg* 1988;**144:**14–19.

59. Mueller PR, van Sonnenberg E, Ferrucci JT. Biliary stricture dilatation: Multicenter review of clinical management in 73 patients. *Radiology* 1986;**160:**17–22.

60. Williams HJ, Bender CE, May GR. Benign postoperative biliary strictures: Dilatation with fluoroscopic guidance. *Radiology* 1987;**163:**629–34.

61. Rossi P, Salvotri FM, Bezzi M. Percutaneous management of benign biliary strictures with balloon dilatation and self expanding metallic stents. *Cardiovasc Intervent Radiol* 1990; **13:**231–9.

62. Maccioni F, Rossi M, Salvatori FM. Metallic stents in benign biliary strictures: Three years' follow-up. *Cardiovasc Intervent Radiol* 1992;**15:**360–6.

63. Menu Y, Vuillerine MP. Non-traumatic abdominal emergencies: Imaging and intervention in acute biliary conditions. *Eur Radiol* 2002;**12:**2397–406.

64. Gulati M. Pancreatic and biliary interventions. In: Berry M, Chowdhury V, Mukhopadhyay S, Suri S (eds). *Gastrointestinal and hepatobiliary imaging*. New Delhi: Jaypee Brothers; 2003:451–64.

65. Van der Valden JJ, Berger MY, Bonjer HJ. Percutaneous treatment of bile duct stones in patients treated unsuccessfully with endoscopic retrograde procedures. *Gastrointest Endosc* 2000;**51:**418–22.

66. Faulkner DJ, Kozarek RA. Gallstones: Fragmentation with a tunable dye laser and dissolution with methyl tert-butyl ether *in vitro*. *Radiology* 1989;**170:**185–9.

67. van Sonnenberg, D' Agostino HB, Casola G, *et al*. Interventional radiology in the gallbladder. Diagnosis, drainage, dissolution and management of stones. *Radiology* 1990;**174:**1–6.

68. Burhenne HJ. Percutaneous extraction of retained biliary tract stones: 661 patients. *AJR Am J Roentgenol* 1980;**134:**888–98.

69. Gulati MS, Srinivasan A, Agarwal PP, Paul SB, Garg P, Rao NDLV. Percutaneous management of malignant biliary obstruction: The Indian perspective. *Trop Gastroenterol* 2003;**24:**47–58.

CHAPTER 4

Endoscopic management of obstructive jaundice

RANDHIR SUD, MANDHIR KUMAR, RAJESH PURI

Endoscopic retrograde cholangiopancreaticography (ERCP), which was first described by McCune et al.[1] in 1968, has traversed a long way from being a diagnostic procedure. Since the 1980s, there has been a dramatic advancement in the management of biliary diseases using this technique. Traditional surgery has become refined but so have non-operative techniques; these have supplanted surgery in many situations. ERCP and its related procedures have now become the mainstay in the management of benign and malignant obstructions of the biliary tract. In benign conditions, it may be curative or palliative, while in malignant conditions, the procedures are only palliative.

Aetiology of obstructive jaundice in malignant conditions	
Primary malignancy	*Metastatic*
Periampullary carcinoma	Porta hepatis
Duodenal carcinoma	Peripancreatic lymph nodes
Papillary carcinoma	
Cholangiocarcinoma	
Pancreatic carcinoma	
Gallbladder carcinoma	

Malignancies causing obstructive jaundice have a poor outcome and curative surgery is possible in only 15%–20% of cases. For unresectable lesions, endoscopic management forms the mainstay of treatment as it is cheaper, involves a much shorter initial hospital stay, has decreased mortality and morbidity, and a success rate comparable to that of surgery.[2,3] The largest trial by Smith et al.[3] randomly assigned 101 patients to biliary bypass and 100 patients to plastic stent placement during ERCP. The rates of technical success (94% v. 92%) and functional success (95% v. 92%) were comparable, although procedure-related mortality was 14% for the group treated with surgery versus 3% for the group treated with endoscopy (p=0.01). Complications were 2.5 times higher (29% v. 11%, p=0.02) for the group treated with surgery. Patients who underwent surgical decompression had a statistically significant longer hospitalization. In contrast, recurrent obstructive jaundice was noted in 36 out of 92 patients with stents as a consequence of stent occlusion, but in only 2 of 92 surgically treated patients. Moreover, gastric outlet obstruction developed in 7% of patients in the surgical group versus 17% in the group with stents. The decrease was a consequence of the concomitant gastrojejunostomies that were undertaken in approximately half the patients who underwent laparotomy (such patients can now be taken care of by endoscopic enteral stenting and the number of repeat procedures can be reduced by the use of metal stents). Finally, the median survival rates for the two groups were comparable (approximately 5–6 months).

It has also been seen that endoscopic techniques are superior to percutaneous treatment.

INDICATIONS FOR ENDOSCOPIC MANAGEMENT

The indications for endoscopic management are as follows:

1. *Preoperative stenting:* Randomized trials do not show any advantage of preoperative biliary tract decompression.[4,5] However, it may be done in exceptional circumstances such as cholangitis, severe pruritus, general debility temporarily contraindicating surgery and incidental discovery of carcinoma during ERCP to prevent iatrogenic cholangitis.[6]
2. *Palliative:* Palliation is indicated for pruritus and cholangitis. Stenting also improves the quality of life, increases the appetite and decreases malabsorption.

Endoscopic therapy involves the use of plastic or metal stents as biliary endoprosthesis. The issues in management are: (i) the type of stent to be used and (ii) single- or double-sided stenting in hilar strictures.

Plastic stents

Polyethylene stents have been in use since they were introduced by Soehendra and Reynders-Frederix in 1980.[7] Despite advances in technology, patency has remained a major problem, with 10 F stents becoming occluded after 3–6 months. Thus, they may be preferred over metal stents if the projected life expectancy due to peritoneal/liver metastasis is less than 3–6 months.

The advantages of plastic stents are:

1. They are cheap,
2. They are retrievable,
3. Their use has shown high success rates of over 90% in distal blocks and about 70% in proximal blocks,[8,9] and
4. They are the therapy of choice in cases of incidental discovery of carcinoma during ERCP.

The disadvantages of plastic stents are:

1. Early post-procedure complications related to endoscopic sphincterotomy or stent-related cholangitis (10%–15%),[10,11] and
2. Stent occlusion within 3–6 months.

Attempts to increase the patency by increasing the size of the stent beyond 10 F, changing the composition of bile with choleretic agents (ursodeoxycholic acid [UDCA]), antibiotics to reduce the bacterial load, aspirin, and changing stent material and design have all been unhelpful.[12–14] Occluded stents need to be replaced if symptoms recur or if there is cholangitis. Randomized trials comparing scheduled stent change revealed no difference in the number of ERCPs per patient, number of stents per patient, mortality rate, need for metal stenting, frequency of surgery, mean stent survival, frequency of cholangitis and time to death.[15–17]

Metal stents

Metal stents have been a major development in stent technology. These are available from a number of companies and are made of steel/nitinol. They can be successfully deployed over the guidewire in more than 95% of cases.

The advantages of metal stents are:

1. Improved biliary drainage because of their large diameter (10 mm) and smaller surface area;
2. Longer patency (9–11 months) that leads to reduced requirement for hospitalization for cholangitis and stent change, which offsets the initial high cost;[18–21]
3. In a small group of patients who suffer rapid and repeated obstruction of plastic stents, it is an absolute indication.

The disadvantages of metal stents are:

1. They are non-retrievable, hence they should not be deployed in potentially resectable tumours;
2. Stent occlusion, though infrequent, may occur because of tumour ingrowth or biliary epithelial hyperplasia induced by the stent. Such patients may be treated by the insertion of a plastic or another metal stent through the original stent.[22] To obviate this, covered stents have been introduced but these are to be used only in case of a distal block;[23]
3. Complications such as entrapment of the stent delivery system in small or non-dilated intrahepatic ducts, malpositioning of stents, trauma to the duodenal wall opposite the papilla with resultant bleeding or perforation, though rare, have been reported.

SINGLE VERSUS DOUBLE DUCT DRAINAGE

There is considerable debate regarding decompression of one or both intrahepatic systems in patients with bifurcation strictures.[24] Advocates of single-stent drainage argue that single-lobe drainage leads to a decrease in jaundice and cholestasis, while proponents of both-side drainage point to a 30%–40% incidence of cholangitis, and increased mortality and death from sepsis if only one lobe is drained.[25,26] The approach should be to pass a guidewire into an intrahepatic duct, aspirate bile and inject a limited amount of contrast to define the anatomy. It is imperative to limit injection of the contrast to the lobe to be drained and avoid manipulation of the other lobe. The other lobe should be drained if there is cholangitis or persistent cholestasis. De Palma *et al.*[27] randomized 157 consecutive patients to undergo unilateral or bilateral hepatic duct drainage. In the intention-to-treat analysis, unilateral drainage was associated with significantly higher rates of successful drainage (defined as decrease in bilirubin to <75% of the pre-treatment values within 1 month) and lower early complication rates (primarily because of lower rates of cholangitis). Thirty-day mortality, late complications and median survival were similar for the two groups. MRCP can help select the liver lobe to be drained, thus avoiding injection of the contrast medium into the contralateral lobe.[28]

ENDOSCOPIC MANAGEMENT OF BENIGN BILIARY OBSTRUCTION

The common causes of benign biliary obstruction are:

1. Choledocholithiasis
2. Stricture due to
   —Postoperative trauma following biliary tract surgery
   —Chronic pancreatitis
   —Sclerosing cholangitis
   —Infestations: biliary ascariasis, *Echinococcus*, *Clonorchis sinensis*, *Fasciola hepatica*
   —Infections: suppurative cholangitis, biliary tuberculosis
3. Others
   —Papillary adenoma
   —Choledochal varices
   —Crohn disease
   —Peptic ulcer disease
   —Haemobilia
   —Sarcoidosis
   —Eosinophilic cholangiopathy

Of these, our discussion will be limited to the relatively common problems of stones and strictures.

Choledocholithiasis

This is seen in 5%–15% of persons suffering from gall stones. Unlike asymptomatic gall stones, asymptomatic CBD stones need to be treated. The introduction of endoscopic sphincterotomy in 1974 by Classen[29] and Kawai[30] has revolutionized the management of bile duct stones from an extensive surgery with its attendant morbidity and mortality to an OPD or day-care procedure.

Following a sphincterotomy, most of the stones can be retrieved using a Dormia basket or stone extraction balloon. Balloons are most useful for extracting relatively small stones (<10 mm) in a non-dilated duct. The major advantage of using a balloon is that it cannot become impacted, although the stone can.

Baskets are preferred over balloons if the stones are large (>10 mm), and for intrahepatic stones, small stones in a dilated duct and stones larger than the downstream duct. The success rate using standard baskets and balloons after sphincterotomy is around 90%.[31,32]

Difficulty or failure to remove the stone can occur due to:

1. Large size of the stone (>15 mm)
2. Shape of the stone
3. Location
4. Consistency
5. Contour of the CBD
6. Diameter of the CBD at the level of and distal to the stones
7. Coexisting pathology such as a stricture/tumour.

In such situations, the options are:

1. *Mechanical lithotripsy:* This is a safe, low-cost procedure and can be performed at the time of initial ERCP. Two types of mechanical lithotripters are available: (i) Soehendra–Metat sheath type and (ii) through the scope model. This procedure leads to the removal of 85%–90% of difficult bile duct stones.[33,34]
2. *Lithotripsy techniques:* These include (i) extracorporeal shock wave lithotripsy (ESWL) and (ii) intracorporeal (laser and electrohydraulic) lithotripsy. These are advanced procedures and are not widely available. They require a nasobiliary tube or a mother–baby scope. Ductal clearance occurs in 80%–90% of patients.[35,36]
3. *Dissolution therapy:* This is no longer an important modality.
4. Stents and nasobiliary drainage.

In failed cases, biliary drainage should be done to prevent stone impaction and cholangitis. This is usually a temporizing measure pending a repeat attempt or surgery.[37,38]

Stenting not only drains the bile duct but may aid in mechanically fragmenting stones, especially in combination with UDCA.[39] Long-term stenting has been believed to be a good palliative measure in elderly and high-risk patients with non-extractable stones, and has a low rate of late complications (cholangitis) of about 12%–15%.[37,40,41] However, recent studies refute this observation.[38,42,43]

This approach should be restricted to patients unfit for elective surgical, endoscopic or percutaneous treatments, and those with a short life expectancy.

Cholecystectomy-related strictures

The risk of CBD injury in open cholecystectomy is 0.5% while in laparoscopic cholecystectomy it varies between 0% and 2%.[44] The majority of cholecystectomy-related strictures are short (<10 mm) and distal to the confluence of the right and left hepatic ducts.[45,46] Most bile duct injuries occur as a result of poorly defined biliary anatomy and attempts to secure haemostasis, while delayed injury is due to ischaemia of the bile duct, especially the right hepatic duct.[47] The distribution of bile duct strictures after laparoscopic cholecystectomy is mid-CBD (42%–50%), confluence (22%–44%), common hepatic duct (28%) and distal CBD (15%).[48] Benign biliary strictures have been classified by Bismuth[45] in relation to their distance from the confluence of the right and left hepatic ducts. This classification has been modified by Bergman *et al.*[49] as follows:

Type A: Leakage from the cystic duct or peripheral hepatic radicle
Type B: Leakage from a major bile duct
Type C: Isolated distal stricture
Type D: Complete transection of the bile duct

Types A and B are most amenable to endoscopic therapy while type D invariably requires surgical correction.

The role of ERCP in the management of patients with strictures is well defined. The preferred treatment is balloon dilatation to 6–10 mm with the ultimate placement of two or three 10 F plastic stents across the stricture. The strictures are redilated and stents exchanged at 3–4-month intervals for 8–12 months till the stricture profile is nearly as open as the downstream duct so that the patient remains symptom- and cholangitis-free. Endoscopic balloon dilatation with stent placement resulted in 70%–80% success rates in some studies.[50–53] A retrospective study comparing surgical with endoscopic therapy concluded that both had similar long-term success rates with recurrence in 17% of patients.[54] These studies indicate that surgery should be reserved for patients with complete transection of the bile duct and failed endoscopic therapy.

Wallstents have also been tried but with poor results.[55]

Chronic pancreatitis-related biliary strictures

Intrapancreatic CBD strictures may occur in 3%–46% of patients with chronic pancreatitis. Most authors report a low stricture resolution rate with plastic stents (11%–30%).[56–58] Metal stents have been tried with a 90% success rate over a follow-up period of 33 months.[59] Plastic stents are useful alternatives for short-term treatment of chronic pancreatitis-induced strictures causing complications and for high-risk surgical patients. However, as a long-term solution, surgery appears to be a better option. Limited data are available on the use of metal stents.

Sclerosing cholangitis

The location and extent of biliary involvement determine the type of treatment for sclerosing cholangitis. Endoscopic balloon dilatation may be beneficial for patients with jaundice secondary to dominant extrahepatic strictures.[60] Cytological brushings to exclude neoplasms[61] should precede dilatation of the dominant stricture. The long-term benefits of biliary dilatation are uncertain in patients with this progressive disease.

Infestation

Biliary ascariasis

Endoscopy is the mainstay of treatment for biliary ascariasis.[62] The worm should be extracted completely using a pair of grasping forceps or a Dormia basket. A polypectomy snare should be avoided as it tends to cut the worm. Endoscopic sphincterotomy should be avoided as the patulous biliary sphincter favours easy entry should re-infection occur. Following endotherapy, the patient should receive antihelminthic therapy.

Echinococcus granulosus

In 25% of cases, the hydatid cyst ruptures into the biliary tree causing obstructive jaundice.[63] In patients with obstructive jaundice or cholangitis, endoscopic biliary sphincterotomy facilitates extraction of the cyst and membranes using a Dormia basket or a biliary occlusion balloon.[64] Saline irrigation of the bile duct may flush out the hydatic sand. Life-threatening episodes of acute cholangitis can be managed by nasobiliary drainage followed by extraction of the cysts.[65,66] Hypertonic saline irrigation of the cyst through nasobiliary drainage ensures sterilization of the germinal layers and remaining daughter cysts. Endoscopic biliary sphincterectomy and ductal clearance followed by internal biliary stenting for 4–6 weeks is used to achieve fistula closure.[67]

REFERENCES

1. McCune WS, Shorb PE, Moscovitz H. Endoscopic cannulation of ampulla of Vater: A preliminary report. Ann Surg 1968;**167**:752–5.
2. Andersen JR, Sorensen SM, Kruse A, Rokkjaer M, Matzen P. Randomised trial of endoscopic endoprosthesis versus operative bypass in malignant obstructive jaundice. Gut 1989;**30**:1132–5.
3. Smith AC, Dowsett JF, Rusell RC, Hatfield AR, Cotton PB. Randomised trial of endoscopic stenting versus surgical bypass in malignant low bile duct obstruction. Lancet 1994; **344**:1655–60.
4. Knyrim K, Wagner HJ, Pausch J, Vakil N. A prospective randomised controlled trial of metal stents for malignant obstruction of the common bile duct. Endoscopy 1993;**25**:207–12.
5. Martignoni ME, Wagner M, Krahenbuhl L, Redaelli CA, Friess H, Buchler MW. Effect of preoperative biliary drainage on surgical outcome after pancreatoduodenectomy. Am J Surg 2001;**181**:52–9.

6. Rey JF, Dumas R, Canard JM, *et al*; French Society of Digestive Endoscopy. Guidelines of the French society of digestive endoscopy: Biliary stenting. *Endoscopy* 2002;**34:**169–73.

7. Soehendra N, Reynders-Frederix V. Palliative bile duct drainage: A new endoscopic method of introducing a transpapillary drain. *Endoscopy* 1980;**12:**12–18.

8. Slivka A, Carr-Locke DL. Therapeutic biliary endoscopy. *Endoscopy* 1992;**24:**100–19.

9. Cheung KL, Lai EC. Endoscopy stenting for malignant biliary obstruction. *Arch Surg* 1995;**130:**204–7.

10. Cotton PB, Lehman G, Vennes J, *et al*. Endoscopic sphincterotomy complications and their management: An attempt at consensus. *Gastrointest Endosc* 1991;**37:**383–93.

11. Motte S, Deviere J, Dumonceau JM, Serruys E, Thys JP, Cremer M. Risk factors for septicemia following endoscopic biliary stenting. *Gastroenterology* 1991;**101:**1374–7.

12. Leung JWC, Banez VP. Clogging of biliary stents: Mechanisms and possible solutions. *Dig Endosc* 1990;**2:**97–101.

13. Halm U, Schiefke I, Fleig WE, Mosner J, Keim V. Ofloxacin and ursodeoxycholic acid versus ursodeoxycholic acid alone to prevent occlusion of biliary stents: A prospective randomized trial. *Endoscopy* 2001;**33:**491–4.

14. Costamagna G, Mutignani M, Rotondano G, *et al*. Hydrophilic hydromer-coated polyurethane stents versus uncoated stents in malignant biliary obstruction: A randomized trial. *Gastrointest Endosc* 2000;**51:**8–11.

15. Tarnasky PR, Miller C, Mauldin P, *et al*. Comparison of prophylactic versus indicated stent exchange for malignant obstructive jaundice using computer modeling. *Gastrointest Endosc* 1996;**43:**399A.

16. Part F, Chapat O, Ducot B, *et al*. A randomized trial of endoscopic drainage methods for inoperable malignant strictures of the common bile duct. *Gastrointest Endosc* 1998;**45:**1–7.

17. Mokhashi M, Rawls E, Tarnsky PR, *et al*. Schedule vs as required stent exchange for malignant biliary obstruction. A prospective randomized study. *Gastrointest Endosc* 2000;**47:**1–6.

18. Davids PH, Groen AK, Rauws EA, Tytgat GN, Huibregtse K. Randomised trial of self-expanding metal stents versus polyethylene stents for distal malignant biliary obstruction. *Lancet* 1992;**340:**1488–92.

19. Carr-Locke DL, Ball TJ, Cannors PJ, *et al*. Multicenter randomized trial of wallstent biliary endoprosthesis versus plastic stents. *Gastrointest Endosc* 1993;**39:**310A.

20. Knyrim K, Wagner HJ, Pausch J, Vakil N. A prospective, randomised, controlled trial of metal stents for malignant obstruction of the common bile duct. *Endoscopy* 1993;**25:**207–12.

21. Yeoh KG, Zimmerman MJ, Cunningham JT, Cotton PB. Comparative costs of metal versus plastic biliary stent strategies for malignant obstructive jaundice by decision analysis. *Gastrointest Endosc* 1999;**49:**466–471.

22. Tham TCK, Carr-Locke DL, Vandervoort J, *et al*. Management of occluded biliary Wallstents. *Gut* 1998;**42:**703–7.

23. Shim CS, Lee YH, Cho YD, *et al*. Preliminary results of a new covered biliary metal stent for malignant biliary obstruction. *Endoscopy* 1998;**30:**345–50.

24. Kozarej RA. Endoscopy in the management of malignant obstructive jaundice. *Gastrointest Endosc Clin North Am* 1996;**6:**153–67.

25. Polydorou AA, Cairns SR, Dowsett JF, *et al*. Palliation of proximal malignant biliary obstruction by endoscopic endoprosthesis insertion. *Gut* 1991;**32:**685–9.

26. Deviere J, Baize M, de Toeuf J, Cremer M. Long-term follow-up of patients with hilar malignant stricture treated by endoscopic internal biliary drainage. *Gastrointest Endosc* 1988;**34:**95–101.

27. De Palma GD, Galloro G, Siciliano S, Lovino P, Catanzano C. Unilateral versus bilateral endoscopic hepatic duct drainage in patients with malignant hilar biliary obstruction: Results of a prospective, randomized and controlled study. *Gastrointest Endosc* 2001; **53**:547–53.

28. Hintze RE, Abou-Rebyeh H, Adler A, Veltzke-Schlieker W, Felix R, Wiedenmann B. Magnetic resonance cholangiopancreatography-guided unilateral endoscopic stent placement for Klatskin tumors. *Gastrointest Endosc* 2001;**53**:40–6.

29. Classen M, Demling L. Endoscopic sphincterotomy of vater and extraction of stones from the choledochal duct. *Dtsch Med Wochenschr* 1974;**99**:496–500.

30. Kawai K, Akasaka Y, Murakami K, *et al*. Complications of endoscopic biliary sphincterotomy of the ampulla of Vater. *Gastrointest Endosc* 1974;**20**:148–56.

31. Fouch PG. Endoscopic management of large common duct stones. *Am J Gastroenterol* 1991;**86**:1561–5.

32. Sherman S, Hawes RH, Lehman GA. Management of bile duct stones. *Semin Liver Dis* 1990;**10**:205–21.

33. Siegel JH, Ben-Zvi JS, Pullano WE. Mechanical lithotripsy of common duct stones. *Gastrointest Endosc* 1990;**36**:351–6.

34. Hintze RE, Adler A, Veltzke W. Outcome of mechanical lithotripsy of bile duct stones in an unselected series of 704 patients. *Hepatogastroenterology* 1996;**43**:473–6.

35. Adamek HE, Maer M, Jakobs R, Wesbecher FR, Neuhauser T, Riemann JF. Management of retained bile duct stones. A prospective open trial comparing extracorporeal and intracorporeal lithotripsy. *Gastrointest Endosc* 1996;**44**:40–7.

36. Neuhaus H, Hoffman W, Gottlieb K, Classen M. Endoscopic lithotripsy of bile duct stones using a new laser with automatic stone recognition. *Gastrointest Endosc* 1994;**40**:708–15.

37. Maxton DG, Tweedle DE, Martin DF. Retained common bile duct stones after endoscopic sphincterotomy: Temporary and long term treatment with biliary stenting. *Gut* 1995;**36**:446–9.

38. Bergman JJ, Rauws EA, Tijssen JG, Tytgat GN, Huibregtse K. Biliary endosprosthesis in elderly patients with endoscopically irretrievable common bile duct stones: Report on 117 patients. *Gastrointest Endosc* 1995;**42**:195–201.

39. Johnson GK, Geenen JE, Venu RP, Schmalz MJ, Hogan JW. Treatment of non-extractable common bile duct stones with combination ursodeoxycholic acid plus endoprostheses. *Gastrointest Endosc* 1993;**39**:528–31.

40. Soomers AJ, Nagengast FM, Yap SH. Endoscopic placement of biliary endoprosthesis in patients with endoscopically unextractable common bile duct stones: A long-term follow up study of 26 patients. *Endoscopy* 1990;**22**:24–6.

41. Peters R, Macmathuna P, Lombard M, Karani J, Westaby D. Management of common bile duct stones with a biliary endoprosthesis: Report on 40 cases. *Gut* 1992;**33**:1412–15.

42. Chopra KB, Peters RA, O'Toole PA, *et al*. Randomized study of endoscopic biliary endoprosthesis versus duct clearance for bile duct stones in high-risk patients. *Lancet* 1996;**348**:791–3.

43. De Palma GD, Catanzano C. Stenting or surgery for treatment of irretrievable common bile duct calculi in elderly patients? *Am J Surg* 1999;**178**:390–3.

44. Macintyre IM, Wilson RG. Laparoscopic cholecystectomy. *Br J Surg* 1993;**80**:552–9.

45. Bismuth H. Postoperative strictures of bile duct. In: Blumgart LH (ed). *The biliary tract: Clinical surgery international*. 5th ed. Edinburgh: Churchill Livingstone; 1982:209–18.

46. David PH, Rauws EA, Coene PP, Tytgat GN, Huibregtse K. Endoscopic stenting for postoperative biliary strictures. *Gastrointest Endosc* 1992;**38**:12–18.

47. Terblanche J, Allison HF, Northover JM. An ischemic basis for biliary strictures. *Surgery* 1983;**94**:52–7.

48. Raute M, Podlech P, Jaschke W, Manegold BC, Trede M, Chir B. Management of bile duct injuries and strictures following cholecystectomy. *World J Surg* 1993;**17**:553–62.

49. Bergman JJ, van den Brink GR, Rauws EA, *et al.* Treatment of bile duct lesions after laparoscopic cholecystectomy. *Gut* 1996;**38:**141–7.
50. Siegel JH, Guelrud M. Endoscopic cholangiopancreatoplasty: Hydrostatic balloon dilatation in the bile duct and pancreas. *Gastrointest Endosc* 1983;**29:**99–103.
51. Huibregtse K, Katon RM, Tytgat GN. Endoscopic treatment of postoperative biliary strictures. *Endoscopy* 1986;**18:**133–7.
52. Berkelhammer C, Kortan P, Haber GB. Endoscopic biliary prostheses as treatment for benign postoperative bile duct strictures. *Gastrointest Endosc* 1989;**35:**95–101.
53. Manoukian AV, Schmalz MJ, Geenen JE, Hogan WJ, Venu RP, Johnson GK. Endoscopic treatment of problems encountered after laparoscopic cholecystectomy. *Gastrointest Endosc* 1993;**39:**9–14.
54. Davids PH, Tanka AK, Rauws EA, *et al.* Benign biliary strictures: Surgery or endoscopy? *Ann Surg* 1993;**217:**237–43.
55. Dumonceau JM, Deviere J, Delhaye M, Cremer M. Plastic and metal stents for post-operative benign bile duct strictures: The best and the worst. *Gastrointest Endosc* 1998;**47:**8–17.
56. Deviere J, Devaere S, Baize M, Cremer M. Endoscopic biliary drainage in chronic pancreatitis. *Gastrointest Endosc* 1990;**36:**96–100.
57. Smits ME, Rauws EA, van Gulik TM, Gouma DJ, Tytgat GN, Huibregtse K. Long-term results of endoscopic stenting and surgical drainage for biliary stricture due to chronic pancreatitis. *Br J Surg* 1996;**83:**764–8.
58. Farnbacher MJ, Rabenstein T, Ell C, Hahn EG, Schneider HT. Is endoscopic drainage of common bile duct stenoses in chronic pancreatitis up-to-date? *Am J Gastroenterol* 2000;**95:**1466–71.
59. Deviere J, Cremer M, Baize M, Love J, Sugai B, Vandermeeren A. Management of common bile duct stricture caused by chronic pancreatitis with metal mesh self expandable stents. *Gut* 1993;**35:**122–6.
60. Marsh JW Jr, Iwatsuki S, Makowka L, *et al.* Orthotopic liver transplantation for primary sclerosing cholangitis. *Ann Surg* 1988;**207:**21–5.
61. Vitale GC, Reed DN Jr, Nguyen CT, Lawhon JC, Larson GM. Endoscopic treatment of distal biliary stricture from chronic pancreatitis. *Surg Endosc* 2000;**14:**227–31.
62. Misra SP, Dwivedi M. Endoscopy-assisted emergency treatment of gastroduodenal and pancreatobiliary ascariasis. *Endoscopy* 1996;**28:**629–31.
63. Rodriguez AN, Sanchez del Rio AL, Alguacil LV, De Dios Vega JF, Fugarolos GM. Effectiveness of endoscopic sphincterotomy in complicated hepatic hydatid disease. *Gastrointest Endosc* 1998;**48:**593–7.
64. Tekant Y, Bilge O, Acarli K, Alper A, Emre A, Ariogul O. Endoscopic sphincterotomy in the treatment of postoperative biliary fistulas of hepatic hydatid disease. *Surg Endosc* 1996;**10:**909–11.
65. Saritas U, Parlak E, Akoglu M, Sahin B. Effectiveness of endoscopic treatment modalities in complicated hepatic hydatid disease after surgical intervention. *Endoscopy* 2001;**33:**858–63.
66. Al Karawi MA, Yasawy MI, el Shiekh Mohamed AR. Endoscopic management of biliary hydatid disease: Report on six cases. *Endoscopy* 1991;**23:**278–81.
67. Dowidar N, El Sayad M, Osman M, Salem A. Endoscopic therapy of fascioliasis resistant to oral therapy. *Gastrointest Endosc* 1999;**50:**345–51.

CHAPTER 5

Interpretation of liver biopsies in jaundice

S. MUKHOPADHYAY, S. DATTA GUPTA

The relationship between liver biopsy and the science and art of medicine is unique. The foundation of many, if not most, liver diseases is based on the liver biopsy. Although a needle biopsy samples about 1/500 000th of the liver, the information it provides is enormous. Liver biopsy remains the gold standard for the evaluation of jaundice in general, and chronic liver diseases in particular. Since a majority of the causes of jaundice are due to non-neoplastic diseases and the histological array of reactions of the liver is limited, liver biopsy may not provide an accurate diagnosis in some cases. The role of biopsy in these cases is to narrow the differential diagnosis and hopefully rule out some considerations. Therefore, liver biopsy is an invaluable tool in the evaluation of the jaundiced patient, provided both the clinician and the pathologist are aware of the usefulness and limitations of the biopsy in a given case.[1–5]

For example, although useful, liver biopsies are usually not required for the diagnosis of acute liver disease. It is only when the diagnosis is unclear despite thorough clinical and laboratory investigations that a liver biopsy must be resorted to. Similarly, in a case of large bile duct obstruction, a liver biopsy may provide histological evidence of cholestasis, but it makes more sense to perform imaging studies, which are more informative. Additionally, although many liver diseases can be suspected or diagnosed by non-invasive methods, many diagnoses in hepatology are clinicopathological, meaning that 'compatible histopathology' is required to validate a clinical or laboratory diagnosis (Boxes 1 and 2).

Therefore, in a given clinical situation, the much awaited report on a liver biopsy, if adequate and assessed properly, invariably has an important bearing on

Box 1	Uses of liver biopsy in the evaluation of jaundice
• Making or confirming a diagnosis	
• Assessing the severity of liver damage	
• Assessing the prognosis in a given case	
• Monitoring the response to therapy	

Box 2	General indications for liver biopsy

- Evaluation, grading and staging of chronic hepatitis—cirrhosis
- Evaluation of the cause of abnormal liver function tests
- Identification and assessment of alcoholic and related non-alcoholic liver disease
- Recognition of systemic inflammatory or granulomatous disease
- Evaluation of fevers of unknown origin
- Evaluation of the type and extent of liver injury caused by therapeutic drugs
- Diagnosis of multisystem infiltrative diseases
- Evaluation of cholestatic liver disease
- Diagnosis of primary and metastatic tumours
- Diagnosis of metabolic liver disease
- Screening of relatives of patients with familial disease
- Evaluation of effectiveness of therapy
- Evaluation of status of the liver before and following liver transplantation
- Provision of tissue for culture and molecular biology tests

Note: A thorough non-invasive investigation must have been carried out before performing a liver biopsy

the overall diagnosis and management of a case of jaundice. However, it must also be emphasized that the decision to do a liver biopsy must be taken judiciously and not merely because of the availability of a needle, a skilled operator and a liver in an ill patient who has full faith in what is being done!

TYPES OF LIVER BIOPSIES

Liver biopsy is most commonly performed on inpatients due to the ease of post-procedure monitoring, but several publications have addressed the issues associated with the performance of this procedure on outpatients.[6–9] The methods in use for performing a liver biopsy are outlined in Box 3. Of all the types of liver biopsy specimens, blind percutaneous needle biopsies are by far the most commonly available to a histopathologist. Imaging is generally reserved and recommended for focal as well as deep-seated lesions. Several centres do liver biopsies under imaging guidance only and this has resulted in liver biopsies being performed more often by radiologists than clinicians in some hospitals.

Box 3	Types of liver biopsies

1. Closed biopsy (not under direct vision, usually synonymous with needle biopsy)
    - Percutaneous (most common)
        - 'Blind'
        - Imaging-guided (ultrasound- or CT-guided)
    - Transjugular (used in patients with ascites or bleeding diatheses)
2. Open biopsy
    - At surgery
        - Laparoscopic biopsy
        - Wedge biopsy
        - Resection specimen
        - Needle biopsy as outlined earlier
    - At transplantation
        - Explants (native liver of the recipient)

Several types of needles are available for percutaneous liver biopsies:

1. Aspiration-type needles: Menghini needle and its variants, Klatskin needles, Jamshidi needle
2. Cutting-type needles: Vim Silverman needle, Trucut needle

The Menghini needle is popular with most clinicians. This is because the needle needs to be in the liver only for a short time, and is thus less likely to tear the liver capsule if the patient breathes while the needle is within the liver. The fact that it bypasses fibrous structures and is thus less likely to damage large intrahepatic blood vessels or bile ducts also makes it safer. This, however, also means that the Menghini needle is not the device of first choice in the estimation of fibrosis in the liver. The needle of choice for this purpose is the Trucut needle, which is relatively more complicated to use, and should therefore be avoided for other indications. Currently, several biopsy 'guns' that contain disposable cutting needles are available. In expert hands, the tissue obtained for diagnosis is equally satisfactory with the needles in common use.[10] The choice of needle generally depends on the convenience of the operator and, in several institutions, is a part of the legacy spanning several generations of trainees.

Transjugular biopsy avoids puncture of the peritoneum and liver capsule. This technique may be used when coagulation parameters are too far deranged to allow a safe percutaneous biopsy. The expertise required to cannulate and negotiate the internal jugular vein precludes the widespread use of this technique, especially in children. There have been criticisms regarding the adequacy of tissue obtained by this route. However, recent reports suggest that, in experienced hands,[11] adequate tissue may be obtained with the Trucut and Ross transjugular needles in up to 91% and 70% of cases, respectively.

In the normal liver, the capsular fibrous tissue dips into the subcapsular parenchyma for a variable distance (around 5 mm).[12] It is therefore recommended that wedge biopsies be taken in such a manner that deep tissue is included. In other words, the wedge should resemble a cup rather than a saucer.

HANDLING A LIVER BIOPSY

Among the frequent reasons for a suboptimal report are inadequate tissue or a badly handled, fixed or processed tissue. Many of these are easily avoidable. First, squeezing the specimen with a pair of forceps should be avoided. The resultant artifacts render interpretation of morphology impossible. A core of tissue (minimum 2.5 cm in length) adequately fixed in 10% neutral buffered formalin is all that is necessary for most indications. For electron microscopy, a 1 cmm piece is fixed in 2.5% glutaraldehyde.

In special circumstances, such as in the diagnosis of metabolic liver disease or obscure infections, additional examinations may be necessary. In such cases, the liver biopsy may either be divided or several passes made with the needle to obtain more than one core of biopsy. It is advisable to always check with the laboratory to determine the most appropriate method for sending the tissue, and clarify the precautions to be adopted. The most convenient method to send tissue for enzyme analysis, fat stains as well as molecular biology studies is to freeze the tissue immediately in liquid nitrogen. If this is not possible, at least for fat staining, the tissue may be rushed to the laboratory and frozen in a cryostat. The tissue can then be divided; half the sections obtained can be used for the appropriate staining and the other half for biochemical analyses. For micro-biological culture, the laboratory should be asked about the container, aseptic precautions and the medium in which the biopsy is to be sent.

As a rule of thumb, the priority should always be to obtain adequate formalin-fixed tissue. All other tests are additional or ancillary to the evaluation of a routine paraffin section. Most laboratories process liver biopsies routinely in automated tissue processors. In some laboratories, hand-processing is done. A preliminary report can be expected only the next day. Processing under vacuum reduces the processing time drastically to a few hours and this is used for rapid reporting, especially of post-transplant biopsies when antirejection or some other therapy is to be instituted urgently.

The mainstay of evaluation of liver biopsies is a haematoxylin and eosin (H&E) stained paraffin section. However, several other stains are used routinely or under special circumstances to augment the findings of H&E staining (Table I). With the advent of immunohistochemistry, the accuracy and ability to characterize several lesions have increased tremendously (Box 4). However, in some circumstances, especially in metabolic liver disease, the role of light microscopy is limited and other tests may be necessary to arrive at a diagnosis.

Adequacy of the sample

As mentioned earlier, a liver biopsy samples only a minute portion of the liver. Therefore, sampling errors are to be expected, especially in diseases that are not diffuse or affect the different components in a patchy manner. This is exemplified in the variation of findings in chronic HCV infection purely on account of sampling.[13,14] An adequate biopsy contains four to six portal tracts, corresponding to approximately a 2.5 cm length core of a needle biopsy.[15,16] This gives an idea regarding the overall architecture of the liver as well as the relationship between the central veins (terminal hepatic venules) and portal tract; it also provides reasonable tissue necessary for the diagnosis of conditions such as cirrhosis and chronic hepatitis. However, for the diagnosis of a diffuse disease such as acute hepatitis, a single lobule may be sufficient to arrive at a diagnosis, and for conditions such as amyloidosis, a biopsy without any portal tract may be sufficient. As mentioned earlier, a subcapsular biopsy is not suitable for the diagnosis of cirrhosis. Further, for unclear reasons, the subcapsular region shows collapse and inflammation out of proportion to the underlying liver disease and hence may not be ideal for the evaluation of conditions such as chronic hepatitis.[12]

Table I. Special stains that may be used on liver biopsy material

Periodic acid Schiff (PAS)	Stains a wide range of glycoproteins; very sensitive but extremely non-specific (PAS-positive: magenta)
*PAS with diastase	Specific for glycogen if diastase sensitive; useful for identifying diastase-resistant α_1-antitrypsin globules and ceroid pigment
*Reticulin (Gordon and Sweet)	Outlines the reticulin framework of the liver (black)
*Masson trichrome	Identifies collagen (blue/green depending on stain used)
Verhoeff van Geison	Stains elastic tissue (Verhoeff stain; black) and collagen (red), bile (green)
Prussian blue	Stains haemosiderin (blue)
Shikata orcein	Stains elastin fibres, HBsAg and copper-associated protein (copper-binding protein) (brown-black)
Victoria blue	Similar to orcein (blue)
Rhodanine or rubeanic acid	Stains copper (rhodanine: red) (not to be confused with rhodamine used for detection of the tubercle bacillus)
Hall stain	Stains bile (green)
Fontana Masson	Stains melanin; pigment of Dubin–Johnson syndrome (black)
Phosphotungstic acid haematoxylin (PTAH)	Stains fibrin and mitochondria (blue)
Congo red	Identifies amyloid; permanganate resistance favours AL over AA amyloid (orange, apple-green birefringence under polarized light)
Crystal violet	Stains amyloid metachromatically (different from the colour of the stain) (pink)
Modified Ziehl–Neelsen	For tubercle bacilli, schistosome eggs and hooklets of hydatid scolices (pink red/magenta)
Warthin–Starry	For spirochetes (black)
Giemsa	For Leishman–Donovan bodies (blue, red)
Oil red O	Stains lipid (red)
Schultz modification of the Lieberman–Burchard reaction	Stains cholesterol
Toluidine blue	Stains mast cells and amyloid metachromatically (different from the colour of the stain) (pink)
Gram stain	Organisms; Gram-positive (blue), Gram-negative (pink)
Methanamine silver	Wall of fungi (black)
Mucicarmine	Mucin, wall of *Cryptococcus* (red)
Alcian blue–PAS	Acid mucin (blue), neutral mucin (magenta)
Luxol fast blue	Sphingolipid (blue)

Colour following staining is indicated in parentheses
* Stains that are routinely performed for every biopsy in some centres
Note: This list is only indicative and may not cover all stains that can be performed

NORMAL LIVER AND SOME ABNORMALITIES

The normal liver is divided into zones depending on the relationship between the three clear landmarks identified on histology (Fig. 1): the portal tract; the terminal hepatic venule (central veins); and the parenchyma of the hepatocytes, sinusoids and the sinusoidal lining cells (endothelial cells, Kupffer cells and hepatic stellate cells). In a lobule, the central veins are considered to be in the middle with the portal tracts at the periphery. According to the acinar concept of Rappaport,[17] the portal tracts are in the middle while the terminal hepatic venules are at the periphery (direction of blood flow in the sinusoids). A lobule as well as the acinus is further divided into three zones. The area around the

Box 4	Special techniques that may be used on liver biopsy material

Immunohistochemistry

Antibodies raised against the following antigens can be used to determine whether the antigen is present in the tissue being studied. Some of the antibodies are used to characterize tumours.

- HBsAg (cytoplasmic staining)
- HBcAg (nuclear staining)
- HCV (problematic due to antigenic variation in the HCV)
- HDV
- Herpesviruses
- Adenovirus
- CMV
- HIV
- Ubiquitin: Mallory bodies
- Cytokeratins (CK)
  - Pan-CK: Mallory bodies
  - 8, 18: Hepatocytes
  - 8, 18, 7, 19: Bile duct epithelium
- Polyclonal carcinoembryonic antigen (CEA): Bile canaliculi
- Alpha fetoprotein (AFP)

- Epithelial membrane antigen (EMA): epithelial cells
- Leucocyte markers
  - Leucocyte common antigen (LCA, CD45 RB): Most leucocytes
  - CD20: B lymphocytes
  - CD3: T lymphocytes
  - CD68: Macrophages
- Endothelial cells: CD34, Factor VIII R Ag
- Marker for mesenchymal cells
  - Vimentin
  - Desmin: Striated muscle
  - Smooth muscle actin: Smooth muscle, stellate cells
  - S-100 protein, neurofilament: Nerve sheath
- Neuroendocrine markers: Synaptophysin, chromogranin, neuron-specific enolase

Electron microscopy

This may be helpful in the following circumstances:

- α_1-antitrypsin deficiency: Granular material in dilated endoplasmic reticulum
- Glycogen storage disorders: Glycogen deposits
- Gaucher disease
- Wilson disease
- Niemann–Pick disease

- Zellweger disease
- Fabry disease
- Drug-induced injury
- Viruses: May identify the causative virus
- Differentiation of Dubin–Johnson pigment from lipofuscin

Fluorescence microscopy

Autofluorescence in erythropoietic protoporphyria and porphyria cutanea tarda

Polarizing microscopy

Polarizing microscopy is another non-routine technique that has been found to be useful in detecting the following substances:

- Talc
- Amyloid

- Malaria pigment
- Uroporphyrin

terminal hepatic venule is the centrizonal area or roughly zone 3 (Rappaport's acinar concept). The area around the portal tract is the periportal area or roughly zone 1 (in Rappaport's acinus). The area in between is the mid-zonal area, roughly corresponding to Rappaport's zone 2. The integrity of the architecture of the liver lies in the unique relationship between the three important components described. Reticulin as well as trichrome stains aid in the evaluation of the overall architecture of the lobule or acinus. Fibrosis as in cirrhosis and extensive necrosis as in bridging and panacinar necroses are common causes of loss of this architectural balance.

The structures in the portal tract or triad consist of the portal venule (the largest structure), hepatic artery and bile duct. Not every portal tract has each of these three structures.[18] Portal dyads are devoid of any one of these structures (usually the portal venule). The ratio of the bile ducts to portal tracts (containing

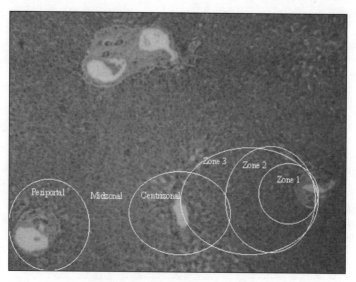

Fig. 1. Normal liver showing three portal tracts and a terminal hepatic venule. The different zones and terminologies used for describing these are indicated. (H&E)

an arteriole) is 0.9–1.8. When this ratio is below 0.5, there is a paucity of the intrahepatic bile ducts (PIBD),[19] which is seen in a variety of conditions ranging from α_1-antitrypsin deficiency to chronic allograft rejection following liver transplantation. A sparse lymphocytic infiltrate may normally be present in the portal tracts. Some experience is required to judge the severity of inflammation, since there is no numerical cut-off value for the normal number of inflammatory cells in the portal tracts. Plasma cells and polymorphs are generally not seen. Inflammatory cells may be found lying in the tract, aggregated as lymphoid follicles, infiltrating the bile ducts (neutrophils indicate histological cholangitis) or extending into the lobule and destroying the adjacent layer of hepatocytes or the limiting plate (piecemeal or interface hepatitis). Abnormal cells, such as an infiltrate from a lymphoma, mimic an inflammatory infiltrate. Granulomas may be identified in tuberculosis, primary biliary cirrhosis (PBC), sarcoidosis and several other conditions. The bile ducts are devoid of intraluminal bile and the presence of bile within the ducts indicates ductular cholestasis. Extravasated bile, foam cells and bile ductular proliferation are typically found in large bile duct obstruction. Bile ductular damage is indicated by vacuolation of the cell cytoplasm, inflammatory infiltrate or necrosis of the lining epithelium. The portal tracts contain collagen and elastic tissue as demonstrated by the orcein stain. Elastic tissue is normally limited to the portal tracts.

Hepatocytes and sinusoidal cells form important components of the lobule and are the site of pathology of several diseases resulting in jaundice. In infants, the liver cell plates are two-cell thick. By 5 years of age, these should be one-cell thick. The cell plates are not parallel to each other and if so, are indicative of abnormal architecture. Two-cell thick plates are seen in regenerating livers. When the plates become three or more cells thick, a neoplastic condition such as a hepatocellular carcinoma (HCC) must be considered. Normally, the ageing liver shows nuclear anisonucleosis and lipofuscin pigment accumulates in the centrizonal (zone 3) areas. Hepatocytes may be enlarged due to hydropic (ballooning) change, fat (fatty change, steatosis) or due to accumulation of other substances such as glycogen. Enlarged hepatocytes may compress the sinusoids. Accumulation of pigments within the lobule is abnormal. Common accumulations include iron (which may be present elsewhere including the portal tracts) and bile. Necrosis of the hepatocytes, often denoted by focal replacement by lymphocytes, should be looked for. Necrosis may be spotty (focal) or confluent, affecting several cells. Confluent necrosis connecting any of the vascular structures (portal tract and central vein) is known as bridging necrosis. Confluent necrosis affecting the entire lobule is termed as panlobular or panacinar necrosis. The sinusoidal cells may contain pigments (malarial pigments and haemosiderin), storage material in metabolic liver disease or may show erythrophagocytosis.

The terminal hepatic venule normally has a rim of collagen all around. This should not be misinterpreted as veno-occlusive disease (VOD). Necrosis and ballooning are very often localized around the central vein.

Viral inclusions and other such abnormalities may be found in any of the structures described above.

It is not possible to detail each and every bit of the procedure for the evaluation of a liver biopsy in this chapter; only the broad principles are outlined. All abnormalities are generally described in relation to their location within the zone (or lobule), extent and severity. Correlation of these changes will provide a guide to the diagnosis. Once this diagnosis is made, the diagnosis and histological observations should explain the clinical picture (clinicopathological correlation). If it does, then the diagnosis is likely to be correct. In many instances, a straight-forward diagnosis may not be forthcoming. At least a reasonable differential diagnosis may be discussed with the clinician. This may help in guiding further evaluation or even therapy. The histopathologist is part of a team that works to treat the patient, and a liver biopsy is one of the several examinations (including clinical) to be performed.

REACTION PATTERNS OF THE LIVER

It must be appreciated that the liver has a limited array of histological changes to a wide variety of diseases. The following major reaction patterns are generally seen:

- Cholestasis
- Hepatocellular damage: hepatitis
- Pigment deposition
- Storage of material within the cells
- Haemorrhage and congestion
- Tumours

A brief list of the common differential diagnosis of major histopathological findings and disease entities for which a liver biopsy is performed are given in Table II and Box 5, respectively. It is obvious that interpretation of liver biopsies

Table II. Differential diagnoses of some common lesions

Lobular mononuclear infiltration with or without necrosis

- Acute hepatitis
- Autoimmune hepatitis
- Primary biliary cirrhosis
- Lymphoma/leukaemia
- Non-specific reactive hepatitis

Lobular lymphocyte/plasma cell infiltration with or without hepatocellular degeneration

- Acute viral hepatitis
  - —Hepatitis A–E
  - —Cytomegalovirus (CMV)
  - —Epstein–Barr virus (EBV)
  - —Others
- Acute drug-induced hepatitis
- Autoimmune (lupoid) hepatitis
- Chronic lobular hepatitis
- Primary biliary cirrhosis
- Leukaemia/lymphoma
- Non-specific reactive hepatitis

Lobular polymorphonuclear cell infiltrate with or without hepatocellular degeneration

- Surgical hepatitis
- Systemic sepsis
- Direct hepatic bacterial or fungal infection
- Viral infections (especially CMV) in the immunocompromised host
- Alcoholic hepatitis
- Non-alcoholic steatohepatitis
- Drug reaction
- Jejunoileal bypass

Confluent hepatocellular necrosis with minimal inflammation

Acute viral infection or massive hepatic necrosis due to

- Hepatotropic viruses (A–E)
- Other hepatitis (non-A, non-B)
- Drug reaction
- Solitary necrotic nodule
- Ischaemia
- Trauma
- Artifact due to poor fixation
- Necrotic tumour

Portal lymphocytic and/or plasma cell infiltrate with minimal lobular inflammation or degeneration

- Hepatitis A
- Resolving acute hepatitis
- Chronic hepatitis
- Primary biliary cirrhosis
- Primary sclerosing cholangitis
- Wilson disease
- Chronic low-grade or intermittent biliary obstruction
- Liver adjacent to a mass lesion
- Malignant infiltrate, particularly lymphoma

Portal polymorphonuclear cell infiltrate with minimal lobular inflammation or degeneration

- Acute biliary obstruction
- Ascending cholangitis
- Sepsis, including toxic shock syndrome
- Drug reactions
- Hyperalimentation
- Viral hepatitis
- Primary biliary cirrhosis

Portal eosinophilic infiltrate (not necessarily predominant but easily identifiable)

- Drug reaction
- Primary biliary cirrhosis
- Primary sclerosing cholangitis
- Parasitic infestation
- Some malignancies, especially Hodgkin disease and mastocytosis
- Extramedullary haematopoiesis
- Langerhans cell histiocytosis

Granulomatous inflammation

- Mycobacterial infection (tuberculosis)
- Fungal infection
- Parasitic infections (schistosomiasis)
- Bacterial infections such as typhoid
- Viral infection
- Rickettsial infection (Q fever)
- Primary biliary cirrhosis
- Sarcoidosis
- Idiopathic granulomatosis
- Drug reaction
- Foreign material
- Lipogranuloma
- Crohn disease
- Malignancy (e.g. Hodgkin disease)
- Chronic granulomatous disease

Table II *(contd.).* Differential diagnoses of some common lesions

Fibrosis
- Cirrhosis
- Non-cirrhotic portal fibrosis
- Congenital hepatic fibrosis
- Alcoholic hepatitis
- Non-alcoholic steatohepatitis
- Chronic venous outflow obstruction
- Heart failure
- Budd–Chiari syndrome
- Veno-occlusive disease
- Focal biliary fibrosis in cystic fibrosis
- Fibrolamellar hepatoma
- Sclerosing hepatocellular carcinoma
- Cholangiocarcinoma
- Metastatic carcinoma
- Congenital syphilis
- Amyloid
- Diabetes mellitus
- Crohn disease

Cholestasis in relative isolation
- Postoperative cholestasis
- Sepsis
- Drugs
- Early bile duct obstruction
- Liver adjacent to mass lesions
- Benign recurrent familial cholestasis
- Cholestasis of pregnancy
- Metabolic diseases

Congestion or haemorrhage, often in association with sinusoidal dilatation
- Hepatic venous outflow obstruction
- Veno-occlusive disease
- Heart failure
- Portal vein or hepatic arterial obstruction
- Infarction
- Drug reaction
- Peliosis hepatis
- Nodular regenerative hyerplasia
- Hepatoportal sclerosis
- Liver adjacent to a mass lesion
- Neoplasms

Sinusoidal dilatation
- Artifact
- Drug reaction
- Hepatic venous outflow obstruction
- Low-grade hepatic blood inflow obstruction
- Peliosis hepatis
- Nodular regenerative hyperplasia
- Adjacent to a mass lesion

Pigments in the liver
- Bile
- Lipofuscin
- Iron
- Formalin
- Dubin–Johnson pigment
- Other exogenous pigments

Intranuclear inclusions
- Glycogenated nuclei
- Prominent nucleoli
- Cytomegalovirus
- Herpes simplex or Varicella zoster
- Adenovirus

Intracytoplasmic inclusions
- Ground-glass cells
- Induction of endoplasmic reticulum
- Fibrinogen
- Drug-associated inclusions
- Lafora disease
- Microvesicular fat
- Mallory hyaline
- Hepatitis B
- α_1-antitrypsin
- Amylopectin
- Cytoplasmic serum protein hyaline inclusions
- Endoplasmic storage disease of the liver
- Hepatic oncocytes
- Giant mitochondria

Extracellular infiltrates
- Amyloid
- Collagen
- Fibrin thrombi

Unusual cells in the liver
- Megakaryocytes
- Extramedullary haematopoiesis
- Metastatic tumour
- Storage cells
- Adipocytes

Table II *(contd.).* Differential diagnoses of some common lesions

The nearly normal biopsy
- Storage or metabolic diseases
- Nodular regenerative hyperplasia
- Non-cirrhotic portal fibrosis

- Carrier state of viral hepatitis
- Drug reactions

Bile duct and ductular proliferation
- Large duct obstruction due to any cause
- Sepsis
- Congenital hepatic fibrosis
- Fibrosis or cirrhosis of any aetiology

- Von Meyenberg complex (bile duct hamartoma)
- Bile duct adenoma
- Focal nodular hyperplasia
- Cholangiocarcinoma

Adapted from Snover DC. Non-neoplastic liver disease. In: Sternberg SS (ed). *Diagnostic surgical pathology.* 2nd ed. New York: Raven Press; 1989.

Box 5	Diagnostic categories in hepatic histopathology
Major disease entities for which liver biopsies are performed:	

- Neonatal cholestasis (neonatal hepatitis syndromes)
- Chronic hepatitis
- Acute viral hepatitis versus drug-induced hepatitis
- Metabolic disorders
- Cirrhosis
- Tumours
- Pyrexia of unknown origin (PUO)

- Hepatosplenomegaly of unknown origin
- Post-transplant evaluation
- Autoimmune hepatitis
- Liver abscesses
- Reye syndrome
- Congenital hepatic fibrosis and infantile polycystic kidney/liver disease
- Budd–Chiari syndrome
- The hyperbilirubinaemias

requires thorough clinicopathological correlation. Information that must be available to the pathologist interpreting a biopsy includes history (including hepatotoxin exposure and potential sources of infection), pertinent examination findings, and the results of LFT, radiology, serology and tests for autoimmunity. The clinician who omits this information and the pathologist who readily accepts such inadequacy is a willing party to the severely limited diagnostic accuracy of the liver biopsy report. In most instances, the consequences of such circumstances affect the patient much more than the reputation of both the clinician and the pathologist (alone as well as combined)! On the other hand, to make sure that the bias of the clinician does not unduly affect the interpretation of the case, it has been recommended that the pathologist attempt to make a diagnosis without clinical information before correlating the case with the clinical information.[5] The latter is best done in conjunction with the clinician.

Cholestasis

Cholestasis to a histopathologist is the presence of visible bile in the tissue section. The bile may be present in the hepatocytes (cellular cholestasis), canaliculi (canalicular cholestasis) and the intrahepatic biliary channels (ductular cholestasis) in various combinations. Failure of excretion of bile may be the consequence of obstruction to the biliary flow through the channels within (intrahepatic cholestasis) or outside the liver (extrahepatic cholestasis) or due to injury to the hepatocytes resulting in non-secretion of bile. Therefore, histo-pathologically, one has to be certain that the pigment is within the canaliculi and other larger bile channels (no other pigment accumulates in these locations). When bile is present within the hepatocytes or Kupffer cells, other pigments may have to be excluded, notably lipofuscin and iron. Bile pigment is yellowish-brown to green in colour. In chronic cholestasis, the evidence for cholestasis may lie only in the form of dilated canaliculi or canalicular rosettes that are identified as hepatocytes arranged in the form of a gland with or without bile within. It must be reiterated that hepatitis is a common cause of cholestasis seen in liver biopsies. Cholestasis may accompany several metabolic liver diseases. The end result of chronic cholestasis due to biliary obstruction and some metabolic liver diseases is fibrosis. Typically, the fibrosis extends from one portal tract to another resulting in so-called secondary biliary cirrhosis (some prefer to use the term secondary biliary fibrosis).[20]

Large bile duct obstruction (extrahepatic) is usually characterized by cholestasis in the interlobar bile ducts (Fig. 2); portal tract changes by way of oedema, ductular proliferation, inflammation, neutrophilic infiltration and ductular infiltration by polymorphs (histological cholangitis); and foam cells. Bile infarcts and bile lakes are helpful features. It must be mentioned that sepsis may also show similar features.[21] However, bile ductular proliferation appears to be less frequent in sepsis. Cholestasis due to hepatitis is predominantly centri-zonal and lacks the portal changes seen in extrahepatic obstruction. Hepatocellular changes by way of ballooning should be looked for. A change similar to ballooning called feathery degeneration has been described in chronic cholestasis. However, the difference between the two is better seen than described. Bland cholestasis can be the result of drugs such as chlorpromazine. It must be mentioned that the centrizonal area is the most frequent site of

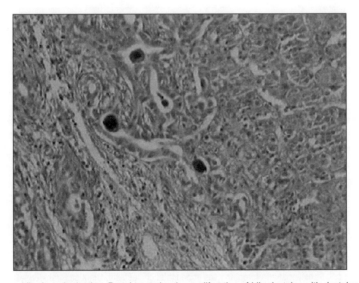

Fig. 2. Large bile duct obstruction. Portal tract showing proliferation of bile ductules with ductular cholestasis. (H&E)

cholestasis, especially in the early stages of cholestasis due to any cause including obstruction. Copper and copper-associated protein is increased in cholestasis of any aetiology or type.[22]

Imaging techniques have practically replaced the need to perform liver biopsy to distinguish between extrahepatic or large duct and intrahepatic cholestasis. However, in certain situations, liver biopsy is important.

Neonatal cholestasis

Neonatal cholestasis (neonatal jaundice lasting >14 days) is an area where liver biopsy is essential. The differential diagnosis is important since it leads to radically different modes of therapy depending on the diagnosis. Extrahepatic biliary atresia (EHBA) is treated surgically whereas neonatal hepatitis is treated medically. Histologically, cholestasis, giant cell transformation of the hepatocytes (Fig. 3) and extramedullary haemopoiesis are features common to many of the conditions that fall under the rubric of neonatal cholestasis.[23-26] Therefore, discriminatory histological features are of great importance and must be actively sought. Indeed, in questionable cases, percutaneous liver biopsy is the most accurate diagnostic test to differentiate neonatal hepatitis from biliary atresia; the caveat is that an experienced paediatric pathologist must interpret the biopsy. However, histology is not foolproof (7%–15% rate of misdiagnoses), and therefore an attempt must be made to include radiological/nuclear scanning features in the final assessment of the pathology. Some of the common aetiologies of neonatal hepatitis are viral hepatitis, the TORCH group of infections, α_1-antitrypsin deficiency, tyrosinaemia, galactosaemia and Niemann–Pick disease. Morphological clues to an aetiology may be found, and include inclusion bodies (CMV, α_1-antitrypsin), fatty change with cirrhosis

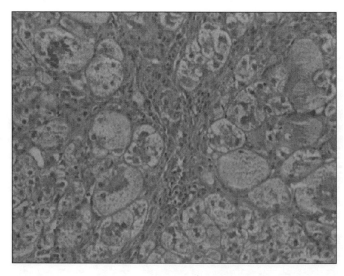

Fig. 3. Giant cell transformation of hepatocytes in neonatal cholestasis. Giant cell transformation may be found in several diseases. Cells with three or more nuclei are identified. In addition, there is ballooning change and fibrosis has set in. (H&E)

(galactosaemia and tyrosinaemia) and whorls on electron microscopy (Niemann–Pick disease). If no aetiology is found, as is often the case, the diagnosis is idiopathic neonatal hepatitis.

There are no unique histological features that distinguish EHBA from neonatal hepatitis. However, it is important to remember that in EHBA, the damage is centred on the portal tracts, and therefore the most severe changes are seen in and around them. In contrast, neonatal hepatitis does not show any regional preference, the lobular disarray and giant cell transformation of hepatocytes being diffuse; portal tract involvement is less than that in EHBA. Bile duct proliferation (i.e. multiple ducts instead of one or two per portal triad) is another feature that favours EHBA over neonatal hepatitis (Fig. 2). Other features that favour a diagnosis of EHBA over neonatal hepatitis include enlarged, fibrotic and inflamed portal tracts, mis-shapen bile ductules and lymphangiectasia of the portal tracts. Fibrosis in EHBA sets in early in the course of the disease with cirrhosis developing as early as within 3 months of age.[27, 28] Loss of bile ducts may accompany EHBA.[29]

Paucity of the intrahepatic bile ducts

A reference to PIBD has already been made. The disease process in PIBD is centred on the portal tracts. The criterion laid down by Alagille is <0.5 inter-lobular ducts per portal tract versus a normal of 0.9–1.8 interlobular ducts per 100 portal tracts.[19] Only true interlobular ducts are to be counted. These accompany the hepatic arterioles in the centre of the portal tracts. Bile ductules must be ignored; or else bile ductular proliferation can grossly alter the counts. Giant cell transformation of the hepatocytes can lead to some confusion with neonatal hepatitis and EHBA. PIBD may occur as a part of the Alagille syndrome,[30] where it is associated with cardiovascular, skeletal and ocular abnormalities, or as a non-syndromic form without these stigmata.[31] α_1-antitrypsin deficiency must always be excluded when PIBD is noted.[32] PIBD has been reported in primary sclerosing cholangitis (PSC),[33] histiocytosis X,[34] CMV infection[35] and chronic allograft rejection,[36] to name a few.[37]

Primary sclerosing cholangitis and primary biliary cirrhosis

PSC exists in large-duct and small-duct forms. The large duct lesions are diagnosed on cholangiography, but the small duct lesions are easily missed unless liver biopsy is resorted to.[38] The basic pathology is fibrosis and stricture formation in the intrahepatic bile ducts. If the biopsy is taken from a point proximal to the stricture, non-specific changes of obstruction to the bile flow are seen. If the biopsy is taken from the point of stricture formation, 'onion-skin' periductal fibrosis (Fig. 4) and loss of the bile ducts are the major histological features. Acute cholangitis and cholangiolitis soon supervene consequent to the obstruction.[39] PBC enters the differential diagnosis in adults but not in children due to overlapping histological features.[40] Granulomas,[41,42] if present (30%–70% of cases), and the relevant antibodies (in PBC)[43] and imaging studies (in PSC) are helpful in doubtful cases. PBC has been described to progress in four different

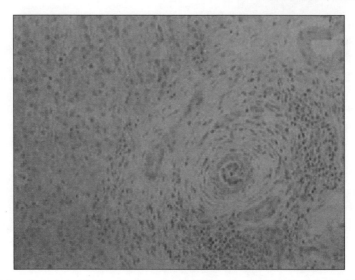

Fig. 4. 'Onion-skinning' of a bile duct. There is portal oedema and lymphocytic infiltrations. Such features are not necessarily seen in primary sclerosing cholangitis and may also be found in large bile duct obstruction. (H&E)

stages ranging from portal inflammation, periportal inflammation, fibrosis and cirrhosis.[42,44] In both PSC and PBC, the histological features may mimic chronic hepatitis. Clinical features, the presence or absence of antimitochondrial antibodies (AMA) granulomas and demonstration of copper-associated proteins are helpful in distinguishing these conditions from the more common chronic viral hepatitis.[22]

Hepatitis

Hepatitis is defined as necrosis and inflammation of the liver. In general, unless qualified, hepatitis is considered to be of viral aetiology and the hepatotropic viruses are most often implicated; these are designated as hepatitis viruses A, B, C, D and E. The GBV-C (considered to be similar to hepatitis virus G) and TT virus (TTV) have been added to this list (*see* pp. 118–19). In addition, especially in the immunocompromised patient, other viruses may cause hepatitis generally as a consequence of a systemic infection.[45] These include CMV, Epstein–Barr virus (EBV), herpesvirus, adenovirus, etc. In some viral infections, such as dengue fever and various viral haemorrhagic fevers, the liver may be affected, although invariably the resulting hepatitis does not alter the prognosis. However, by and large, hepatitis due to known hepatotropic viruses is more common than hepatitis due to other viruses.

A liver biopsy is rarely, if ever, performed to make a diagnosis of acute hepatitis. Liver biopsy is sometimes performed in acute hepatitis as a consequence of a mistaken clinical diagnosis or when the diagnosis is unclear; as a part of the work-up following a liver transplantation (e.g. rejection *v.* hepatitis) and to know the severity of hepatitis. On the other hand, liver biopsy is almost mandatory in chronic hepatitis as a part of the diagnosis, to evaluate the severity of hepatitis and determine the progression to cirrhosis or effect of therapy.

It is essential to remember that histological features of hepatitis, especially acute hepatitis, generally do not suggest the aetiology of the disease. Thus, drug-induced acute hepatitis and acute viral hepatitis (AVH) may be histologically indistinguishable. Similarly, there is considerable overlap between chronic viral hepatitis (CVH), autoimmune hepatitis (AIH) and conditions such as Wilson disease. Therefore, clinical details, biochemical data, and the results of serological and molecular biology tests need to be correlated in each and every case to arrive at a comprehensive diagnosis.

General features

The histological changes in hepatitis[46–48] include hepatocellular damage, inflammatory cell infiltration with or without cholestasis, Kupffer cell prominence, siderosis, endothelialitis, bile ductular damage, bile ductular proliferation and varying regenerative changes of hepatocytes. Chronic hepatitis may progress through fibrosis to cirrhosis.

Hepatocellular damage

Hepatocellular damage is reflected as ballooning degeneration (Figs 3 and 5) and cell death. The hepatocytes may undergo apoptosis[49] characterized by shrunken, rounded, anucleate masses that fragment. Apoptotic bodies may be found in the sinusoids. Apoptotic cells are also known as acidophil or Councilman bodies. Necrosis of the hepatocytes may be identified as a loss of cells. Depending on the severity and location of cell loss, necrosis may broadly be either focal or spotty (single cells) or confluent (groups of cells). Confluent necrosis that connects two vascular landmarks of the liver lobule (especially the central vein

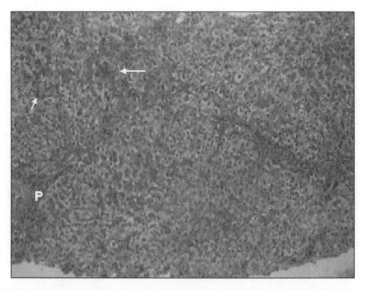

Fig. 5. Diffuse ballooning of the hepatocytes in acute viral hepatitis. There is associated cholestasis (arrow) and portal inflammation (P). (H&E)

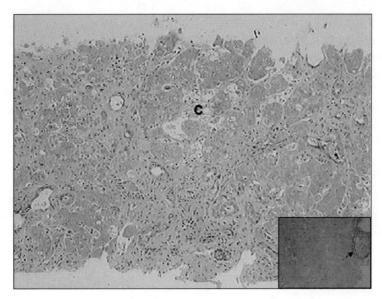

Fig. 6. Bridging necrosis connecting the portal tracts. There is confluent necrosis (C) and intracellular cholestasis. (H&E) The inset shows elastic fibres confined to the portal tract but not in the necrotic areas (orcein).

and portal tract) is called bridging necrosis (Fig. 6). Necrosis that affects the entire lobule is called panlobular or panacinar necrosis (Fig. 7). Piecemeal or interface necrosis (Fig. 8) occurs at the interface between the mesenchyme and parenchyma of the liver. Thus, this refers to necrosis of the periportal hepatocytes (limiting plate). Bridging necrosis is in a way a piecemeal necrosis. Piecemeal necrosis, though an important feature in chronic hepatitis, is also seen in acute hepatitis.

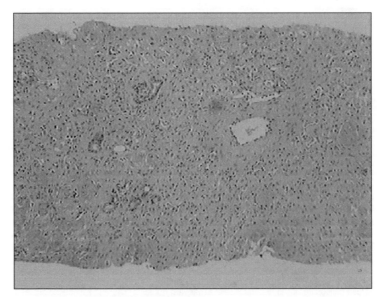

Fig. 7. Panlobular necrosis. The entire lobule shows necrosis of the hepatocytes, and bile ducts in the portal tracts as well as the terminal hepatic venules are drawn closer to each other. (H&E)

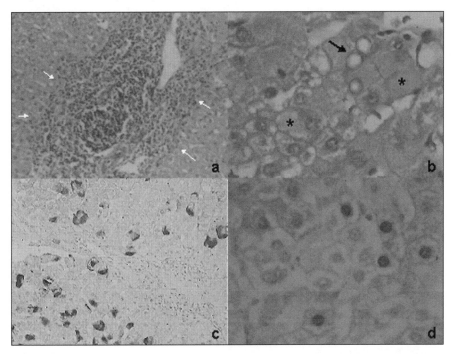

Fig. 8. Liver biopsy in chronic hepatitis. (a) Portal inflammation and lymphoid aggregate in chronic hepatitis C. There is interface hepatitis or piecemeal necrosis (arrows). (H&E) (b) Ground-glass hepatocytes (asterisk) in chronic hepatitis B. A few glycogenated (clear) nuclei can be identified as an incidental finding (arrows). Nuclear glycogeneration is seen in several conditions and is not typical of chronic hepatitis. (H&E) (c) Immunohistochemical localization of HBsAg. The staining is cytoplasmic. (DAB chromogen) (d) HBcAg immunohistochemistry generally shows nuclear localization. (DAB chromogen)

It must be pointed out that that there is often difficulty in distinguishing bridging necrosis from fibrosis. Reticulin and trichrome stains may be misleading for the inexperienced. Orcein staining is helpful in these circumstances.[50] Elastic tissue is normally confined to the portal tract. Therefore, the area of bridging necrosis will not contain any elastic fibres (Fig. 6). On the other hand, in the case of bridging fibrosis, elastic tissue will be demonstrable. Fibrosis in acute hepatitis is seen in the rare histological variant, the fibrosing cholestatic type.[51]

In typical AVH, almost all the lobules are uniformly affected (Fig. 5). In acute hepatitis, hepatocellular changes are usually most pronounced in the centri-zonal/zone 3 area. Thus, ballooning degeneration is predominantly perivenular (zone 3). Areas of spotty and confluent necroses may be present, and apoptotic hepatocytes are seen. The combination of ballooning change of varying degree, unaffected hepatocytes and necrosis gives rise to lobular disarray. In some situations, hepatocytes seem to be arranged in the form of an aggregate with or without a central sinusoid (not a canaliculus). This is known as a hepatitic rosette. Other changes that may be seen include multinucleation of the hepatocytes and formation of giant cells (Fig. 3). These giant cells are especially seen in neonates as a consequence of a variety of conditions. Cholestasis and siderosis may also be identified. Cholestasis is identified mainly within the hepatocytes. Kupffer cells and portal macrophages are prominent. Within the portal tract, there is a lymphocytic infiltration. Fibrosis is not seen.

In the case of typical chronic hepatitis, the lobule shows scattered foci of necrosis. Ballooning change and cholestasis are generally not seen. Portal tracts show variable lymphocytic, plasma cell and macrophage infiltration. Fibrous expansion of the portal tract may be present. There may be portal lymphoid follicle formation with bile duct damage.

Acute hepatitis is characterized by lobular changes while chronic hepatitis typically shows portal inflammation. An exception to this description is acute HAV infection which may present with a portal infiltrate simulating chronic hepatitis.[52] Similarly, in acute HCV infection,[53] the features resemble chronic HCV infection, or the changes may be subtle with a prominent sinusoidal lymphocytic infiltrate simulating infectious mononucleosis. The history and serology should help in arriving at a diagnosis.

Bile duct changes

Infiltration of the portal bile duct by lymphocytes and degenerative changes by way of vacuolation are reported in HCV infection.[54] Ductular cholestasis and bile ductular proliferation may be observed only in severe hepatitis[55] but these features generally suggest an obstruction.

Kupffer cell changes

Kupffer cells are activated and engulf the debris of necrosis and inflammation in hepatitis. A diastase PAS stain brings these out elegantly. Siderosis may also be demonstrated. Kupffer cell activation is common in acute hepatitis and during exacerbation of chronic hepatitis. In the resolving phase of acute hepatitis, Kupffer cells laden with cellular debris, as highlighted by the diastase PAS stain, may be the only evidence of recent hepatitis.

Inflammation

The predominant inflammatory infiltrate in hepatitis is the lymphocyte. Macrophages and plasma cells (especially in hepatitis) may be present; inflammatory infiltrate is found at the site of necrosis and in the portal tracts. A sinusoidal lymphocytic infiltrate and portal lymphoid follicles are seen in HCV infection.[56] Polymorphs and eosinophils may be present in the portal tracts but are not common.

Aetiological diagnosis

In AVH, it is not possible to identify the hepatitis virus in the liver on routine histological examination. The features that suggest HAV infection include a chronic hepatitis-like picture. In HEV infection, some cases of HAV infection and, in our experience, in several cases of HBV infection, prominent cholestasis is identified. Fatty change and severe necrosis is reported in acute HDV infection. Immunohistochemical localization[57] of HBsAg (cytoplasmic) and HBcAg (nuclear) is usually not demonstrable in acute HBV infection. Exceptions to this are immunohistochemical localization of HBsAg in immunosuppressed individuals (post-transplantation and following HIV infection) and in fibrosing cholestatic hepatitis. Immunohistochemistry for HDV (nuclear) also helps in identifying this virus in acute hepatitis. Identification of HAV, HEV and HCV in liver tissue is possible by molecular biology techniques. Acute HCV infection resembles chronic HCV infection histologically and detection of the virus is currently done by molecular biology techniques. Fortunately, simple and standard serological tests permit the diagnosis of a majority of acute hepatitides caused by the common hepatotropic viruses. In general, liver biopsy is not required to make a diagnosis of AVH. A combination of clinical features and serological tests suffices to indicate the pathology in most cases. Similarly, the management of AVH does not call for an assessment of the histopathology in the vast majority of cases.

In chronic hepatitis, HBV infection is identified by the presence of ground-glass hepatocytes (Fig. 8). These cells can be stained by the orcein stain (Shikata cells) and also by immunohistochemistry for HBsAg. Immunohistochemical localization of HBcAg is seen as a replicative HBV infection (Fig. 8). HDV infection can be identified by immunohistochemistry as mentioned earlier. Special stains or immunohistochemistry on tissue sections do not permit the localization of HCV in a routine laboratory. Histological features that suggest chronic hepatitis C[56] include fatty change, portal lymphoid follicle formation (Fig. 8) and bile duct damage. There are apoptotic bodies in the lobule with sinusoidal lymphoid infiltrate. Granulomas[58] and Mallory bodies have also been reported in chronic hepatitis C. It is difficult to distinguish acute and chronic hepatitis C histologically. In the carrier state (only HBV infection without inflammation), inflammation and fibrosis do not develop. Fatty change is not exclusive to HCV infection. This can be seen in a fair proportion of cases with HBV infection also. In both chronic hepatitis B and C, loss of virus is associated with reduction in inflammatory changes. A reactivation of hepatitis should arouse the suspicion of superinfection with another virus. Superinfection of chronic hepatitis B with HCV tends to reduce the expression of HBV antigens in tissue[59] while the converse is the case in superinfection of chronic hepatitis C by HBV.[60]

In addition to morphological clues such as ground-glass hepatocytes (HBV), lymphoid follicles (HCV) and inclusion bodies (herpesviruses and CMV), the aetiology of infectious hepatitis can often be established by immunohisto-chemical means. Antibodies are now available against the hepatitis viruses, herpesviruses, CMV, adenovirus and many other pathogens. The more uncommon entities (such as syphilis, leptospirosis and Q fever) also have characteristic, but not pathognomonic, histological features.

Distinguishing between acute and chronic hepatitis

In general, changes in acute hepatitis are similar from lobule to lobule whereas in chronic hepatitis the changes are more variable (Fig. 5). Ballooning change is frequent in acute hepatitis. In chronic hepatitis, ballooning change accompanies reactivation of the illness. Necrosis and inflammation in acute hepatitis occur predominantly in the lobule with an accentuation around the central vein (zone 3). On the other hand, the portal and periportal areas are the site of inflammation in chronic hepatitis (Fig. 8). In the lobule, areas of necrosis are scattered without a specific pattern in chronic hepatitis, unlike the predominantly centrizonal location in acute hepatitis. It is very unusual to observe panlobular or wide bridging necrosis in chronic hepatitis (Figs 6 and 7). Hepatitic rosettes (group of hepatocytes without a central canaliculus) are often seen in AIH. Cholestasis is invariable in acute hepatitis and distinctly rare, both histologically and clinically, in chronic hepatitis (in chronic hepatitis the serum bilirubin levels generally do not rise beyond 3.5 mg/dl). Giant cell transformation is seen in acute hepatitis, especially in neonates (Fig. 3). Prominence of the Kupffer cells is obvious in acute hepatitis. Fatty change is seen in chronic hepatitis, more so with HCV infection. In the recovery phase, diagnosis may rest on the identification of Kupffer cells and prominent portal macrophages stained by the diastase PAS reaction. Finally, demonstration of fibrosis adds to confirmation of a diagnosis of chronic hepatitis.

Differential diagnosis

Differential diagnosis of acute hepatitis due to hepatitis virus includes acute hepatitis due to other viruses. In CMV infection, there are scattered foci of neutrophilic infiltration. Granulomas, foci of coagulative necrosis and portal karyorrhexis have been described. Typical nuclear inclusions in hepatocytes, endothelial cells and bile duct epithelium may be found. These inclusions are large, eosinophilic, intranuclear with a peri-inclusion 'halo'. Cytoplasmic inclusions are rare. Immunohistochemistry is helpful in doubtful cases.

In EBV infection, sinusoidal lymphocyte infiltration is prominent. The portal tract is infiltrated by a large number of lymphocytes, plasma cells and immuno-blasts. In herpes and adenovirus infections, areas of confluent necrosis, varying from a few foci to massive necrosis, are invariable. Nuclear inclusions are usually found in hepatocytes adjacent to the necrotic foci.

In herpes simplex virus (HSV) and Varicella zoster (VZV) hepatitis, the nuclear inclusion is eosinophilic (more than in CMV infection), and typically occupies the entire nucleus giving a ground-glass appearance. Adenovirus inclusions are large and basophilic. Acute hepatitis with cholestasis may mimic bile duct obstruction. The presence of ductular cholestasis, bile duct prolifera-tion and other portal changes without the lobular changes in acute hepatitis allows a reasonable differentiation.

Drug-induced hepatitis is sometimes indistinguishable from AVH.[61–63] Features suggestive of drug-induced or toxic injury to the liver include demonstrated or bland zone 3 necrosis, lack of inflammation especially in the portal tracts, cholestasis, numerous neutrophils, eosinophils and epithelioid cell granulomas. Antituberculosis drugs, NSAIDs, anaesthetics and herbal medicines may be the offending agents. Toxic injury such as due to mushroom poisoning may give a similar appearance.

AIH may give rise to a picture similar to acute hepatitis. Numerous plasma cells, hepatitic rosettes, bile duct damage and marked necrosis are suggestive features. Identification of autoantibodies and a response to steroids are helpful.

CVH needs to be distinguished from AIH, Wilson disease, α_1-antitrypsin deficiency, PBC, PSC and drug-induced hepatitis. Changes adjacent to a space-occupying lesion and a lymphoma are other differential diagnoses. The clinical history, appropriate laboratory tests and special stains are necessary to make these distinctions.

Grading and staging of chronic hepatitis

Over the years, classification of chronic hepatitis into chronic persistent hepatitis, chronic lobular hepatitis, chronic active hepatitis and chronic septal hepatitis have been rendered obsolete. Piecemeal necrosis was the earlier defining feature of chronic hepatitis, but is no longer so. It was realized that prognosis was not only related to necrosis and inflammation but also to the type of virus and recently to its genotype. With the availability of effective therapy, there was a need to objectively assess the severity of liver changes and determine the response to such therapy. In the current scenario, the main histological issues in chronic hepatitis are:

1. What is the severity of the liver damage? Has it increased or decreased compared to the previous biopsy? Has it changed with therapy?
2. What is the cause of the liver damage?
3. Has cirrhosis set in?

The first set of questions is tackled objectively by grading and staging the liver damage. Grading assesses the extent of liver parenchyma that is involved by the necroinflammatory process, and staging attempts to semiquantify the fibrosis, such as may be present. This information can be used clinically to assess the efficacy of current therapy, and the need for further therapy. Clinical trials currently in progress are using this liver biopsy-based information to assess the efficacy of drugs undergoing evaluation.

Several schemes for grading and staging are available. Currently used grading and staging systems have evolved from the original histological activity index (HAI) of Knodell *et al.*[64] (*see* Chapter 7, Table II, p. 126) The HAI included the severity of both necroinflammatory changes and fibrosis. The grading and staging systems of the International Liver Group[65] and the METAVIR algorithm[66] for chronic HCV hepatitis are popular. In the International Liver Group system,[65] four parameters are scored for necroinflammation: interface hepatitis, confluent necrosis, spotty necrosis and portal inflammation; to a maximum score of 18. Fibrosis is scored on a scale of 0 to 6 (cirrhosis). These systems are of value in comparing serial biopsies. Intraobserver variations are low and interobserver variations among experts or between pathologists who have agreed upon the variables beforehand are also within acceptable limits.[67,68]

The second question, regarding aetiology, has invariably been answered by clinical or serological means by the time biopsy is performed. Nevertheless, histology can often suggest which virus (or other organism) may have caused the hepatitis, as mentioned earlier. Immunohistochemistry, using antibodies against common liver pathogens, is a powerful technique to confirm clinical/laboratory data, or to make a diagnosis when these data are inconclusive.

Whether cirrhosis has set in or not is reflected by the staging mentioned earlier. Stains such as a reticulin stain or Masson trichrome stain are routinely performed to aid in this assessment.

A few pitfalls must be recognized. First, a liver biopsy specimen represents only about 1/500 000th of the entire liver, and therefore a possibility of sampling error always exists. Second, subcapsular samples over-represent liver damage and must always be interpreted with caution.

Autoimmune hepatitis

There are no histological features to reliably distinguish autoimmune chronic hepatitis from CVH, especially hepatitis C, which closely mimics this condition. However, the index of suspicion for this entity should be high if the pathologist encounters a predominance of plasma cells in the portal areas, or hypocellular areas of collapse, or microacinus formation (rosettes). Similarly, multinucleated hepatocytes are more frequently encountered in AIH as compared to CVH. Serological and immunological tests aid in the diagnosis.[69,70]

ALCOHOLIC AND NON-ALCOHOLIC STEATOHEPATITIS

Fatty change or the accumulation of fat within the hepatocytes[71] is one of the most frequent lesions seen in a liver biopsy. The causes of fatty change in the liver span the entire gamut of lesions or diseases described in any book on hepatology. The causes range from alcohol, obesity, diabetes, metabolic diseases, malnutrition, CVH (especially HCV), tuberculosis, toxic injury, drugs and ischaemia, to name a few. Fat in the hepatocytes is usually due to an accumulation of triglycerides. The fat accumulates as a large vacuole that displaces the nucleus to the periphery: the macrovesicular fatty change or macrovesicular steatosis (Fig. 9). In some cases, such as fatty liver of pregnancy, Reye syndrome, tetracycline toxicity, Wolman disease and nucleoside analogue toxicity, the fat droplets are small and dispersed, often giving the appearance of a ballooned hepatocyte. Fat stains (oil red O) best demonstrate this microvesicular steatosis (Fig. 9), which is associated with deranged mitochondrial beta-oxidation of fatty acids[72] and generally with severe liver disease. The location of steatosis is typical in some conditions. Thus, zone 3 (centrizonal) fatty change is seen in alcoholic liver disease (ALD), non-alcoholic fatty liver disease (NAFLD) and chronic venous congestion of the liver, while zone 1 (periportal) fatty change is seen in kwashiorkor, total parenteral nutrition and AIDS. An inflammatory response comprising histiocytes and polymorphs around a ruptured hepatocyte containing fat results in the formation of lipogranulomas. Incidentally, fat may accumulate in the hepatic stellate cells, especially as a consequence of hypervitaminosis A.[73]

Steatohepatitis is a condition that is associated with fatty change. The terminology is self-explanatory. There is inflammation of the liver with steatosis. Characteristically, steatohepatitis is seen in ALD[74] and its counterpart non-alcoholic steatohepatitis (NASH).[75] In both these conditions, the changes are typically located in zone 3 (centrizonal area). Early changes are characterized by ballooning of the hepatocytes. Hepatocytes contain Mallory hyaline (Fig. 9).[76] An inflammatory

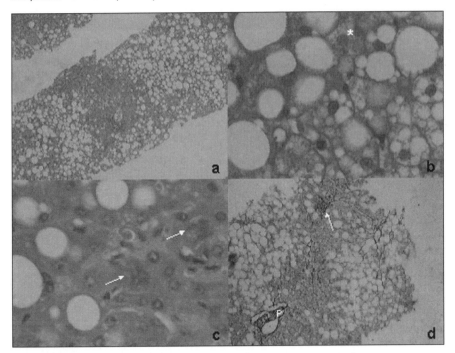

Fig. 9. Steatohepatitis. (a) Fatty change in a needle biopsy. (H&E) (b) Microvesicular (asterisk) and macrovesicular fatty change. (H&E) (c) Mallory hyaline seen as eosinophilic ropy material (arrows) in a case of alcoholic hepatitis. (H&E) (d) Increased reticulin in zone 3 (arrow) from a case of non-alcoholic steatohepatitis. The portal tract is indicated (P). (reticulin stain)

infiltrate composed predominantly of neutrophils is identified around the hepatocytes especially those with Mallory hyaline. In chronic alcoholics, hyaline globular or spindle-shaped intracytoplasmic inclusions (2–10 µ) representing megamitochondria[77] may be identified. There is associated pericellular and perivenular fibrosis. This pattern of fibrosis around the cells is known as chicken-wire fibrosis. The end result is extensive fibrosis and cirrhosis.

In an alcoholic, the severity of histological changes ranges from steatosis (usually without any severe clinical manifestation), alcoholic steatohepatitis, fibrosis and cirrhosis (all with variable clinical presentation including jaundice). Microvesicular steatosis in alcoholics (alcoholic foamy degeneration)[78] and alcoholic steatohepatitis with prominent zone 3 perivenular fibrosis (alcoholic sclerosing hyaline necrosis)[79] are special histological types associated with a poor prognosis. It must be emphasized that alcoholics may present with jaundice due to alcoholic pancreatic disease that results in changes of large bile duct obstruction on liver biopsy.

The association of fatty liver alone and fatty liver with steatohepatitis, histologically simulating ALD but due to causes other than alcohol is known as NAFLD and NASH.[80] In fact, NAFLD[81] has been used to encompass all such lesions of which the more severe forms associated with steatohepatitis, fibrosis or cirrhosis are known as NASH. While alcoholic and non-alcoholic liver diseases are similar histologically, Mallory hyaline and neutrophils are reported to be more frequent in alcoholics, whereas fatty change and nuclear glycogenation (clear nuclei, especially in diabetes; also found in Wilson disease and glycogen storage disease) are generally more marked in non-alcoholics (Fig. 8).[80–82] Currently, a grading and staging system, similar to that for chronic hepatitis, is in use for the evaluation of liver biopsies of NASH.[83]

INHERITED METABOLIC DISORDERS

Inherited metabolic disorders (IMD) of the liver present in a variety of forms. They may present either as a primary liver disease or as a biochemical defect, or affect some other organ. The age at presentation can vary from the neonatal period to adulthood and, in some instances, the affected individuals may not be symptomatic during their entire lifetime. Often the presentation differs depending on the age at manifestation. Thus α_1-antitrypsin deficiency presents as 'neonatal hepatitis' in the period following birth or may manifest as chronic hepatitis or cirrhosis in childhood or adulthood. It is therefore necessary to correlate clinical and biochemical features before arriving at a diagnosis. Unfortunately, facilities for a satisfactory work-up of metabolic disorders are not available even in the best of institutions and liver biopsy can at best suggest certain diagnostic possibilities.

In metabolic diseases, liver biopsy is performed when there is liver dysfunction (clinically or otherwise) to obtain tissue that may confirm a presumptive diagnosis and to stage the disease prior to therapy such as bone marrow transplantation. Since several techniques and stains may be necessary to arrive at a diagnosis, liver biopsies from suspected cases should be divided into at least three portions: one for routine processing, one for electron microscopy and one snap frozen. It may be necessary to fix some tissue in alcohol in certain metabolic diseases (e.g. cystinosis). If the quantity of tissue obtained is small then all attempts should be made to preserve it for paraffin sections. This is the most important aspect of the evaluation of liver biopsies for IMD.

Approach to diagnosis

The following account gives the approach to the diagnosis of IMD based on the light microscopy findings.[84,85] The predominant tissue reaction determines the probable diagnosis.

Cholestasis

Some metabolic diseases present with histological cholestasis.
1. *Presence of 'bland' cholestasis:* Benign recurrent intrahepatic cholestasis
2. *Cholestasis associated with giant cell transformation:* Neonatal hepatitis-like picture in IMD includes Niemann–Pick disease, familial cholestasis of North American Indians and arteriohepatic dysplasia
3. *Cholestasis associated with pseudoglands and fatty change:* This is typical of three conditions—early stages of galactosaemia, tyrosinaemia and

hereditary fructose intolerance. All these conditions may progress to cirrhosis[86]

4. *Chronic cholestasis with foam cells, bile plugs and increased copper storage:*
   - *Associated with PIBD:* Arteriohepatic dysplasia (Alagille syndrome) should be suspected (cirrhosis is rare in this condition), and α_1-antitrypsin deficiency
   - *Associated with cirrhosis:* End result of chronic progressive intrahepatic cholestasis or Byler disease; familial cholestasis of North American Indian children and several other rare, improperly characterized, heredofamilial diseases.[25]

Storage diseases

Storage disease/disorder is the term used for the accumulation of different substances in the cells as a result of a metabolic disorder. The accumulation may involve either one or more components of the hepatic parenchyma. In general, diseases involving the lysosomal enzymes affect the reticuloendothelial cells or sinusoidal cells of the liver.

1. *Clear hepatocyte cytoplasm:* Glycogen storage diseases are the commonest cause. The PAS stain with and without diastase digestion is helpful but does not indicate if the amount of glycogen is increased. Glycogen storage disease type IV and type II may lead to cirrhosis.[87] Diabetes mellitus may also lead to glycogen accumulation.

2. *Hepatocyte and sinusoidal cell clearing:* Mucopolysaccharidoses (Hunter, Hurler disease) have an appearance similar to that of glycogenosis. However, the Kupffer cells are also affected and the colloidal iron stain is helpful in diagnosis.[88] In glycoproteinosis (sialidosis, fucosidosis, mannosidosis) as well as mucolipidoses, cytoplasmic vacuolation is irregular and lacks neutral lipids. The diagnosis is based on the identification of the biochemical defect since both light and electron microscopy are not diagnostic.

3. *Cytoplasmic vacuolation due to neutral lipids ('fatty change'):* This may be seen in urea cycle disorders, carnitine deficiency and as a manifestation of several metabolic diseases such as porphyria cutanea tarda (PCT), glycogenosis type I, diabetes mellitus, galactosaemia, hereditary fructose intolerance, tyrosinaemia, homocystinuria, Wilson disease, abetalipoproteinaemia, cholesterol ester storage disease, Wolman disease, cystic fibrosis, Refsum disease, Schwartzmann syndrome, etc.

4. *A foamy cytoplasm especially of the Kupffer cells* is typical of the sphingolipidoses. Pale basophilic to tan Kupffer cells characterize the prototype Niemann–Pick disease. The nuclei are pyknotic or irregular. On paraffin section, these cells stain with luxol fast blue that is routinely used for the demonstration of myelin. Niemann–Pick disease may present in adulthood with portal hypertension.[89] In GM1 gangliosidosis, the foamy cells contain acid mucopolysaccharides. Membrane-bound cytoplasmic bodies are observed on electron microscopy.

5. *Cytoplasmic striations of enlarged Kupffer cells* and similar cells in the portal

tract is characteristic of Gaucher disease.[90] The cells have a crinkled tissue paper appearance. Unfortunately, striations may not be appreciable on routine H&E stains. Masson trichrome and PAS stains are helpful. Iron deposition may be demonstrated. A marked acid phosphatase activity is seen on enzyme histochemistry. On transmission electron microscopy, 30–60 mm membrane-bound, spindled or rod-shaped inclusions are identified. Unlike Niemann–Pick disease, Gaucher disease is often associated with pericellular fibrosis that may be progressive.

6. *Cytoplasmic inclusions* that resemble ground-glass hepatocytes are seen in Lafora disease and type IV glycogenosis.

7. *Rounded eosinophilic globules* are characteristic of α_1-antitrypsin deficiency[91] (PAS-positive, diastase-resistant, immunohistochemistry is helpful), and other less common conditions such as fibrinogen storage disease. Incidentally, megamitochondria have a similar appearance.

8. *The identification of cytoplasmic crystals* requires examination of frozen sections or unstained paraffin sections under polarized light. Electron microscopy may be helpful. Accumulation of cysteine crystals (hexagonal, rectangular and birefringent) is seen in cystinosis. Alcohol fixation is recommended. Cholesterol crystals accumulate in the Kupffer cells in Tangier, Niemann–Pick and Fabry diseases. In Wolman and cholesterol ester diseases, cholesterol and triglycerides accumulate in the Kupffer cells as well as hepatocytes. Frozen sections examined under polarized light reveal birefringent cholesterol crystals. The Liebermann–Burchard reaction confirms the nature of these crystals. Triglycerides are demonstrated by oil red O or Sudan B black stains. Uroporphyrin crystals in PCT are needle shaped and seen in unstained sections. Associated fatty change, haemosiderosis and fibrosis are invariably present. A brilliant red birefringence of canalicular casts (generally brown in colour) of protoporphyrin are identified in erythropoietic porphyria.

9. *Accumulation of pigments* is associated with a host of metabolic disorders. In addition to bile and protoporphyrin, brown granular pigments may accumulate predominantly in the hepatocytes which may be lipofuscin, lipomelanin and haemosiderin. Of these, hemosiderin and lipomelanin granules are coarse; haemosiderin is distinctly refractile. Haemosiderin is stained by the Perls reaction. Both lipofuscin and lipomelanin are PAS positive. However, lipofuscin can also be seen with the long Ziehl–Neelsen stain. Lipomelanin is argentaphilic (Fontana Masson positive) and autofluorescent on frozen section. Lipofuscin is found in the hepatocytes in Gilbert disease, and also in the Kupffer cells in chronic granulomatous disease, ceroid lipofuscinosis, Niemann–Pick disease, Fabry disease and cholesterol ester disease. Lipomelanin accumulates in the zone 3 (centrizonal) hepatocytes in the Dubin–Johnson syndrome.[92] On gross examination, a needle biopsy is black in colour.

Haemosiderin is deposited in the hepatocytes and other liver cells as a consequence of primary haemochromatosis (also known as genetic or

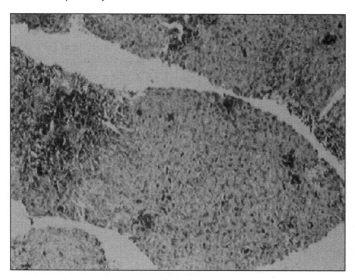

Fig. 10. Extensive haemosiderosis in post-transfusion chronic hepatitis C affecting a thalassaemic patient. Note the predominantly portal localization of the haemosiderin (Perls stain).

hereditary haemochromatosis) or secondary haemosiderosis.[93] Primary haemochromatosis is a disorder with an inherited propensity for iron overload in contrast to conditions in which the source of iron overload is known to fall under the rubric of secondary haemochromatosis (Fig. 10). Although in hereditary haemochromatosis hepatocyte siderosis overshadows reticulo-endothelial siderosis, the histological features in both situations are those of iron overload and its consequences. The two conditions are, therefore, histologically identical and must not be interpreted without knowledge of the clinical context. Genetic haemochromatosis is diagnosed on the basis of a combination of clinical features, cirrhosis on liver biopsy and evidence of increased iron stores (serum iron studies or quantification of hepatic iron stores). The liver shows extensive deposition of iron as haemosiderin (which stains blue with the Perls/Prussian blue stain) in the hepatic parenchyma as well as in the Kupffer cells and bile duct cells. The normal liver does not contain any demonstrable iron except in the first few weeks of life. The biochemical determination of hepatic iron, therefore, is of importance in establishing a diagnosis of haemochromatosis. The normal iron content of liver tissue is <1 mg/g dry weight of liver. Levels in genetic haemochromatosis commonly exceed 10 mg/g dry weight of liver. Levels >22 mg/g dry weight of liver are associated with the development of fibrosis and cirrhosis.

In addition to haematological disorders, iron overload is often found in the liver in conditions such as PCT, galactosaemia, tyrosinaemia and Zellweger syndrome. There is associated fibrosis, and cirrhosis may be seen.

It must be mentioned that copper storage has no recognizable crystalline deposition. The common copper storage disease due to a metabolic defect—Wilson disease—is characterized by a chronic hepatitis-like picture that progresses to cirrhosis.[94] Unlike some of the other metabolic disorders, a diagnosis of Wilson disease implies that effective therapy can be instituted. This disease can mimic all forms of liver disease in childhood. This diagnosis, therefore, should be assiduously sought in all children with hepatic or neurological involvement, or with other characteristic findings such as Kayser–Fleischer corneal rings. Serum caeruloplasmin measurement is the mainstay of diagnosis. The liver pathology is not specific. Some of the more common features are fatty change, vacuolation or glycogenation of nuclei, Mallory hyaline, chronic hepatitis and cirrhosis. Ideally, liver copper stores should be assessed in any patient suspected of having this disorder. The normal liver does not contain any demonstrable copper except in the first few weeks of life. Concentrations fall to the adult value of about 30 mg/g of dry tissue within 6 months of birth. Although any level >40 mg/g is suspicious, patients with Wilson disease typically have levels >250 mg/g. The hepatic copper concentration can also be assessed qualitatively with stains for copper such as rubeanic acid and rhodamine stains. The latter is preferred since it is able to distinguish bile from copper deposits. Increased copper-associated protein (copper-binding protein) has a direct relationship with the accumulation of copper and its demonstration is sufficient to suggest the diagnosis. The orcein stain (black granules) is generally used for this purpose. However, the assessment of hepatic copper by these methods is fraught with technical difficulties and a negative result by no means precludes a diagnosis of Wilson disease. To further complicate the situation, copper also accumulates in the liver in chronic cholestasis, in the normal foetus and in other diseases such as Indian childhood cirrhosis. Quantitative copper determination is therefore the best indicator of Wilson disease. Electron microscopy shows increased mitochondrial matrix density, dilatation of the tips of the cristae and separation of the liver membranes. Enlarged peroxisomes appear flocculent.

10. *Storage of sulphatide* in metachromatic leukodystrophy is recognized by the PAS stain and metachromasia by the cresyl violet or toluidine blue stains. In Fabry disease, ceramide trichexoside is stored in both hepatocytes and reticuloendothelial cells. The cells are PAS positive. Electron microscopy reveals lamellar inclusions that are typically concentric with a periodicity of 5–6 nm.

11. *In cystic fibrosis,*[95] PAS-positive material is found inspissated in the periportal bile ductules. Mucin stains are negative. There is associated portal fibrosis (focal biliary fibrosis).

Non-specific changes

In certain peroxisome disorders, such as the Zellweger disease, there may be subtle or non-specific changes. Demonstration of an absence of peroxisomes is necessary to make the diagnosis.

Hepatitis-like picture

Morphological changes simulating acute or chronic hepatitis are seen in some metabolic disorders. This finding is not diagnostic, but heightens the suspicion of these conditions. In most instances, it may be necessary to exclude common causes of hepatitis such as viral/drug-induced hepatitis. It needs to be emphasized that other features characteristic of these diseases help to substantiate the diagnosis.

Focal necrosis is reported in PCT, galactosaemia, hereditary fructose intolerance, tyrosinaemia, primary haemochromatosis and Wilson disease. Acute hepatitis with or without severe necrosis is often a presenting feature of Wilson disease. Neonatal giant cell hepatitis may be the result of α_1-antitrypsin deficiency. Chronic hepatitis-like features are described in α_1-antitrypsin deficiency and Wilson disease.

Cirrhosis

IMD that commonly lead to cirrhosis are glycogenosis type IV, galactosaemia, tyrosinaemia, α_1-antitrypsin deficiency, Wilson disease and primary haemochromatosis. Of these, galactosaemia, primary haemochromatosis and some cases of glycogenosis type IV are usually associated with micronodular cirrhosis and the rest with mixed or macronodular cirrhosis.

Tumours

HCC is generally reported in metabolic disorders in the setting of a cirrhotic liver. Therefore, diseases that result in cirrhosis are those that will be associated with HCC. Of these, tyrosinaemia is considered to be one of the more common causes. Hepatocellular adenoma is rarely associated with galactosaemia, glycogenosis type I and familial diabetes mellitus.

Cystic fibrosis

The diagnosis is made by estimation of sweat chloride concentration. However, a percentage of cases show typical features, namely proliferating bile ducts containing inspissated PAS-positive material.[95] It has been shown that histology may demonstrate marked liver disease in cystic fibrosis well before the LFT become abnormal.

Hyperbilirubinaemias

Liver biopsy is used to substantiate the diagnosis in certain hyperbilirubinaemic states in childhood.[92] The histology of the liver must be shown to be normal (both by light as well as electron microscopy) in Gilbert syndrome, while a defect in canalicular transport leads to pigment accumulation in the hepatocytes in the Dubin–Johnson syndrome. The pigment that accumulates in the Dubin–Johnson syndrome is a dark, golden-brown substance that resembles lipofuscin. This similarity extends to the histochemical level. However, electron microscopy is useful in making the distinction between these two pigments. The Dubin–Johnson pigment (which is found within lysosomes) differs from lipofuscin electron microscopically in being more pleomorphic and of variable electron density.

Therefore, certain common IMD may be reasonably diagnosed on light microscopy of paraffin sections with or without special stains. These include α_1-antitrypsin deficiency, cystic fibrosis, Gaucher disease, glycogenosis type IV, mucopolysacharidoses, PCT, erythropoietic protoporphyria and Lafora disease. In the case of Niemann–Pick disease, Wolman disease, Zellweger syndrome, gangliosidosis and Wilson disease, electron microscopy is often required for confirmation. However, in some of these conditions, such as Niemann–Pick and Wilson diseases, light microscopy may be sufficient to provide the diagnosis. In tyrosinaemia, galactosaemia, hereditary fructose intolerance and glycogen storage disease type I, light microscopy is relatively characteristic but diagnostic confirmation rests on biochemical studies.

Nevertheless, in IMD the diagnosis rests on a combination of clinical, biochemical, histological and other studies. Histology is invariably necessary but obviously does not provide an unequivocal diagnosis in several conditions. It must be noted that in some metabolic liver disorders, the purpose of the biopsy is to make a histological diagnosis while in others the major purpose is to obtain tissue for biochemical evaluation.

FIBROSIS AND CIRRHOSIS

The end result of several liver diseases is fibrosis and, by and large, cirrhosis is irreversible. It is for this reason that liver biopsy is the paramount investigation in the confirmation of fibrosis and cirrhosis. The stages of fibrosis ultimately resulting in cirrhosis have already been mentioned in the staging of chronic hepatitis.

Increased fibrosis can be appreciated even in the routine H&E stain and easily confirmed on stains for collagen, reticulin and elastin. The fibrosis is generally more prominent at the site of injury and proceeds to involve other areas. In general, the fibrosis begins either around the portal tract or central vein and extends to the adjacent portal tract or central vein, as the case may be. Thus, in chronic hepatitis of viral or other aetiology, in parasitic infections such as schistosomiasis, and in non-cirrhotic portal fibrosis (NCPF), obstructive cholangiopathic liver diseases, haemosiderosis and haemochromatosis, etc., the fibrosis begins around the portal areas. It must be mentioned that portal-to-portal fibrosis is typical of biliary and metabolic liver disease. When the disease affects the centrizonal (zone 3) areas such as in long-standing chronic venous congestion of the liver, toxic liver damage resulting in veno-occlusive disease, NASH and alcoholic liver disease (ALD), the fibrosis is predominantly around these areas. In wedge biopsies, interpretation of fibrosis and fibrosis versus cirrhosis should be made with caution. The subcapsular region (Fig. 11), as mentioned earlier, may give an erroneous diagnosis of cirrhosis unless the biopsy is deep enough. In some cases, both a wedge and a needle biopsy are recommended.[12,96]

The main histological features of cirrhosis are fibrous septa, parenchymal nodules and disruption of liver architecture. Cirrhosis is a diffuse process

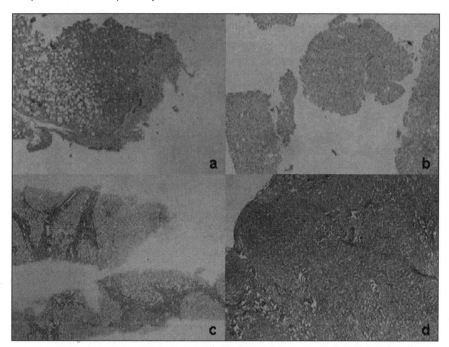

Fig. 11. Liver biopsy in cirrhosis. (a) Subcapsular areas need to be avoided for interpreting cirrhosis. (H&E) (b) Fragmentation of cores of liver biopsy in cirrhosis. (H&E) (c) Reticulin staining showing nodules. (reticulin stain) (d) Jigsaw puzzle-shaped nodules seen in secondary biliary cirrhosis and cirrhosis due to metabolic disorders. (Masson trichrome)

affecting the entire liver and resulting in the formation of nodules.[97] Both the fibrosis and nodularity are diffuse. Thus, diffuse nodularity unaccompanied by fibrosis (nodular regenerative hyperplasia) and diffuse fibrosis unaccompanied by nodularity (NCPF) do not qualify as cirrhosis. If a majority of the nodules are <3 mm in size, the cirrhosis is micronodular (as in ALD); if the nodules are >3 mm, the cirrhosis is termed macronodular (as in metabolic liver disease), while a mixed micro–macro nodular cirrhosis is typical of post-hepatitic cirrhosis. The biopsy is usually fragmented when an aspiration type of needle is used (Fig. 11). However, reticulin stains will reveal a rim of fibres at the periphery. It is recommended that a diagnosis of cirrhosis be made when at least 75% of the nodule is rimmed by fibrosis. A practical problem that often arises in these cases is that the pathologist cannot assess the presence or absence of nodules because of the limited size of the biopsy specimen and biopsy of large nodules. Some clinicians prefer to use cutting type needles over aspiration needles[98] to obtain a satisfactory specimen from a cirrhotic liver, although others do not find any such advantage.[10]

Besides the diagnosis, the other information that may be gleaned from the biopsy in this condition includes:

- the aetiology of the cirrhosis;
- the activity of the disease process. This activity refers to the degree to which the antecedent condition that caused the cirrhosis still exists. Histologically,

activity is assessed by examining the interface between the nodules and septa. A clear interface indicates minimal activity, whereas an interface obscured by inflammatory cells indicates residual activity;
- the presence or absence of HCC.

In the vast majority of cases, a perusal of the biopsy offers no clues as to what has, in the past, caused liver damage. However, occasionally, there may be histological clues to the aetiology of the cirrhosis. For example, special stains and/or immunohistochemistry may reveal HBV or HCV in the hepatic parenchyma. Routine stains may reveal loss of the intrahepatic bile ducts secondary to PBC, PSC or PIBD. Stains for copper or copper-binding protein may reveal Wilson disease; the Prussian blue stain may reveal haemochromatosis; and the PAS stain with and without diastase may reveal α_1-antitrypsin deficiency. It is worthwhile to note that once cirrhosis has set in, treatment is unlikely to alter the prognosis, whatever the aetiology. Nevertheless, an aetiological diagnosis may help in other ways, such as offering genetic counselling to the family of the patient.

The enigmatic entity known as Indian childhood cirrhosis has unusual histological features that resemble those of ALD. These include the presence of Mallory hyaline, prominent inflammatory infiltrates and the deposition of marked fibrous tissue throughout the liver parenchyma. However, in contrast to ALD, steatosis is minimal and there is a distinct lack of regenerative nodules. Copper and copper-binding protein levels in the liver are markedly elevated.[99] The disease typically progresses to a micronodular cirrhosis.

The most helpful stain in cirrhosis is the reticulin stain (Fig. 11). However, to differentiate the collapse engendered by hepatic necrosis from true cirrhosis, the orcein stain is helpful. Masson trichrome (Fig. 11) reveals the presence of collagen fibrosis, and can also reveal characteristics not seen on reticulin staining, for example, pericellular fibrosis in steatohepatitis.

An important consideration in the differential diagnosis of cirrhosis in children is congenital hepatic fibrosis. As opposed to cirrhosis, congenital hepatic fibrosis is characterized by the absence of inflammation and regenerative nodules, and the presence of anastomosing biliary channels rather than proliferating bile ductules.[100] A note of caution is warranted because in congenital hepatic fibrosis, the liver shows prominent fibrosis and numerous spaces lined by bile duct epithelium. These spaces may become cystic and the histological picture is then indistinguishable from polycystic kidney/liver disease. NCPF enters into the clinical differential diagnosis of portal hypertension. In this condition, the histology is normal. It is important to demonstrate the absence of cirrhosis.

SYSTEMIC INFECTIONS AND MISCELLANEOUS CONDITIONS

Liver biopsies are often performed to evaluate abnormal LFT and fevers of unknown origin.[101] In most instances, an infection is suspected. Indeed, the liver is frequently affected by various infections since this is a filter that receives both systemic and portal blood. The changes that subsequently occur in the liver are

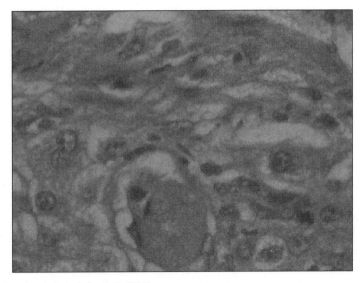

Fig. 12. Ductular cholestasis in sepsis (H&E)

varied. The organism may be identified in some cases, whereas in others the diagnosis is at best presumptive or even conjectural, since the changes may be non-specific. It is beyond the scope of this chapter to describe the features associated with the many organisms that can infect the liver, and only a salient diagnostic approach is discussed. Histopathology of the liver in viral hepatitis has been discussed in an earlier section.

The liver in sepsis

A non-specific but typical change is described in liver biopsies from patients with sepsis. These changes do not indicate the nature of the infection (bacterial or fungal) but are sufficient to warrant a search for an infection (blood culture, etc.). Recognition of these features is essential, especially in an ill patient ('ICU jaundice') or following transplantation. Prompt therapy is needed since sepsis, unless treated early and adequately, may be fatal.

The liver biopsy shows canalicular and bile ductular cholestasis (Fig. 12).[102,103] Kupffer cells are prominent with or without erythrophagocytosis and there may be associated fatty change. The portal tracts show lymphocytic infiltration. Typically, there is little or no hepatocellular necrosis.

Hepatitis-like changes

Liver biopsies with changes simulating conventional viral hepatitis are commonly associated with systemic viral infections. The histological features have been mentioned in the section on hepatitis. The patient may be immuno-compromised. It must be pointed out that in some cases granulomas may be found. Further, in immunocompetent patients, especially those with CMV infection, typical inclusions and antigens may not be demonstrable.

Granulomatous inflammation

It is estimated that about 10% of liver biopsies show granulomas and most systemic granulomatous diseases will also involve the liver to some extent.[104] Therefore, in suspected granulomatous inflammation that may be systemic or associated with an abnormal LFT, a liver biopsy is a common investigation.

Morphologically, several types of granulomas may be identified.

Microgranulomas: These are clusters of Kupffer cells that are non-specific.

Epithelioid granulomas: These comprise nodular aggregates of macrophages with or without necrosis. This is the type of granuloma that is implied whenever the unqualified term of granuloma is used. There are numerous conditions associated with epithelioid granulomas.

Lipogranulomas: These are deposits of lipids and vacuolated macrophages with inflammation and fibrosis, as in mineral oil granulomas and steatohepatitis.

Fibrin ring granulomas: A fibrin band encircling a vacuolated centre with surrounding histiocytes and inflammatory cells[105] is typically seen in Q fever.

By and large, it is the epithelioid cell granuloma that needs to be evaluated in a liver biopsy. In some instances, the diagnosis is obvious—ova of *Schistosoma* or fungal profiles may be identified within the granuloma, and acid-fast bacilli in a necrotizing granuloma. In others, the diagnosis can be compatible with a condition that is common or prevalent in that population, e.g. necrotizing granuloma and tuberculosis. In the remaining cases, the pathologist may not be able to provide a reasonable clue to the aetiology of the granuloma.

The location of a granuloma is important. Portal/periportal granulomas are characteristic of sarcoidosis and PBC; the association with bile ducts and autoantibodies help to distinguish the two conditions. Lipogranulomas in the portal/perivascular regions are almost diagnostic of mineral oil granulomas.

Non-necrotizing granulomas are seen in a variety of conditions. In India, tuberculosis is the commonest cause (Fig. 13). There may be associated fatty change.[106] Acid-fast bacilli are unfortunately demonstrable in less than 10% of cases. Confluent granulomas generally suggest tuberculosis. Sarcoidosis[107] and idiopathic granulomatous disease of the liver may be considered in the differential diagnosis. In sarcoidosis the granulomas are clustered but discrete and are associated with central hyalinization and fibrosis (reticulin-rich granulomas). However, it may be difficult to differentiate tuberculosis from sarcoidosis. An exclusively portal/periportal granuloma with the features described above should warrant an investigation of sarcoidosis (provided the biopsy is not from a proven case of tuberculosis!). Non-necrotizing granulomas with eosinophils are found in fungal and parasitic infections, and in drug-induced granulomas. Fortunately, in fungal infections, it is invariably possible to identify the fungus with special stains (PAS/methanamine silver). Several serial sections may be required to demonstrate the fungus or the parasite ova (*Schistosoma*, helminthic and biliary nematode infection). In schistosomiasis,[108] a black pigment and fibrosis is present. A similar pigment within the Kupffer cells is characteristic of malaria.[109] In *falciparum* malaria, the Kupffer cells may additionally show erythrophagocytosis. If non-necrotizing granulomas are associated with cholestasis or bile duct injury/loss,

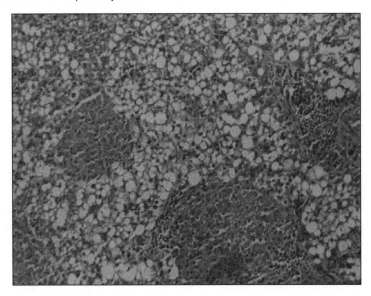

Fig. 13. Granulomatous hepatitis due to tuberculosis. There is associated fatty change. (H&E)

PBC or drug-induced disease must be considered. Sarcoidosis is a less likely possibility. The presence of birefringent material on polarized microscopy, suggestive of starch or talc, is seen in intravenous drug abusers.

Small or microgranulomas associated with a prominence of the Kupffer cells and sinusoidal plasma cell infiltrate should prompt a search for organisms within the Kupffer cells. Visceral leishmaniasis[110] is one condition that may show these features. *Histoplasma*, although rare in India, is another. In histoplasmosis, necrotizing granulomas may also be identified. Both leishmaniasis and histoplasmosis result in similar-sized structures within the sinusoidal cells. The PAS and methanamine silver stains help in distinguishing these organisms by staining the *Histoplasma*. Typhoid fever[111] is another cause of microgranulomas and Kupffer cell proliferation.

Necrotizing granulomas could show suppuration or caseation. Suppurative necrosis is commonly encountered in fungal infections, especially candidiasis, and in bacterial infections such as listeriosis. Tuberculosis is the commonest cause of a caseating granuloma in India. Unless proven otherwise, a caseating granuloma in a liver biopsy is considered to be due to tuberculosis. Unfortunately, only 30% of tuberculosis granulomas in the liver biopsy show caseous necrosis. Some of the other features are described in the section on non-necrotizing granulomas. Necrotizing granulomas indistinguishable from tuberculosis are found in brucellosis and histoplasmosis.

Suppurative inflammation

In suppurative inflammation, there is a pronounced neutrophilic infiltrate and parenchymal necrosis. The lesions may vary from tiny microabscesses to a huge abscess. Bacterial infection is the commonest cause.

Suppurative inflammation must be distinguished from focal aggregates of neutrophils that occur in the subcapsular sinusoidal parenchyma following a prolonged hepatic or abdominal surgical procedure ('surgical hepatitis'). Similar aggregates are also found in CMV infection and steatohepatitis (alcoholic and non-alcoholic). The clinical setting and other histological findings should help in sorting out these differential diagnoses.

The diagnosis of an abscess is not difficult. Identification of the aetiology is challenging for the histopathologist. Several serial sections and special stains (and cultures) may be necessary. Common causes include bacteria, actino-mycosis, aspergillosis and mucormycosis. The necrotic material should be thoroughly examined in the case of amoebic abscess.[112] The term 'abscess' may not be histologically accurate in this case as a neutrophilic response is rare. Typically organisms measuring 15–40 μ in diameter are identified in a nondescript background of coagulative necrosis.

Amyloidosis

The principle for diagnosis of amyloidosis in the liver is similar to that elsewhere.[113] The condition may be suspected on H&E sections. Either one or more of the following—metachromasia on crystal violet staining, apple-green birefringence on Congo red staining and thioflavin T fluorescence—are required for confirmation. The amyloid is generally deposited in the space of Disse and compresses the hepatocytes (Fig. 14), or in the wall of the arterioles in the portal tract.

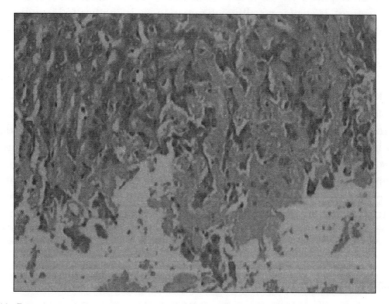

Fig. 14. Extensive amyloid deposition in the liver. The hepatocytes appear compressed and atrophic. (H&E)

Reye syndrome

Reye syndrome can be suspected clinically by the combination of a history of a prodromal illness (often treated symptomatically with aspirin, which is implicated in the aetiopathogenesis of this syndrome) with hepatic and central nervous system dysfunction. However, characteristic liver biopsy findings are mandatory for a definitive diagnosis. These features are microvesicular fatty change and mild-to-absent hepatocellular necrosis.[114]

Budd–Chiari syndrome

The confirmatory diagnostic test for this condition is hepatic venography, but needle biopsy often yields characteristic histological features. The essential feature is marked congestion of the central veins and sinusoids. Coagulative necrosis is frequent in the acute stage. Progressive sinusoidal dilatation is accompanied by atrophy of the hepatocytes, frequently followed by zone 3 fibrosis. The pathologist must not term the condition Budd–Chiari syndrome unless the precise anatomical location of the obstruction is known.[115] A more accurate pathological diagnosis would be hepatic venous outflow tract obstruction (HVOTO). In VOD, there is toxic necrosis around the central veins with resultant thrombosis and fibrosis.

Acquired immune deficiency syndrome

Hepatic lesions in AIDS[116] are generally related to a variety of opportunistic infections associated with immune deficiency. Patients may suffer from conventional hepatitis. It may be reiterated that HBsAg may be demonstrated in the liver by immunohistochemistry even in acute hepatitis B infection; unlike what is observed in the immunocompetent host. Cryptosporidia and microsporidia are generally the aetiological agents implicated in AIDS cholangiopathy, a condition that simulates sclerosing cholangitis. Peliosis hepatis (blood-filled cysts) and an unrelated condition bacillary peliosis hepatis (dilated vascular spaces in a myxoid stroma containing numerous bacteria demonstrable by the Warthin–Starry stain) are other lesions that have been described. In addition, non-specific changes such as fatty change, focal inflammation and amyloidosis may be found.

Liver disease in pregnancy

Four lesions are unique to liver disease in pregnancy.[117] Acute fatty liver is characterized by microvesicular fatty change. In intrahepatic cholestasis of pregnancy, there is severe zone 3 (perivenular) cholestasis. Pre-eclampsia and eclampsia are characterized by fibrin thrombi in the portal vessels and periportal sinusoids. In severe cases, periportal necrosis and haemorrhage are present. In the HELLP syndrome (haemolysis, elevated liver enzymes and low platelets), changes ranging from non-specific inflammation to those similar to pre-eclampsia may be seen. Liver diseases found in the non-pregnant state may also manifest during pregnancy.

TUMOURS AND TUMOUR-LIKE CONDITIONS

In India, space-occupying lesions (SOLs) in the liver or liver masses (tumours and tumour-like lesions) are uncommon as compared to hepatitis. Nevertheless, in a referral centre, the hepatologist or surgeon is likely to encounter a relatively large number of such cases. In many instances, these lesions pose diagnostic difficulties and late presentation, especially of malignant lesions, make satisfactory therapy difficult.

Whenever a diagnosis of a liver mass is made, the following steps are generally undertaken.

- Identification of an underlying lesion that can account for the mass
- Characterization of the mass by a non-invasive method to determine the subsequent course of action—diagnostic procedure and therapeutic approach
- Pre-treatment aspiration/biopsy wherever necessary
- Treatment options: wait and watch, ablation, excision, liver transplantation
- Further evaluation of the lesion after excision
- Follow-up as indicated with or without biopsy

The pathologist is thus involved at various stages of these decision-making steps.

Classification

In the absence of an underlying liver disease, metastatic tumours are up to 30 times more common than primary tumours. In those with cirrhosis, HCC is relatively frequent. For the purpose of diagnosis, a histogenetic classification of tumours and tumour-like lesions of the liver (Table III) is used.

Histological appearance

From the histogenetic classification it is obvious that the histological appearances of these lesions[118,119] have some resemblance to the parent tissue. Details of individual tumours have not been described here.

Of the benign tumours, haemangiomas are the commonest. The diagnosis is fortunately relatively easy, as these are characterized by blood-filled vascular channels. Imaging modalities have virtually reduced the need for biopsies to a bare minimum. Focal nodular hyperplasia (FNH) is characterized by large blood vessels in a central scar. Small, uniform bile ducts with or without mononuclear cells and polymorphs are seen in fibrous bands that radiate from the central stellate scar. Hepatocellular adenomas consist of usually pale (glycogen-containing) hepatocytes arranged in trabeculae that are two-cell thick and compress the sinusoids. Portal triads are absent but blood vessels may be

Table III. Histogenetic classification of liver tumours

Benign	Malignant
Epithelial tumours and tumour-like lesions	
Hepatocellular adenoma	Hepatoblastoma
Nodular regenerative hyperplasia	Hepatocellular carcinoma (HCC)
Focal nodular hyperplasia	Fibrolamellar HCC
	Other variants of HCC
	Combined HCC and cholangiocarcinoma (CCA)
Biliary	
Bile duct adenoma	CCA
Solitary unilocular cyst	Combined HCC and CCA
Ciliated foregut cyst	Biliary cystadenocarcinoma
Biliary cystadenoma	
—Mucinous	
—Serous	
Biliary papillomatosis	
Mixed epithelial and mesenchymal tumours and tumour-like lesions	
Mixed hamartoma	Carcinosarcoma
Mesenchymal hamartoma	
Mesenchymal tumours and tumour-like lesions	
Vascular	
Infantile haemangioendothelioma	Angiosarcoma
Cavernous haemangioma	Epithelioid haemangioendothelioma
Lymphangioma/lymphangiomatosis	Kaposi sarcoma
Hereditary haemorrhagic telangiectasia	
Lipomatous	
Lipoma	Liposarcoma
Angiomyolipoma	
Focal fatty change	
Pseudolipoma	
Fibrous	
Fibroma (fibrous tumour/mesothelioma)	Fibrosarcoma
Inflammatory pseudotumour	
Myomatous	
Leiomyoma	Leiyomyosarcoma
	Embryonal rhabdomyosarcoma
Neural	
Neurofibroma	Neurofibrosarcoma
Others	
	Undifferentiated (embryonal) sarcoma
	Malignant fibrous histiocytoma
	Osteosarcoma
Miscellaneous tumours and tumour-like lesions	
Adrenal rest tumour	Adenosquamous carcinoma
Pancreatic heterotopia	Mucoepidermoid carcinoma
Endometrial cyst	Squamous carcinoma
Epidermoid cyst	Neuroendocrine tumours (carcinoids)
Benign teratoma	Malignant teratoma
Hepatic pregnancy	Endodermal sinus (yolk sac) tumours
Congenital cysts	Primary lymphoma
Parasitic cysts (hydatid cyst)	
Abscesses	
Metastatic tumours	

numerous. Thick-walled vessels are usually found at the periphery of the tumour, which often does not have a distinct capsule. While benign epithelial tumours including cysts (especially mucinous biliary cysts) may become malignant, the same is not true for benign mesenchymal tumours. Distinguishing hepatocellular adenomas and biliary adenomas from their malignant counterparts is often difficult. Some benign tumours are age-specific (such as infantile haemangioendothelioma) while others may be seen more often in females (biliary cystadenoma).

HCC and metastatic tumours account for the vast majority of liver tumours. Multiple lesions in a non-cirrhotic liver are likely to be metastatic tumours in a given clinical setting. A majority of adenocarcinomas resemble the tumours at the primary site. However, when the tumours are poorly differentiated, special stains to demonstrate mucin and immunohistochemistry are helpful. There are no reliable histological features to distinguish metastatic adenocarcinomas from peripheral cholangiocarcinomas with certainty, although immunohistochemistry may be helpful. A combination of clinical features, imaging, operative findings and exclusion of a metastasis is the surest way of making this diagnosis. Hilar cholangiocarcinoma, by way of its location, is more easily diagnosed.

Microscopically, HCCs resemble thickened cords of liver tissue (three or more cells thick) which has a strong resemblance to hepatocytes (Fig. 15) with varying degrees of differentiation.[120] Generally, the tumours are poor in reticulin. Acinar differentiation may be found. Demonstration of bile secretion by the tumour cells is a definite indication of hepatocellular differentiation. Immunohistochemistry for alpha-fetoprotein is usually unhelpful. Polyclonal, but not monoclonal, carcinoembryonic antigen (CEA) stains the canalicular membrane of the tumour cells. Problems arise in distinguishing well-differentiated HCCs from hepatic adenomas, and HCCs from an adenomatous nodule in a cirrhotic liver.[121]

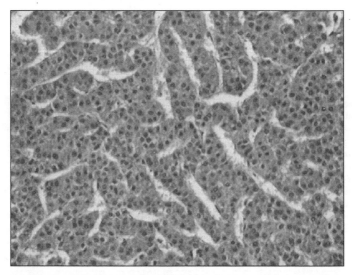

Fig. 15. Hepatocellular carcinoma showing a thickened cord of cells. The tumour cells resemble hepatocytes with nuclear pleomorphism. (H&E)

Reticulin staining may be helpful in such cases. Variants of HCC[118-120] such as fibrolamellar HCC are characterized by lamellae of fibrosis separating the hepatocytes. These cells have an oncocytic appearance at places and may also show perinuclear vacuoles. These tumours have a better prognosis than conventional HCCs. The clear cell variant of HCC is rich in glycogen. The clear cells mimic metastasis from other clear cell tumours, especially renal cell carcinoma.

Hepatoblastomas are seen in children below 4 years of age. The tumour attempts to recapitulate the embryonal and foetal development of the liver. Some tumours are purely epithelial while others consist of a mixture of epithelial and mesenchymal elements such as primitive mesenchyme, osteoid, cartilage or rhabdomyoblasts. An undifferentiated or anaplastic type has been described. The epithelial cells may be of the foetal type resembling adult hepatocytes of a small size or the embryonal type of even smaller round cells with a high nuclear:cytoplasmic ratio. Extramedullary haemopoiesis is common.

Other malignant tumours are relatively rare. Nevertheless lymphomas, leukaemias and other haematopoietic malignancies may involve the liver.

Abscesses and cysts also present as tumour-like lesions. In addition to abscesses due to bacterial infections, amoebae are an important aetiological agent in India. Parasites are found more often in the wall than in the centre of the abscess. Patients with an inflammatory pseudotumour often present with fever that responds to excision of the lesion. Histological examination shows myofibroblasts, plasma cells, lymphocytes, foamy histiocytes with collagen bundles and blood vessels.

In general, the histological diagnosis of hepatic tumours is done by light microscopy with the help of a few special stains. Immunohistochemistry is required to characterize poorly differentiated tumours.

Role of histopathology

Advances in imaging have permitted non-invasive diagnosis of liver tumours fairly accurately. However, prior to resection of malignant tumours, a preoperative tissue diagnosis is often sought. An imaging-guided FNAC or biopsy is recommended. In some institutions, because of the fear of needle-track seedlings, HCCs may not be biopsied;[122] even FNAC is avoided! The reported incidence of needle-track seedlings is as high as 3.4% for HCCs.[112] Hence, in resectable tumours, it is argued that a preoperative biopsy is not mandatory. Frozen sections are performed in those cases wherein a preoperative diagnosis has not been obtained and an immediate therapeutic decision needs to be taken. Evaluation of the resection margins is done to ensure a mandatory 1 cm tumour-free margin after excision. However, the role of positive margins in HCC appears to be controversial, as there are reports to suggest that the outcome may not be dependent on tumour-free margins. The resected specimen should be examined with a view to enable accurate staging and grading (where necessary) of the tumours. Grading of HCC is not common practice although it is recommended that this be recorded.

It is essential to carefully examine the histology of the liver adjacent to the tumour. Diseases affecting the adjacent parenchyma may have a bearing on the tumour, e.g. chronic hepatitis and cirrhosis in HCC, PSC in cholangiocarcinoma, etc. Further, a diffuse disease of the liver has a bearing on the outcome following resection (which depends on the functional reserve of remaining parenchyma). The parenchyma immediately adjacent to a mass in the liver may show non-specific changes such as cholestasis and inflammation.[123] This must be borne in mind while interpreting biopsies that may have missed the lesion.

Finally, the histopathologist is in a unique position to study tissues from the lesion and adjacent areas with colleagues from other specialties to identify markers that may have a bearing on the future outcome and biology of such conditions. The role of the histopathologist is to help in the diagnosis, provide prognostic attributes and contribute to research when assessing tumours and tumour-like lesions of the liver.

POST-TRANSPLANT EVALUATION

Liver biopsy is the modality of choice, in addition to pretransplant work-up, for monitoring complications following from hepatic transplantation. In brief, the settings in which evaluation of the liver histology is essential are diagnosis of rejection,[124] sepsis, recurrence of disease and other causes of post-transplant jaundice such as viral hepatitis, biliary obstruction, vascular blockage, post-transplant lymphoproliferative disease, and so on. The general principles of diagnosis of such conditions are the same as in the non-transplant setting. The prospective graft may be biopsied to determine its suitability for grafting since excessive steatosis and preservation injury or ischaemic damage may result in early graft loss.

Hepatic allograft rejection is of three types: hyperacute (humoral, antibody mediated), acute (cellular) and chronic (ductopenic). The terminology suggests the time-frame of occurrence. Although protocol biopsies were in vogue because immunosuppressive therapy was generally biopsy driven, with the availability of excellent immunosupprsessive agents, the frequency of graft biopsies for this purpose has reduced worldwide. Hyperacute rejection of the liver is rare and is due to preformed antibodies. Histologically, the condition is characterized by haemorrhagic necrosis of the graft. Acute cellular rejection[125] is fairly common and the diagnosis rests on the identification of portal inflammation (large lymphoid cells, macrophages, plasma cells, neutrophils and eosinophils), bile duct damage (infiltration of the epithelium, nuclear changes, vacuolation of the cytoplasm) and endothelialitis or endothelitis (attachment of lymphoid cells to the endothelium and subendothelial inflammation) (Fig. 16). Acute rejection is invariably graded and this has therapeutic implications. Moderate and severe rejection may require an increase in immunosuppressive therapy. A semiquantitative grading system that gives a score—the Rejection Activity Index (RAI)—has been proposed. Often there is a doubt of associated sepsis, especially when there is ductular cholestasis. The clinician needs to be warned of this

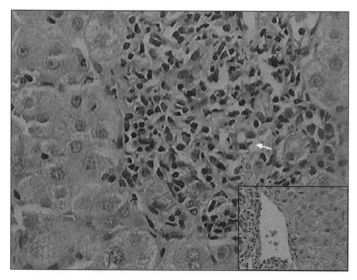

Fig. 16. Acute cellular rejection following orthotopic liver transplantation. Allograft liver biopsy 7 days post transplant showing portal inflammation and bile duct damage (arrow). Inset shows endothelialitis characterized by subendothelial inflammation in a portal vein branch. (H&E)

possibility since an increase in immunosuppression under such circumstances would be disastrous. Chronic rejection[126] usually occurs 60 days post-transplant. The characteristic features are a loss of more than 50% of the bile ducts (vanishing bile duct syndrome) and the often histologically elusive foamy arteriopathy or the subintimal accumulation of foam cells in the arteries.

Nowhere else is the value of a team approach more appropriate than in the post-transplant setting. The combination of liver diseases that occurs in this setting is complex. The liver biopsy provides only clues to the possible cause of the problem. Other members of the team, including the radiologist, work on this lead to arrive at a reasonable diagnosis so that prompt and appropriate therapy can be instituted.

If the value and limitations of the role of liver biopsy are respected and a proper clinicopathological correlation made, then the liver biopsy is not only one of the most powerful tools in the hands of the entire team that looks after the ailing liver but a boon to the sick patient.

REFERENCES

1. Riely CA. Liver biopsy shown useful in work up of patients with chronically abnormal 'LFTs'—still. *Gastroenterology* 1990;**98**:797–8.
2. Van Ness MM, Deihl AM. Is liver biopsy useful in the evaluation of patients with chronically elevated liver enzymes? *Ann Intern Med* 1989;**111**:473–8.
3. Van Leeuwen DJ, Wilson L, Crowe DR. Liver biopsy in the mid 1990s: Questions and answers. *Semin Liver Dis* 1995;**15**:340–59.
4. Grant A, Neuberger J. Guidelines on the use of liver biopsy in clinical practice. *Gut* 1999;**45** (Suppl):IV 1–IV 11.
5. Desmet VJ. What more can we ask from the pathologist? *J Hepatol* 1996;**25** (Suppl):25–9.

6. Lebrec D. Various approaches to obtaining liver tissue—choosing the biopsy technique. *J Hepatol* 1996;**25** (Suppl):20–4.

7. Fox VL, Cohen MB, Whitington PF, Colletti RB. Outpatient liver biopsy in children: A medical position statement of the North American Society for Pediatric Gastroenterology and Nutrition. *J Pediatr Gastroenterol Nutr* 1996;**23**:213–16.

8. Janes CH, Lindor KD. Outcome of patients hospitalized for complications after outpatient liver biopsy. *Ann Intern Med* 1993;**118**:96–8.

9. Garcia-Tsao G, Boyer JL. Outpatient liver biopsy: How safe is it? *Ann Intern Med* 1993;**118**:150–3.

10. Bateson MC, Hopwood D, Duguid HL, Bouchier IA. A comparative trial of liver biopsy needles. *J Clin Pathol* 1980;**33**:131–3.

11. Maciel AC, Marchiori E, Barros SG, *et al.* Transjugular liver biopsy: Histological diagnosis success comparing the Trucut to the modified Ross needle. *Arq Gastroenterol* 2003;**40**:80–4. Epub 2004.

12. Petrelli M, Scheuer PJ. Variation in subcapsular liver structure and its significance in the interpretation of wedge biopsies. *J Clin Pathol* 1967;**20**:743–8.

13. Siddique I, El Naga HA, Madda JP, Memon A, Hasan F. Sampling variability on percutaneous liver biopsy in patients with chronic hepatitis C virus infection. *Scand J Gastroenterol* 2003;**38**:427–32.

14. Regev A, Berho M, Jeffers LJ, *et al.* Sampling error and intraobserver variation in liver biopsy in patients with chronic HCV infection. *Am J Gastroenterol* 2002;**97**:2614–18.

15. Holund B, Poulsen H, Schilichting P. Reproducibility of liver biopsy diagnosis in relation to the size of the specimen. *Scand J Gastroenterol* 1968;**15**:329–35.

16. Soloway RD, Baggenstoss AH, Schoenfield LJ, Summerskill WH. Observer errors and sampling variability tested in evaluation of hepatitis and cirrhosis by liver biopsy. *Am J Dig Dis* 1971;**16**:1082–6.

17. Rappaport AM. The microcirculatory acinar concept of normal and pathological hepatic structure. *Beitr Pathol* 1976;**157**:215–43.

18. Crawford AR, Lin X-Z, Crawford JM. The normal adult human liver biopsy: A quantitative reference standard. *Hepatology* 1998;**28**:323–31.

19. Alagille D. Intrahepatic biliary atresia (hepatic ductular hypoplasia). In: Berenberg SR (ed). *Liver disease in infancy and childhood.* Netherlands: Martinus Nijhoff Medical Division; 1976:129–42.

20. Poupon R, Chazouillìres O, Poupon RE. Chronic cholestatic diseases. *J Hepatol* 2000;**32** (Suppl):129–40.

21. Christoffersen P, Poulsen H. Histological changes in human liver biopsies following extrahepatic biliary obstruction. *Acta Pathol Microbiol Scand* 1970;**212**:150–7.

22. Guarascio P, Yentis F, Cevikbas U, Portmann B, Williams R. Value of copper-associated protein in diagnostic assessment of liver biopsy. *J Clin Pathol* 1983;**36**:18–23.

23. Watson S, Giacoia GP. Cholestasis in infancy: A review. *Clin Pediatr* 1983;**22**:30–6.

24. Balistreri WF. Neonatal cholestasis. *J Pediatr* 1985;**106**:171–84.

25. Riely CA. Familial intrahepatic cholestatic syndromes. *Semin Liver Dis* 1987;**7**:119–33.

26. Lefkowitch JH. Biliary atresia. *Mayo Clin Proc* 1998;**73**:90–5.

27. Balistreri WF, Grand R, Hoofnagle JH, *et al.* Biliary atresia: Current concepts and research directions. Summary of a symposium. *Hepatology* 1996;**23**:1682–92.

28. Mowat AP. Biliary atresia into the 21st century: A historical perspective. *Hepatology* 1996;**23**:1693–5.

29. Raweily EA, Gibson AAM, Burt AD. Abnormalities of intrahepatic bile ducts in extrahepatic biliary atresia. *Histopathology* 1990;**17**:521–7.

30. Kahn EI, Daum F, Markowitz Jaiges HW, *et al.* Arteriohepatic dysplasia. Hepatobiliary morphology. *Hepatology* 1983;**3**:77–84.

31. Ludwig J, Wiesner RH, La Russo NF. Idiopathic adulthood ductopenia: A cause of chronic cholestatic liver disease and biliary cirrhosis. *J Hepatol* 1988;**7**:193–9.
32. Allagile D. Alpha-1-antitrypsin deficiency. *Hepatology* 1984;**4**:115–45.
33. Harrison RF, Hubscher SG. The spectrum of bile duct lesions in end-stage primary scelorsing cholangitis. *Histopathology* 1991;**19**:321–7.
34. Leblanc A, Hadchouel M, Johan P, Odievre M, Alagille D. Obstructive jaundice in children with histiocytosis X. *Gastroenterology* 1981;**80**:134–9.
35. Finegold MJ, Carpenter RJ. Obliterative cholangitis due to cytomegalovirus: A possible precursor of paucity of intrahepatic bile ducts. *Hum Pathol* 1982;**13**:662–5.
36. International Working Party. Terminology for hepatic allograft rejection. *Hepatology* 1995;**22**:648–54.
37. Ludwig J. Idiopathic adulthood ductopenia: An update. *Mayo Clin Proc* 1998;**73**:285–91.
38. Ludwig J. Small-duct primary sclerosing cholangitis. *Semin Liver Dis* 1991;**11**:11–17.
39. Ludwig J. Surgical pathology of the syndrome of primary sclerosing cholangitis. *Am J Surg Pathol* 1989;**13** (Suppl):43–9.
40. Scheuer PJ. Primary biliary cirrhosis. *Proc R Soc Med* 1967;**60**:1257–60.
41. Lee RG, Epstein O, Jauregul H, Sherlock S, Scheuer PJ. Granulomas in primary biliary cirrhosis: A prognostic feature. *Gastroenterology* 1981;**81**:983–6.
42. Nakanuma Y, Ohta G. Quantitation of hepatic granulomas and epithelioid cells in primary biliary cirrhosis. *Hepatology* 1983;**3**:423–7.
43. Leung PSC, Coppel RL, Ansari A, Munoz S, Gershwin ME. Antimitochondrial antibodies in primary biliary cirrhosis. *Semin Liver Dis* 1997;**17**:61–9.
44. Ludwig J, Dickson ER, McDonald GS. Staging of chronic non-suppurative destructive cholangitis (syndrome of primary biliary cirrhosis). *Virchows Arch Pathol Anat* 1978; **379**:103–12.
45. Pessoa MG, Terrault NA, Ferrel LD, Hepatitis after transplantation: The role of the known and unknown viruses. *Liver Transplant Surg* 1998;**4**:461–8.
46. Peters RL. Viral hepatitis: A pathologic spectrum. *Am J Med Sci* 1975;**270**:17–31.
47. Philips MJ, Purcell S. Modern aspects of the morphology of viral hepatitis. *Hum Pathol* 1981;**12**:1060–84.
48. Bianchi L. Liver biopsy interpretation in hepatitis. Part II. Histopathology—classification of acute and chronic viral hepatitis/differential diagnosis. *Pathol Res Pract* 1983:**178**:180–213.
49. Lau Jyn, Xie X, Lai MMC, Wu PC. Apoptosis and viral hepatitis. *Semin Liver Dis* 1998;**18**:169–76.
50. Scheuer PJ, Maggi G. Hepatic fibrosis and collapse: Histological distinction by orcein staining. *Histopathology* 1980;**4**:487–90.
51. Davies SE, Portmann BC, O'Grady JG, *et al.* Hepatic histological findings after transplantation for chronic hepatitis B virus infection, including a unique pattern of fibrosing cholestatic hepatitis. *Hepatology* 1991;**13**:150–7.
52. Okuno T, Sano A, Deguchi T, *et al.* Pathology of acute hepatitis A in humans. Comparison with acute hepatitis B. *Am J Clin Pathol* 1984;**81**:162–9.
53. Kobyayashi K, Hashimoto E, Ludwig J, Hisamitsu T, Obata H. Liver biopsy features of acute hepatitis C compared with hepatitis A, B and non-A, non-B, non-C. *Liver* 1993;**13**:69–73.
54. Kaji K, Nakanuma Y, Sasaki M, *et al.* Hepatic bile duct injuries in chronic hepatitis C: Histopathologic and immunohistochemical studies. *Mod Pathol* 1994;**7**:937–45.
55. Schmid M, Cueni B. Portal lesions in viral hepatitis with submassive hepatic necrosis. *Hum Pathol* 1972;**3**:209–16.
56. Scheuer PJ, Ashrafzadeh P, Sherlock S, Brown D, Dusheiko GM. The pathology of hepatitis C. *Hepatology* 1992;**15**:567–71.

57. Gerber MA, Thung SN. The diagnostic value of immunohistochemical demonstration of hepatitis viral antigens in the liver. *Hum Pathol* 1987;**18**:771–4.

58. Goldin RD, Levine TS, Foster GR, Thomas HC. Granulomas and hepatitis C. *Histopathology* 1996;**28**:265–7.

59. Guido M, Thung SN, Fattovich G, *et al*. Intrahepatic expression of hepatitis B virus antigens: Effect of hepatitis C virus infection. *Mod Pathol* 1999;**12**:599–603.

60. Guido M, Rugge M, Colombari R, *et al*. Prompt hepatitis C virus suppression following hepatitis B virus superinfection in chronic untreated hepatitis C. *J Gastroenterol Hepatol* 1998;**30**:414–17.

61. Review by International Group (no authors listed). Guidelines for diagnosis of therapeutic drug-induced liver injury in liver biopsies. *Lancet* 1974;**1**:854–7.

62. Aithal PG, Day CP. The natural history of histologically proved drug induced liver disease. *Gut* 1999;**44**:731–5.

63. Larrey D. Drug induced liver diseases. *J Hepatol* 2000;**32** (Suppl):77–88.

64. Knodell RG, Ishak KG, Black WC, *et al*. Formulation and application of a numerical scoring system for assessing histological activity in asymptomatic chronic active hepatitis. *Hepatology* 1981;**1**:431–5.

65. Ishak K, Baptista A, Bianchi L, *et al*. Histological grading and staging of chronic hepatitis. *J Hepatol* 1995;**22**:696–9.

66. Bedossa P, Paynand T. The METAVIR cooperative study group. An algorithm for the grading of activity in chronic hepatitis C. *Hepatology* 1994;**20**:15–20.

67. Westin J, Lagging LM, Westjal R, Norkrane G, Dhillon AP. Interobserver study of liver histopathology using the Ishak score in patients with chronic hepatitis C virus infection. *Liver* 1999;**19**:183–7.

68. Rozario R, Ramakrishna B. Histopathological study of chronic hepatitis B and C: A comparison of two scoring systems. *J Hepatol* 2003;**38**:223–9.

69. Czaja AJ. Autoimmune liver disease. *Curr Opin Gastroenterol* 1998;**14**:242–9.

70. Obermayer-Straub P, Strossburg CP, Manns MP. Autoimmune hepatitis. *J Hepatol* 2000;**32** (Suppl):181–97.

71. Hoyumpa AM, Greene HL, Dunn GD, Schenker SS. Fatty liver: Biochemical and clinical considerations. *Dig Dis* 1975;**20**:1142–70.

72. Fromenty B, Berson A, Pessayre D. Microvesicular steatosis and steatohepatitis: Role of mitochondrial dysfunction and lipid peroxidation. *J Hepatol* 1997;**26** (Suppl):13–22.

73. Russell RM, Boyer JL, Bagheri SA, Hruban Z. Hepatic injury from chronic hypervita-minosis A resulting in portal hypertension and ascites. *N Engl J Med* 1974;**291**:435–40.

74. French SW, Nash J, Shitabata P, *et al*. Pathology of alcoholic liver disease. *Semin Liver Dis* 1993;**13**:154–69.

75. Seth SG, Gordon FD, Chopra S. Nonalcoholic steatohepatitis. *Ann Intern Med* 1997;**126**:137–45.

76. Denk H, Stumptner C, Zatloukal K. Mallory bodies revisited. *J Hepatol* 2000;**32**:689–702.

77. Chedid A, Mendenhall CL, Tosch T, *et al*. Significance of megamitochondria in alcoholic liver disease. *Gastroenterology* 1986;**90**:1858–64.

78. Uchida T, Kao H, Quispe-Sjogren M, Peters RL. Alcoholic foamy degeneration—a pattern of acute alcoholic injury of the liver. *Gastroenterology* 1983;**84**:683–92.

79. Edmondson HA, Peters RL, Reynolds TB, Kuzuma OT. Sclerosing hyaline necrosis of the liver in the chronic alcoholic. *Ann Intern Med* 1963;**59**:646–73.

80. Ludwig J, Viggiano TR, McGill GB, Oh BJ. Nonalcoholic steatohepatitis: Mayo Clinic experiences with a hitherto unnamed disease. *Mayo Clin Proc* 1980;**55**:434–8.

81. Matteoni CA, Younossi ZM, Gramlich T, Boparai N, Liu YC, McCullogh AJ. Nonalcoholic fatty liver disease: A spectrum of clinical and pathological severity. *Gastroenterology* 1999;**116**:1413–19.

82. Brunt EM. Nonalcoholic steatohepatitis: Definition and pathology. *Semin Liver Dis* 2001;**21**:3–16.

83. Brunt EM, Janney CG, Di Bisceglei AM, Neuschwander-Tetri BA, Bacon BR. Nonalcoholic steatohepatitis: A proposal for grading and staging the histological lesions. *Am J Gastroenterol* 1999;**94**:2467–74.

84. Ishak KG Hepatic morphology in the inherited metabolic disease. *Semin Liver Dis* 1986;**6**:246–58.

85. Portmann BC. Liver biopsy in the diagnosis of inherited metabolic disorders. In: Anthony PP, MacSween RNM (eds). *Recent advances in histopathology. Vol. 14.* Edinburgh: Churchill Livingstone; 1989:139–59.

86. Mieles LA, Esquivel COO, Van Theil DH, *et al.* Liver transplantation for tyrosinemia: A review of 10 cases from the University of Pittsburg. *Dig Dis Sci* 1990;**35**:153–7.

87. McAdams AJ, Heg G, Bone KE. Glycogen storage disease, types 1 to X: Criteria for morphologic diagnosis. *Hum Pathol* 1974;**5**:463–87.

88. Resnick JM, Whitley CB, Loonard AS, Krivit W, Snover DC. Light and electron microscopic features of the liver in mucopolysaccharidosis. *Hum Pathol* 1994;**25**:276–86.

89. Tassoni JP, Fawaz KA, Johnston DE. Cirrhosis and portal hypertension in a patient with adult Niemann–Pick disease. *Gastroenterology* 1991;**100**:567–9.

90. James SP, Stromeyer FW, Chang C, Barranger JA. Liver abnormalities in patients with Gaucher's disease. *Gastroenterology* 1981;**80**:126–33.

91. Deutsch J, Becker H, Aubock L. Histopathological features of liver disease in alpha-1-antitrypsin deficiency. *Acta Paediatr* 1991;**393** (Suppl):8–12.

92. Berthelot P, Dhumeaux D. New insights into the classification and mechanisms of hereditary, chronic, non-haemolytic hyperbilirubinemias. *Gut* 1978;**19**:474–80.

93. Deugnier YM, Loréal O, Turlin B, *et al.* Liver pathology in genetic hemochromatosis: A review of 135 homozygous cases and their bioclinical correlations. *Gastroenterology* 1992;**102**:2050–9.

94. Ferenci P, Gilliam TC, Gitin JD, *et al.* An international symposium on Wilson's and Menke's disease. *Hepatology* 1996;**24**:952–8.

95. Nagel RA, Westaby D, Javaid A, *et al.* Liver disease and bile duct abnormalities in adults with cystic fibrosis. *Lancet* 1989;**16**:1422–5.

96. Imamura H, Kawasaki S, Bandari Y, Sanjo K, Idezuki Y. Comparison between wedge and needle biopsies for evaluating the degree of cirrhosis. *J Hepatol* 1993;**17**:215–19.

97. Anthony PP, Ishak KG, Nayak NC, Poulsen HE, Scheuer PJ, Sobin LH. The morphology of cirrhosis: Definition, nomenclature and classification. *Bull World Health Organ* 1977;**55**:521–40.

98. Colombo M, Del Ninno E, de Franchis R, *et al.* Ultrasound-assisted percutaneous liver biopsy: Superiority of the Tru-Cut over the Menghini needle for diagnosis of cirrhosis. *Gastroenterology* 1988;**95**:487–9.

99. Popper H, Goldfisher S, Sternleib I, Nayak NC, Madhavan TV. Cytoplasmic copper and its toxic effects. Studies in Indian Childhood Cirrhosis. *Lancet* 1979;**1**:1205–8.

100. Hodgson HJF, Davies DR, Thompson RPH. Congenital hepatic fibrosis. *J Clin Pathol* 1976;**29**:11–16.

101. Holtz T, Moseley RH, Scheiman JM. Liver biopsy in fevers of unknown origin: A reappraisal. *J Clin Gastroenterol* 1993;**17**:29–32.

102. Lefkowitch JH. Bile ductular cholestasis: An ominous histopathologic sign related to sepsis and 'cholangitis lenta'. *Hum Pathol* 1982;**13**:19–24.

103. Banks JG, Foulis AK, Ledingham IM, MacSween RN. Liver function in septic shock. *J Clin Pathol* 1982;**35**:1249–52.

104. Lefkowitch JH. Hepatic granulomas. *J Hepatol* 1999;**30**:40–5.

105. Marazuela M, Moreno A, Yebra M, Cerezo E, Gomez-Gesto C, Vargas JA. Hepatic fibrin-granulomas. A clinicopathologic study of 23 patients. *Hum Pathol* 1991;**22**:607–13.
106. Alvarez SJ, Carpio R. Hepatobiliary tuberculosis. *Dig Dis Sci* 1983;**28**:193–200.
107. Ishak KG. Sarcoidosis of the liver and bile ducts. *Mayo Clin Proc* 1998;**73**:467–72.
108. Dunn MA, Kamel R. Hepatic schistosomiasis. *Hepatology* 1981;**1**:653–61.
109. Pounder DJ. Malarial pigment and hepatic anthracosis. *Am J Surg Pathol* 1983;**7**:501–2.
110. Daneshbod K. Visceral leishmaniasis (kala-azar) in Iran: A pathologic and electron microscopic study. *Am J Clin Pathol* 1972;**87**:156–66.
111. Khosla SN. Typhoid hepatitis. *Postgrad Med J* 1990;**66**:923–5.
112. Stanley SL Jr. Amebiasis. *Lancet* 2003;**361**:1025–34.
113. Falk RH, Comenzo RL, Skinner M. The systemic amyloidoses. *N Engl J Med* 1997; **337**:898–900.
114. Kimura S, Kobayashi T, Tanaka Y, Sasaki Y. Liver histopathology in clinical Reye syndrome. *Brain Dev* 1991;**13**:95–100.
115. Ludwig J, Hashimoto E, McGill DB, van Heerden JA. Classification of hepatic venous outflow obstruction; ambiguous terminology of the Budd–Chiari syndrome. *Mayo Clin Proc* 1990;**65**:51–5.
116. Lefkowitch JH. The liver in AIDS. *Semin Liver Dis* 1997;**17**:335–44.
117. Riely CA. Liver disease in the pregnant patient. *Am J Gastroenterol* 1999;**94**:1728–32.
118. Okuda K, Ishak KG (eds). *Neoplasms of the liver.* Tokyo: Springer; 1987.
119. Anthony PP. Liver tumours: An update. In: Anthony PP, MacSween RNM (eds). *Recent advances in histopathology. Vol. 14.* Edinburgh: Churchill Livingstone; 1989.
120. Nayak NC. Hepatocellular carcinoma—a model of human cancer; clinicopathological features, etiology and pathogenesis. *Indian J Pathol Microbiol* 2003;**46**:1–16.
121. International Working Party. Terminology of nodular hepatocellular lesions. *Hepatology* 1995;**22**:983–93.
122. Durand F, Regimbeau JM, Belghiti J, *et al.* Assessment of the benefits and risks of percutaneous biopsy before surgical resections of hepatocellular carcinoma. *J Hepatol* 2001;**35**:254–8.
123. Gerber MA, Thung SN, Boderheimer HC Jr, Kapelmas B, Schaffner F. Characteristic histologic trial in liver adjacent to metastatic neoplasms. *Liver* 1986;**6**:85–8.
124. Batts KP. Acute and chronic hepatic allograft rejection: Pathology and classification. *Liver Transplant Surg* 1999;**5** (Suppl):521–9.
125. International Panel, Banff Schema for grading liver allograft rejection. An international consensus document. *Hepatology* 1997;**25**:658–63.
126. International Panel, Update of the International Banff Schema for liver allograft rejection: Working recommendations for the histopathologic staging, reporting of chronic rejection. *Hepatology* 2000;**31**:792–9.

RECOMMENDED READING
(For all aspects and details of liver biopsy interpretation)

1. Macsween RNM, Burt AD, Portmann BC, Ishak KG, Scheuer PJ, Anthony PP (eds). *Pathology of the liver.* 4th ed. Edinburgh: Churchill Livingstone; 2002.
2. Scheuer PJ, Lefkowitch JH (eds). *Liver biopsy interpretation.* 6th ed. Edinburgh: WB Saunders; 2000.
3. Lee RG (ed). *Diagnostic liver pathology.* St Louis: Mosby; 1994.
4. Patrick RS, McGee JOD (eds). *Biopsy pathology of the liver.* London: Chapman and Hall; 1988.

CHAPTER 6

Acute viral hepatitis

P. KAR, ANIL JAIN, ARUN KUNDRA

Acute viral hepatitis (AVH) is a disease known since antiquity. Epidemic jaundice has been mentioned in the *Talmud,* and Hippocrates is credited with the first description of the disease in the fourth century BC.[1]

Acute viral hepatitis is a systemic infection predominantly affecting the liver. It has been defined as an acute self-limiting disease with a serum AST elevation of at least five-fold or clinical jaundice or both.[2] The differentiation of AVH from chronic viral hepatitis is based on the duration of the disease; the duration being 6 months or more in chronic hepatitis.

AETIOLOGY

Almost all cases of AVH are caused by one of five viral agents, either alone or in concert: hepatitis A virus (HAV), hepatitis B virus (HBV), hepatitis C virus (HCV), the HBV-associated delta agent or hepatitis D virus (HDV) and hepatitis E virus (HEV). While four of these are RNA viruses (HAV, HCV, HDV and HEV), one is a DNA virus (HBV) (Tables I–IV).

Table I. The major agents causing hepatitis

Genome	Faecal–oral transmission	Parenteral transmission
DNA virus	–	Hepatitis B virus
RNA virus	Hepatitis A virus	Hepatitis C virus
	Hepatitis E virus	Hepatitis D virus

Table II. Virology of agents causing hepatitis

Characteristics	HAV	HBV	HCV	HDV	HEV
Family	*Picornaviridae*	*Hepadnaviridae*	*Flaviviridae*	Viroid	*Caliciviridae/ Flaviviridae/* alpha supergroup
Size (nm)	27–32	42	55	35	32
Shape	Icosahedral	Spherical	Spherical	Spherical	Icosahedral
Envelope	Absent	Present	Present	Present (HBsAg)	Absent
Genome	7.5 kb ssRNA	3.2 kb dsDNA	9.4 kb ssRNA	1.7 kb ssRNA	7.5 kb ssRNA

Table III. Clinical features of hepatitis caused by different agents

Feature	HAV	HBV	HCV	HDV	HEV
Transmission					
Oral	Common	Not likely	No	No	Common
Percutaneous	Rare	Common	Common	Common	Unknown
Sexual	No	Common	Yes, rare	Yes, rare	No
Perinatal	No	Common	Yes, low frequency	No	Yes, unknown frequency
Incubation period (days)	15–49 (average 25)	60–180	14–160	21–45	15–60
Clinical illness at presentation	Paediatric 5%; Adults 70%–80%	10%–15%	5%–10%	10%, higher with super-infection	Adults 70%–80%
Jaundice	Adults 30%; Children <5%	5%–20%	5%–10%	Unknown	Common
Fulminant	<1%	<1%	Rare	2%–7.5%	<1%, up to 30% in pregnancy
Case-fatality rate	0.1%–2.7%	1%–3%	1%–2%	Coinfection <1%; Super-infection >5%	0.5%–4% (1.5%–21% in pregnant women)
Chronic infection	None	Adults <5%; Infants >90%	80%–90%	Superinfection >80%; Co-infection ≤5%	None

Table IV. Interpretation of different serological tests in viral hepatitis

Agent	Serological test	Interpretation
HAV	IgM anti-HAV	Current or recent infection
	IgG anti-HAV	Previous infection; indicates immunity
HBV	HBsAg	Acute or chronic infection
	HBeAg	High levels of viral replication; indicates infectivity
	Anti-HBe	No or low levels of viral replication and infectivity
	IgM anti-HBc	Recent HBV infection
	IgG anti-HBc	Recovered or chronic HBV infection
	Anti-HBs	Immunity to HBV infection
HCV	Anti-HCV (by EIA)	Positive 2–3 weeks after clinical onset; remains positive with chronicity or with clearance of virus
	Anti-HCV (by RIBA)	Confirmatory test for a positive anti-HCV by EIA
	HCV RNA by PCR	Positive earlier in the course of infection (as early as a week after exposure); persists during chronic infection
HDV	IgM anti-HDV	Current or chronic infection
	IgG anti-HDV (high titre>1:1000)	Ongoing viral replication—chronic infection
	IgG anti-HDV (low titre)	Past infection
HEV	IgM anti-HEV	Current or recent infection
	IgG anti-HEV	Previous infection; indicates immunity

RIBA: recombinant immunoblot assay; EIA: enzyme-linked immunoassay

HEPATITIS A VIRUS

Virology

HAV is an icosahedral, non-enveloped, hepatotropic virus, 27–32 nm in diameter, which belongs to the genus Hepatovirus within the *Picornaviridae* family.[3] There are at least four distinct genotypes and most of the strains that infect humans belong to genotypes I and III.

Incidence and prevalence

HAV has a worldwide distribution and is the most common cause of viral hepatitis. Three different patterns of prevalence have been recognized. In countries with poor sanitary conditions, such as those in Africa, Asia (including India), and Central and South America, HAV infection is highly endemic, with most persons being infected within the first few years of life, and the prevalence of protective antibodies to HAV in adults approaches 100%.[4] In areas of intermediate endemicity (Eastern Europe, republics of the former Soviet Union, parts of the Americas and Asia), sanitary conditions are variable and some children escape infection in early childhood.[4] Hence, the peak rates of clinically apparent infection occur in older children and adolescents. In low-endemic areas (northern and western Europe, the United States, Canada and Australia), peak infection rates occur among adolescents and young adults, with outbreaks occasionally occurring in day-care centres and residential institutions.[4]

Modes of transmission

The major mode of transmission is person-to-person via the faecal–oral route. Individuals from a low socioeconomic backgound have a higher rate of infection because of the greater exposure to risk factors such as large families, household crowding, inadequate systems for disposal of human waste and lack of clean drinking water. Water-borne transmission is another important mode of spread of infection. Food-borne hepatitis A is also well described and the consumption of contaminated, uncooked or undercooked food such as shellfish, has led to large outbreaks of the disease.

Transmission of HAV via the sharing of non-sterile needles and blood-borne biological products has been described[5] but such transmission occurs only rarely.

Clinical manifestations

HAV results only in acute infection and does not produce chronic disease. The clinical spectrum of the disease ranges from silent, asymptomatic infection to fulminant hepatitis. Atypical manifestations include cholestasis, relapse after recovery, extrahepatic symptoms and the possible triggering of autoimmune diseases.

The incubation period is 15–49 days (average 25 days). The preicteric phase is characterized by non-specific prodromal symptoms that last for 1–2 weeks and abate with the onset of jaundice, although weakness and malaise may persist for a longer period. The duration of jaundice is less than 2 weeks in the majority of patients; complete clinical and biochemical recovery is seen in 60% of patients within a period of 2 months and in nearly 100% of patients by 6 months. Overall, the prognosis in acute HAV infection is excellent, and chronic hepatitis does not occur. Fulminant hepatitis (acute liver failure) is rare and case-fatality rates for hepatitis A are only 0.14% in hospitalized patients. The severity of the illness is age-dependent. Patients over 50 years of age have the most severe disease, whereas infection in children is usually asymptomatic or, if symptomatic, non-icteric.[6]

Two atypical courses of acute infection have been described: (i) prolonged cholestasis; and (ii) relapsing hepatitis.[7] In patients with prolonged cholestasis, the duration of jaundice exceeds 12 weeks.

Diagnosis

The detection of anti-HAV in the serum by radioimmunoassay (RIA) or enzyme-linked immunoassay (EIA) is the gold standard for diagnosis. The presence of IgM anti-HAV in a patient who presents with clinical features of hepatitis, or in an asymptomatic person with elevated serum aminotransferase levels, is diagnostic of acute HAV infection. IgG anti-HAV indicates previous exposure and immunity to HAV; a rising titre of IgG anti-HAV is indicative of recent exposure.

Natural history

Hepatitis A is typically a benign, self-limiting infection, with the majority of patients exhibiting complete recovery within 2 months of the onset of illness. The severity of hepatitis A infection increases with age; acute liver failure and death are increasingly prevalent in persons above 40 years of age.[8] Fulminant HAV infection is rare and chronic HAV infection does not occur.

Treatment

Supportive measures are the only treatment necessary in most cases of acute HAV infection. Sedatives and narcotics should be avoided. There are no mandatory dietary restrictions. Hospitalization is advised in patients with severe or persistent anorexia or vomiting, and in those who show signs of developing acute liver failure.

Prevention

Prevention requires attention to public and personal health measures. Travellers to endemic areas should be advised to avoid drinking water or beverages with ice from sources of unknown purity, eating uncooked shellfish, or eating uncooked and unpeeled fruits and vegetables.

Passive immunization

Postexposure prophylaxis should be given to household and sexual contacts of infected individuals, attendees of day-care centres where cases of hepatitis A have been reported, or in settings with the potential for repeated exposure, such as institutional facilities. A single intramuscular dose of immune globulin (0.02–0.06 ml/kg) containing IgG anti-HAV should be given as soon as possible, preferably within 2 weeks, to individuals exposed to hepatitis A.

Active immunization

For active immunoprophylaxis, both live-attenuated and inactivated virus vaccines are available. The live-attenuated vaccine induces the development of anti-HAV in 100% of vaccinees but, because of the potential risk of reversion of a live vaccine to a virulent strain, inactivated virus vaccines have been developed. The latter are also highly immunogenic, with 90%–98% sero-conversion rates after a single dose and a 100% seroconversion rate after 3 doses.[9,10] Immunity after a 2-dose vaccination series (at 0 and 6–12 months) is likely to last for at least 10 years and may last for as long as 50 years.

HEPATITIS B VIRUS

Virology

HBV is a DNA virus of the family *Hepadnaviridae*, 42 nm in diameter. Its genome has 4 open reading frames (ORF) (S, P, C and X) that encode 4 major proteins: HBsAg or surface or S protein (major envelope protein), polymerase, viral core protein, or hepatitis B core antigen (HBcAg) and X protein, respectively. There is remarkably little genomic variability in HBV, although 4 major serological types (adw, ayw, adr and ayr) have been described based on the serological responses to minor differences in the proteins encoded by the surface gene. Mutant forms of HBV with mutations in the precore, surface and X genes, as well as the core promoter region, have also been described.

Incidence and prevalence

It is estimated that there are approximately 400 million carriers of HBV worldwide. Hyperendemic regions include Southeast Asia, China, the western Pacific and sub-Saharan Africa, where infection is almost universal and about 10%–20% of the population are chronic carriers. Areas with intermediate prevalence include North Africa, the Middle East and South America, where 1%–5% of the population are chronic carriers. North America, western Europe, Australia and New Zealand have low levels of endemicity, with HBsAg carrier rates of about 0.1%–2% of the population. The incidence of acute HBV infection in developed countries is falling due to changes in behaviour (e.g. an increase in safe sexual practices) as well as effective vaccination programmes.[11]

Modes of transmission

HBV is parenterally transmitted via blood or blood products, sharing needles for injectable drugs or by sexual or perinatal exposure—the same routes as for HIV. Viral particles are detectable in the body secretions, including semen and saliva. Thus, contact with mucous membranes and their secretions is likely to be a mode of transmission of HBV.[11] Other risk factors for HBV infection include working in a healthcare setting, undergoing transfusions and dialysis, acupuncture, tattooing, travel abroad and residence in an institution.[12]

In high-prevalence areas, the major means of spread is perinatal transmission or horizontal spread during the first 2 years of life. In contrast, most HBV infections in low-prevalence areas are acquired in early adult life through unprotected sexual activity, drug injection, occupational exposure, or receipt of contaminated organs or blood products.

Clinical manifestations

The incubation period from acute exposure to clinical symptoms ranges from 60 to 180 days. About 70% of patients have subclinical, anicteric hepatitis, whereas 30% develop icteric hepatitis. The prodromal period consists of non-specific constitutional symptoms that could be followed by anorexia, myalgias, fatigue, jaundice and right upper quadrant abdominal pain. Symptoms usually resolve within 2–3 months. Biochemical abnormalities usually commence with the prodromal phase of the acute illness and may persist for several months.

HBsAg and markers of viral replication (HBeAg and HBV DNA) become detectable before the onset of clinical symptoms or biochemical abnormalities. HBc antibody (anti-HBc) becomes positive with the onset of symptoms and can be detected throughout the course of the infection.

Extrahepatic findings are common in patients with acute HBV infection. Arthralgias and rashes occur in 25% of cases. Other manifestations include serum sickness-like syndrome with immune complex deposition, polyarteritis nodosa with systemic vasculitis, neuropathy (mononeuritis), renal disease, cutaneous vasculitis, arthritis, Raynaud phenomenon, Guillain–Barré syndrome and membranoproliferative glomerulonephritis.

The most serious complication of acute HBV infection is fulminant hepatic failure, which occurs in less than 1% of cases.

Diagnosis

The serological EIAs for the diagnosis of acute HBV infection (IgM anti-HBc, HBsAg and HBeAg) are both sensitive and specific. The detection of IgM anti-HBc indicates acute HBV infection, and the detection of HBeAg indicates active viral replication and increased infectivity. Diagnostic modalities based on molecular biology, such as the polymerase chain reaction (PCR) for the detection of HBV DNA, can also be employed.

Natural history

Two major factors influence the development of chronic infection: the age of the individual at the time of infection and the immune status of the host.

While the risk of chronicity after acute HBV infection is low (<5%) in immunocompetent adults,[13,14] it is greatly increased in immunosuppressed patients (e.g. those on chronic haemodialysis, exogenous immunosuppression, HIV infection and cancer chemotherapy). The risk of chronicity following an infection acquired in the neonatal period is extremely high (up to 90%), presumably because neonates have an immature immune system.

Treatment

Treatment of acute HBV infection is largely supportive and antiviral therapy is not indicated. Attention should be paid to the indices of hepatic synthetic function (prothrombin time, and serum bilirubin and albumin levels). Evidence of significant impairment should prompt close monitoring, preferably in a hospital setting and, if hepatic failure is progressive, liver transplantation should be considered.

Prevention

HBV infection can be prevented by three main strategies: (i) behaviour modification to prevent disease transmission; (ii) passive immunoprophylaxis; and (iii) active immunization.

Passive immunoprophylaxis is used in four situations: (i) neonates born to HBsAg-positive mothers; (ii) after needle-stick exposure; (iii) after sexual exposure; and (iv) after liver transplantation in patients who were HBsAg-positive pretransplantation.

The current recommendations for active immunization are universal vaccination, especially in areas highly endemic for HBV. Although yeast-derived recombinant vaccines are the most widely available, both plasma-derived and recombinant HBV vaccines are safe and highly effective. Both vaccines are administered intramuscularly in a 3-dose schedule (at 0, 1–2 and 6–12 months) and the protective efficacy rates approach 95%. Protection is demonstrated by the production of anti-HBs, and levels of 10 million units/ml or higher are considered seroprotective. Immunity can last for more than 10 years and may be lifelong. Although not recommended routinely, postvaccination testing for the development of anti-HBs may be a reasonable strategy for individuals at high risk, such as healthcare workers. Those who do not respond to the vaccine should be revaccinated with 3 additional doses.

HEPATITIS C VIRUS

Virology

This enveloped virus is approximately 50 nm in diameter and belongs to the family *Flaviviridae*. It consists of a positive-strand RNA surrounded by the core (nucleocapsid), which is surrounded by two envelope proteins (E1 and E2).[15] The genome of HCV has approximately 9600 nucleotides.

HCV has an inherently high mutation rate, which results in considerable heterogeneity throughout the genome.[16] The first designation used to describe genetic heterogeneity is the genotype, which refers to genetically distinct groups of HCV isolates that have arisen during the evolution of the virus.[16] The second component of genetic heterogeneity is discussed on page 140.[16,17]

Incidence and prevalence

The worldwide seroprevalence of HCV infection, based on the detection of antibody to HCV (anti-HCV), is estimated to be 3%. However, marked geographical variation exists and three different epidemiological patterns can be identified: (i) in countries such as the United States and Australia, HCV infection is mostly found among persons between 30 and 49 years of age, indicating that HCV transmission occurred largely in the relatively recent past, primarily among young adults infected through intravenous drug use; (ii) in areas such as Japan or southern Europe, the prevalence of HCV infection is highest in older persons, suggesting that the risk of HCV transmission was greatest in the distant past (>30 years ago); and (iii) in countries such as Egypt, high rates of infection are observed in all age groups, suggesting that there is an ongoing high risk of acquiring HCV.

Modes of transmission

The major modes of transmission of HCV infection can be divided into percutaneous (blood transfusion and needle-stick inoculation) and non-percutaneous (sexual contact, perinatal exposure). Overall, blood transfusion from unscreened donors and injecting drug use are the two best documented risk factors. Available evidence indicates that, in contrast to the percutaneous modes of transmission, transmission by non-percutaneous routes is inefficient; this is particularly true for sexual transmission. The source of transmission remains unknown in up to 10% of cases.[18]

Clinical manifestations

HCV accounts for approximately 20% of cases of acute hepatitis. Acute infection is, however, rarely seen in clinical practice, because the vast majority of patients have no clinical symptoms.[19] Jaundice may develop in 25% of these patients, whereas 10%–20% may present with non-specific symptoms, such as fatigue, nausea and vomiting, indistinguishable from the symptoms of other types of AVH. HCV RNA appears in the blood within 2 weeks of exposure and is followed by an increase in serum aminotransferase levels several weeks later. Serum aminotransferase levels may exceed 1000 U/L in 20% of cases and generally follow a fluctuating pattern during the first month. Fulminant hepatitis is rare.

Reported extrahepatic manifestations of HCV infection include membrano-proliferative glomerulonephritis, essential mixed cryoglobulinaemia, porphyria cutanea tarda, leucocytoclastic vasculitis, focal lymphocytic sialadenitis, Mooren corneal ulcers, lichen planus, rheumatoid arthritis, non-Hodgkin lymphoma and diabetes mellitus.

Diagnosis

Immunological or serological tests, such as third-generation EIA and recombinant immunoblot assay (RIBA), identify the presence of anti-HCV, which indicates exposure to the virus without differentiating among acute, chronic and resolved infection.[20] In contrast, molecular or virological assays such as PCR-based methods or branched DNA assays detect specific viral nucleic acid sequences (HCV RNA), which indicate persistence of the virus.[20] Therefore, serological assays are typically used for screening and first-line diagnosis, and virological assays are needed to confirm active infection.

Natural history

HCV infection is self-limiting in only 15% of patients in whom HCV RNA in the serum becomes undetectable and ALT levels return to normal. Approximately 85% of infected patients do not clear the virus by 6 months and chronic hepatitis develops. Progression of the disease is largely silent and patients are often identified only on routine biochemical screening or blood donation. The factors that are associated with progression to liver disease include age (>40 years), male gender and increased alcohol intake (>50 g daily).[21]

Treatment

If detected, treatment of acute HCV infection was considered till recently to be largely supportive and antiviral therapy was not given. However, recent data support the treatment of acute hepatitis C, although firm guidelines regarding which patient to treat, when to treat and what therapy to use are not yet available.

Prevention

As there is no effective vaccine and postexposure prophylaxis against HCV, a major effort should be made to counsel both HCV-infected patients and those at risk of infection. Adequate sterilization of medical and surgical equipment is mandatory. HCV-infected patients should be instructed to avoid sharing razors and toothbrushes, and cover any open wounds. In addition, safe sexual practices, such as the use of latex condoms, should be encouraged.

HEPATITIS D VIRUS

Virology

HDV or the delta agent, discovered by Rizzetto and colleagues in 1977, is a small (36 nm) defective RNA virus that requires the helper function of another virus (HBV). Its genome consists of a single-stranded, positive-sense RNA molecule of 1679–1683 bases. Although the replication of HDV can occur within hepatocytes in the absence of HBV, HBV is necessary for coating the HDV virions and allowing their spread from cell to cell.

Incidence and prevalence

Worldwide, there are about 15 million persons infected with HDV. Areas of high prevalence include Italy, certain parts of Eastern Europe, the Amazon basin, Colombia, Venezuela, western Asia and some Pacific Islands. The prevalence of HDV infection in patients with HBV infection is low in the general population, as represented by blood donors, and highest among persons with percutaneous exposures, such as injecting drug users (20%–53%) and haemophiliacs (48%–80%).[22]

Modes of transmission

The modes of transmission of HDV are similar to those of HBV infection, and percutaneous exposure is the most efficient. Intravenous drug use is among the commonest modes of HDV transmission in areas of low prevalence. Haemophiliacs and other persons who receive large amounts of pooled blood products are also at increased risk of acquiring HDV infection. Sexual transmission of HDV is less efficient than that of HBV, and perinatal transmission is rare.

Clinical manifestations

Acute HDV infection can occur in a patient with established HBV infection (superinfection) or concurrently with HBV infection (coinfection). In general, patients with hepatitis D seem to suffer from a more serious and progressive disease than those with other forms of viral hepatitis.

Diagnosis

IgM anti-HDV (EIA/RIBA) is detectable during the early phase of acute infection and therefore serves as a useful marker of acute disease. However, it is not useful in distinguishing between coinfection (HBV and HDV acquired simultaneously) and superinfection (HDV acquired in a chronic HBV carrier), and this distinction is made by the presence or absence of IgM anti-HBc. In acute coinfection with HDV and HBV, IgM anti-HDV and HDV RNA are present in the serum together with IgM anti-HBc, whereas in patients with superinfection, HDV markers are present in the absence of IgM anti-HBc.

HDV RNA is an early marker of acute infection and a useful marker of HDV replication in patients with chronic infection. In acute HDV infection, serum HDV RNA is detectable in up to 90% of cases during the symptomatic phase of the illness and becomes undetectable after clinical resolution.[23] Because only a few regions of the HDV genome are highly conserved among different genotypes of HDV, the efficiency of reverse trancriptase (RT)-PCR is dependent on the choice of primers for amplification.

Natural history

Acute hepatitis caused by coinfection with HDV and HBV is associated with a higher risk of severe or fulminant liver disease than is hepatitis caused by HBV alone. In coinfected persons, HDV infection has little impact on the natural history of HBV infection, and the rate of chronicity following coinfection with HBV and HDV is equal to that of HBV infection alone. In contrast, in superinfection with HDV, the presence of established HBV infection provides the ideal substrate for HDV and, as a consequence, chronic progressive liver disease develops in more than 90% of patients. HBsAg-positive patients with anti-HBe who are superinfected with HDV usually develop chronic disease, whereas HBsAg-positive patients with HBeAg who become superinfected with HDV develop fulminant disease.

Treatment

The management of acute HDV infection is supportive. There have been no studies of antiviral therapy in this context. The frequency of fulminant hepatic failure is greater with HDV infection than with HBV infection alone, and patients should be monitored closely for evidence of encephalopathy, coagulopathy and other signs of liver failure. Liver transplantation is the treatment of choice for patients with fulminant disease secondary to HDV superinfection.

Prevention

HDV replication is dependent on HBV replication, and thus vaccination against HBV is a safe and efficacious prophylaxis against hepatitis D. However, hepatitis B immunoglobulin and HBV vaccine are of no value in preventing HDV super-infection. Prevention of HDV superinfection depends primarily on behaviour modification, such as the use of condoms to prevent sexual transmission and needle-exchange programmes to prevent transmission by intravenous drug use.

HEPATITIS E VIRUS

Virology

HEV is an icosahedral, non-enveloped virus (approximately 27–34 nm in diameter), which was initially grouped into the family *Caliciviridae* but subsequently shifted to the alpha-like supergroup of positive-strand RNA viruses. Geographically distinct isolates of HEV have been classified roughly into four genotypes: genotype 1 (Asian isolates: Myanmar, China, Pakistan and the former Soviet Union); genotype 2 (a single isolate from Mexico); genotype 3 (isolates from North America); and genotype 4 (isolates from some parts of China and Taiwan). Despite the presence of genetically different isolates of HEV, there appears to be only one serotype.

Incidence and prevalence

HEV is the most common cause of epidemic enterically transmitted hepatitis. Worldwide, two geographical patterns can be differentiated: endemic areas of HEV prevalence, in which major outbreaks and a substantial number of sporadic cases occur; and non-endemic regions, in which HEV accounts for a few cases of AVH, mainly among travellers to endemic regions. Endemic disease is geographically distributed around the equatorial belt, including Central America, Africa and the Middle East, India, Asia and the Southeast Pacific.

Modes of transmission

HEV is transmitted by the faecal–oral route, and the most common vehicle of transmission during epidemics is the ingestion of water contaminated with faeces.

Clinical manifestations

HEV infection is self-limiting and not different from other causes of viral hepatitis. The incubation period after exposure to HEV is 15–60 days (average 40 days). Two phases of illness have been described, a prodromal and preicteric phase characterized by fever and malaise, and an icteric phase characterized by jaundice, dark urine, clay-coloured stools, anorexia, nausea, vomiting and abdominal pain. Peak serum aminotransferase levels coincide with the onset of the icteric phase and generally return to normal within 1–6 weeks.[24] Fulminant hepatitis has been described in association with HEV infection. Pregnant women are at increased risk for a fulminant course and the maternal case-fatality rate increases with the duration of pregnancy.[25]

Diagnosis

Acute infection is diagnosed by the detection of the IgM antibody by EIA/Western blot using recombinant-expressed or synthetic proteins. In the majority of patients, IgM anti-HEV is undetectable 5–6 months after the onset of illness. IgG anti-HEV is detectable shortly after IgM anti-HEV becomes detectable and remains detectable in most patients 1 year after acute infection. Because HEV RNA is not detectable in the serum during the symptomatic phase of the illness, diagnostic tests based on the detection of HEV RNA in the serum have limited application.

Natural history

Acute HEV infection is usually mild and self-limiting, and symptoms generally resolve within 6 weeks. Chronic HEV infection does not occur.

Treatment

Supportive care is the cornerstone of therapy and no specific interventions are required. Uncommonly, fulminant hepatitis occurs, which should prompt consideration for liver transplantation.

Prevention

Effective prevention relies primarily on improved sanitation because no immunoprophylaxis is currently available. Provision of a clean source of water is one of the principal preventive measures. Travellers to endemic areas should be advised to avoid drinking water or beverages with ice from sources of unknown purity, eating uncooked shellfish, or eating uncooked and unpeeled fruits and vegetables.

ACUTE VIRAL HEPATITIS OF UNKNOWN AETIOLOGY

Although hepatitis viruses A, B, C, D and E are all well characterized and molecularly defined agents with an unequivocal association with AVH, the aetiology of a small, yet significant, proportion of AVH cases remains unknown. Hepatitis of unknown aetiological origin, typically referred to as non-A, non-E or NANE or cryptogenic hepatitis, has been reported to constitute about 10%–20% of both acute community-acquired and transfusion-associated hepatitis. Non-viral causes (e.g. toxic, immunological, metabolic) may be responsible for some of these cases. However, evidence obtained after the rigorous application of criteria to exclude drug exposure, alcohol abuse, autoimmune diseases and other conditions that cause liver damage strongly suggests that there may be some still unidentified hepatotropic (i.e. hepatitis) viruses.

POTENTIAL HEPATOTROPIC VIRUSES: PRETENDERS AND CONTENDERS[26]

The intense search for newer hepatitis agents bore fruit in the mid-1990s with the discovery of a putative blood-borne hepatitis virus called the hepatitis G virus (HGV) and three so-called GB viruses. Recently, two novel DNA viruses, the TT and SEN viruses, have also been identified as possible agents of NANE hepatitis.

Hepatitis G virus

In the mid-1990s, two different groups, namely, the Virus Discovery Group at Abbott Laboratories and researchers at Genelabs Technologies Inc., announced the discovery of a new hepatitis virus, isolated from the serum of a patient with community-acquired non-A, non-B hepatitis, and called the isolate hepatitis GB virus-C (GBV-C) and HGV, respectively.[27,28] Subsequently, when the genomes of HGV and GBV-C were compared, a high degree of sequence homology was found, and it was concluded that GBV-C and HGV are independent isolates of the same virus.

HGV/GBV-C is a member of the *Flaviviridae* family. It possesses a single-stranded RNA genome (approximately 9362 nucleotides long) capable of encoding a single polyprotein of 2873 amino acids. Even though HCV belongs to the same virus family, there is only a limited amino acid sequence homology (25%), showing that no close relationship exists.

HGV/GBV-C infection is widespread and the carrier frequency in the general community is high. A close examination of HGV/GBV-C prevalence using suitable controls shows that there is little evidence that could support the direct involvement of HGV/GBV-C in the aetiology of NANE hepatitis. It is true that

HGV/GBV-C is found in a proportion of cases of NANE hepatitis but the virus does have multiple modes of transmission and it may merely be an 'accidental tourist' transmitted along with the real agent(s) of NANE hepatitis. The virus does not appear to be hepatotropic.

TT virus

By using representational differential analysis, Nishizawa *et al.*[29] reported the isolation of a novel DNA virus, named the TT virus, from the serum of a Japanese patient (initials TT) who developed post-transfusion hepatitis of unknown aetiology. Further characterization of the virus showed that it possesses a negative-sense, single-stranded, circular DNA genome comprising approximately 3800 nucleotides with three conserved ORF and sequence motifs consistent with a rolling circle mode of replication. The size of the virion has been estimated to be 30–50 nm. The TT virus has been tentatively classified as the only member of a new virus family *Circoviridae*.

Based on the current prevalence data, the virus appears to be ubiquitous with a global distribution and the extraordinarily high frequency of infection suggests that it is unlikely to have a direct link with a specific disease. The consensus from many studies is that TT virus infection is unlikely to be a cause of NANE hepatitis. It has been mooted that perhaps a specific TT virus variant may have some disease association, but even this must be considered unlikely.

SEN virus

Recently, scientists working at the DiaSorin Biomolecular Research Institute in Italy claimed to have discovered a new virus that may be the primary cause of most cases of NANE hepatitis.[30] The virus has been provisionally named the SEN virus (SEN-V) after the source patient, and preliminary information suggests that the original isolate is a representative of a virus cluster containing at least eight members (SEN-V A through H). SEN-V is a single-stranded DNA virus, which lacks an envelope. The genome is linear and contains approximately 3900 nucleotides with at least three ORF. The characteristics of SEN-V revealed so far show a remarkable parallel with those of the TT virus and it may be that the viruses share a common ancestor.

Information available on SEN-V and liver disease is very limited, and there is no convincing evidence to date which would suggest that SEN-V causes significant liver disease. Moreover, it appears that the baseline prevalence of SEN-V in the healthy population is fairly high and its presence in patients with NANE liver disease may be a mere reflection of its high level of prevalence in the general population. The lessons learnt from the hepatitis virus pretenders (HGV/GBV-C and TT virus) need to be kept in mind while evaluating any future contenders, including SEN-V.

REFERENCES

1. Giangranade G. Hippocrates in hepatitis. In: Lee CA, Thomas H (eds). *Classical papers in viral hepatitis*. London: Sci Press; 1988:1–3.
2. Smedile A, Farci P, Verme G, *et al*. Influence of delta infection on severity of hepatitis B. *Lancet* 1982;**2**:945–7.
3. Wimmer E, Murdin A. Hepatitis A and the molecular biology of picornaviruses: A case for a new genus of the family *Picornaviridae*. In: Hollinger FB, Lemon SM, Margolis HS (eds). *Viral hepatitis and liver disease*. Baltimore: Williams & Wilkins; 1991:1–41.
4. Melnick J. History and epidemiology of hepatitis A virus. *J Infect Dis* 1995;**171** (Suppl):S2–S8.
5. Manucci PM, Gdovin S, Gringeri A, *et al*. Transmission of hepatitis A to patients with hemophilia by factor VIII concentrates treated with organic solvent and detergent to inactivate viruses. *Ann Intern Med* 1993;**20**:1–7.
6. Romero R, Lavine J. Viral hepatitis in children. *Semin Liver Dis* 1994;**14**:289–302.
7. Schiff E. Atypical clinical manifestations of hepatitis A. *Vaccine* 1992;**10** (Suppl):S18–S20.
8. Hu M, Kang L, Yao G. An outbreak of hepatitis A in Shanghai. In: Bianchi L, Gerok W, Maier K, Deinhardt F (eds). *Infectious diseases of the liver*. London: Kluwer; 1990:361–72.
9. Werzberger A, Mensch B, Ketter R, *et al*. A controlled trial of formalin-inactivated hepatitis A vaccine in healthy children. *N Engl J Med* 1992;**327**:453–7.
10. Innis BL, Snitbhan R, Kunasol P, *et al*. Protection against hepatitis A by an inactivated vaccine. *JAMA* 1994;**271**:1328–34.
11. Alter MJ, Mast E. The epidemiology of viral hepatitis in the United States. *Gastroenterol Clin North Am* 1994;**23**:437–55.
12. Margolis H, Alter M, Hadler S. Hepatitis B: Evolving epidemiology and implications for control. *Semin Liver Dis* 1991;**11**:84–92.
13. Seeff LB, Beebe GW, Hoofnagle JH, *et al*. A serological follow-up of the 1942 epidemic of post-vaccination hepatitis in the United States Army. *N Engl J Med* 1987;**316**:965–70.
14. Hyams KC. Risks of chronicity following acute hepatitis B virus infection: A review. *Clin Infect Dis* 1995;**20**:992–1000.
15. Choo QL, Richman K, Han J, *et al*. Genetic organization and diversity of the hepatitis C virus. *Proc Natl Acad Sci USA* 1991;**88**:2451–5.
16. Bukh J, Miller R, Purcell R. Genetic heterogeneity of hepatitis C virus: Quasispecies and genotypes. *Semin Liver Dis* 1995;**15**:41–63.
17. Farci P, Purcell RH. Clinical significance of hepatitis C virus genotypes and quasispecies. *Semin Liver Dis* 2000;**20**:103.
18. National Institutes of Health. Consensus development conference panel statement: Management of hepatitis C. *Hepatology* 1997;**26** (Suppl):2S–10S.
19. Alter HJ, Seeff LB. Recovery, persistence and sequelae in hepatitis C virus infection: A perspective on long-term outcome. *Semin Liver Dis* 2001;**20**:17–35.
20. Morishima C, Gretch DR. Clinical use of hepatitis C virus tests for diagnosis and monitoring during therapy. *Clin Liver Dis* 1999;**3**:717–40.
21. Poynard T, Bedossa P, Opolon P, for the OBSVIRC, METAVIR, CLINIVIR and DOSVIRC groups. Natural history of liver fibrosis progression in patients with chronic hepatitis C. *Lancet* 1997;**349**:825–32.
22. Ponzetto A, Forzani B, Parravicini PP, *et al*. Epidemiology of hepatitis delta virus (HDV) infection. *Eur J Epidemiol* 1985;**1**:257–63.
23. Smedile A, Rizzetto M, Denniston K, *et al*. Type D hepatitis: The clinical significance of hepatitis D RNA in serum as detected by a hybridization-based assay. *Hepatology* 1986;**6**:1297–1302.
24. Chauhan A, Jameel S, Dilawari J, Chawla Y, Kaur U, Ganguly N. Hepatitis E virus transmission to a volunteer. *Lancet* 1993;**341**:149–50.

25. Balayan M, Usamov R, Zamyatina N, *et al.* Experimental hepatitis E infection in domestic pigs. *J Med Virol* 1990;**132:**58–9.
26. Bowden S. New hepatitis viruses: Contenders and pretenders. *J Gastroenterol Hepatol* 2001;**16:**124–31.
27. Linnen J, Wages J, Zhang-Keck ZY, *et al.* Molecular cloning and disease association of hepatitis G virus: A transfusion-transmissible agent. *Science* 1996;**271:**505–8.
28. Lisitsyn N, Lisitsyn N, Wigler M. Cloning the differences between two complex genomes. *Science* 1993;**259:**946–51.
29. Nishizawa T, Okamoto H, Konishi K, *et al.* A novel DNA virus (TTV) associated with elevated transaminase levels in posttransfusion hepatitis of unknown etiology. *Biochem Biophys Res Commun* 1997;**241:**92–7.
30. Primi D, Sortini A. Identification and characterization of SEN virus, a family of novel DNA viruses [Abstr]. *Antiviral Ther* 2000;**5** (Suppl):G.7.

CHAPTER 7

Chronic hepatitis

MANOJ KUMAR, S.K. SARIN

The spectrum of chronic inflammatory diseases of the liver extends from acute to chronic hepatitis, and finally to cirrhosis. Chronic hepatitis comprises several diseases having common clinical manifestations and are marked by chronic necroinflammatory injury that can lead insidiously to cirrhosis and end-stage liver disease (Box 1). The disease is defined as chronic if there is evidence of ongoing injury of 6 months' duration or more. This definition is rather arbitrary, and conditions affecting the liver that are chronic are well defined, even though they may present acutely. Common conditions that present acutely in spite of being chronic in character are autoimmune and metabolic liver diseases.

The strict definition of chronic hepatitis is based on histological features of hepatocellular necrosis and chronic inflammatory cell infiltration in the liver, but the diagnosis can usually be made from the clinical features and results of blood tests alone. Chronic hepatitis has multiple causes including viruses, medications, metabolic abnormalities and autoimmune disorders. The most common forms are chronic hepatitis B and C, and autoimmune hepatitis (AIH). Drug-induced or metabolic liver diseases, and alcoholic and non-alcoholic steatohepatitis can also cause chronic necroinflammatory lesions of the liver. Despite extensive testing, some cases cannot be attributed to any known cause.

CLINICAL FEATURES

The clinical symptoms of chronic hepatitis are typically non-specific, intermittent and mild; a large proportion of patients have no symptoms of liver disease at all.

Box 1	Major causes of chronic hepatitis
• Chronic hepatitis B • Chronic hepatitis D • Chronic hepatitis C • Autoimmune hepatitis	• Drug-induced chronic hepatitis • Wilson disease • Cryptogenic hepatitis (non-A, non-E hepatitis)

The most common symptom is fatigue, which may be intermittent. Some patients have sleep disorders or difficulty in concentrating. Pain in the right upper quadrant, if present, is usually mild, intermittent and aching in character.

In many cases, the diagnosis of chronic hepatitis is made after abnormalities are identified in the results of LFT. Such abnormalities may be detected on routine health evaluation, during assessment for an unrelated health problem or at the time of voluntary blood donation. Symptoms of advanced disease or an acute exacerbation include nausea, poor appetite, weight loss, muscle weakness, itching, dark urine and jaundice. Once cirrhosis is present, weakness, weight loss, abdominal swelling, oedema, easy bruisability, gastrointestinal bleeding and hepatic encephalopathy with mental confusion may arise.

The most common physical finding is liver tenderness. In patients with severe or advanced disease, other findings may include a firm liver or mild enlargement of the spleen, spider angiomata and palmar erythema. Once cirrhosis is present, signs may include muscle wasting, ascites, oedema, skin excoriations or bruises and hepatic fetor.

BIOCHEMICAL FEATURES

Although symptoms and signs are not particularly useful in identifying chronic hepatitis, the results of biochemical and haematological blood tests are fairly reliable. Most typical are elevations in ALT and AST levels with little elevation in ALP levels. The elevations are usually in the range of 1–5 times the upper limit of normal, and the ALT level is generally somewhat higher than the AST level unless cirrhosis is present. Serum aminotransferase levels can be normal when the disease is mild or inactive, but can also be markedly elevated in the range typical of acute hepatitis (10–25 times the upper limit of normal) during acute exacerbations. Although there may be major discrepancies between the extent of liver enzyme elevations and histological estimates of activity as shown by liver biopsy, monitoring these values over time generally provides a reasonable estimate of the severity of the disease. Serum aminotransferase levels can be used for an approximate grading as shown below:

- Mild: <100 IU/L (up to 3 times the upper limit of normal)
- Moderate: 100–400 IU/L (up to 10 times the upper limit of normal)
- Severe: >400 IU/L (more than 10 times the upper limit of normal)

In general, elevation of ALP and GGT levels is mild in chronic hepatitis, unless cirrhosis is present.

Serum bilirubin and albumin levels as well as PT are normal in patients with chronic hepatitis, unless the disease is severe or advanced. Any elevation in serum direct bilirubin level or decrease in albumin level should be considered as evidence of serious disease activity or injury. Serum immunoglobulin levels are mildly elevated or normal in chronic viral hepatitis but may be strikingly elevated in chronic AIH.

Blood counts are normal in chronic hepatitis, unless cirrhosis or portal hypertension is present with an associated decrease in white blood cell and platelet counts. Serial determination of the platelet count may provide the earliest clinical evidence of progression of chronic hepatitis to cirrhosis.

RADIOLOGICAL FEATURES

USG imaging can define hepatic texture and size, determine the presence of hepatic masses, assess the gallbladder and intrahepatic bile ducts, define the size of the spleen, and determine the presence of collateral vessels and portal venous flow. CT scan and nuclear magnetic imaging of the liver are not helpful unless a mass or abnormality is detected on USG.

HISTOLOGY

Chronic hepatitis, regardless of the cause, is characterized by several pathological changes that are present to a variable extent in all cases. These include the following: portal inflammation, periportal injury and inflammation, several forms of degeneration and death by apoptosis of intra-acinar hepatocytes with an associated inflammatory response and fibrosis, which may involve only the portal and periportal areas or may form septa.[1]

Portal inflammation: In all forms of chronic hepatitis, the portal areas are variably infiltrated by lymphocytes and plasma cells. Lymphoid aggregates or follicles with germinal centres may be present, typically in chronic hepatitis C. In patients with AIH, a large number of plasma cells are often present in the portal inflammatory infiltrate.

Hepatitis-associated bile duct lesions: This is characterized by swelling, vacuolation, nuclear irregularity and sometimes pseudostratification of the biliary epithelial cells. The basement membrane may appear to be ruptured, and lymphocytes, and occasionally plasma cells and neutrophils, infiltrate the ducts. However, the ducts are not destroyed, as in primary biliary cirrhosis (PBC), so that portal areas without ducts are seldom seen. Duct lesions have been seen in all forms of hepatitis but most often in chronic hepatitis C.[2]

Interface hepatitis: Formerly known as piecemeal necrosis, this condition can be recognized as irregularity of the limiting plate, caused by extension of the portal infiltrate through the plate to the surrounding parenchyma. The limiting plate becomes irregular and may disappear as the portal area expands.

Parenchymal injury: Intra-acinar necroinflammatory changes are present to some degree in all forms of chronic hepatitis. It is typically multifocal (spotty) in distribution and consists mainly of areas of apoptosis. More severe intra-acinar injury, including changes typical of acute hepatitis, is generally seen when biopsy is done during an acute exacerbation of chronic hepatitis, even if the patient is asymptomatic. Some degree of steatosis may be present, most often in chronic hepatitis C but also in other cases.

Fibrosis: Fibrosis is invariably a component of chronic hepatitis, though the degree of fibrous deposition varies from patient to patient. Fibrosis occurs insidiously during the course of chronic hepatitis and typically begins in the periportal regions. Ultimately, bands of fibrosis can link adjacent portal areas, or portal and central areas, distort the hepatic architecture, and lead to cirrhosis and portal hypertension.

Hepatic histological analysis is useful for grading the severity of and staging chronic hepatitis, and is usually done to confirm a diagnosis made on the basis of the patient's history, physical examination and the results of blood tests. Hepatic histological evaluation may help to confirm the diagnosis of AIH and clarify the role of α_1-antitrypsin deficiency or Wilson disease. Most importantly, histological analysis of the liver can exclude other diagnoses that occasionally mimic chronic hepatitis clinically or cause similar patterns of liver enzyme level elevations, including fatty liver, alcoholic liver disease, steatohepatitis, drug-induced liver disease, sclerosing cholangitis, iron overload and veno-occlusive disease.

CLASSIFICATION

Classification is based on the aetiology, clinical grade, and histological grade and stage.

Aetiology

Chronic hepatitis can be caused by several diseases that are similar clinically but respond differently to therapy, and must be managed individually. Patients with suspected chronic hepatitis should be carefully evaluated for fatty liver, alcohol- or drug-induced liver disease, metabolic liver diseases, autoimmune markers, and specific and appropriate serological tests for viral hepatitis (Table I).

Table I. Aetiological classification of chronic hepatitis

Diagnosis	Sex	Associations	Diagnostic tests
Chronic hepatitis B	Male	Healthcare workers, homosexuals, drug abusers, blood transfusion, parenteral exposure, born to infected mother	HBsAg, HBV DNA, HBeAg or HBcAg in the liver
Chronic hepatitis C	Equal	Blood transfusion, blood products, drug abusers	Anti-HCV, HCV RNA (using PCR)
Chronic hepatitis D	Male	Healthcare workers, homosexuals, drug abusers, blood transfusion, parenteral exposure	Anti-HDV, HDV RNA or HDV antigen in the liver
Autoimmune hepatitis	Female	Multisystem involvement (diabetes, arthralgia, haemolytic anaemias, nephritis and others)	Antinuclear antibodies (ANA), anti-smooth muscle antibody (ASMA), anti-liver kidney microsome antibody (LKM)
Drug-induced liver disease	Female	Isoniazid, methyl dopa, nitrofurantoin, dantrolene, propylthiouracil, etc.	History, rechallenge if necessary
Wilson disease	Equal	Family history, haemolysis, neurological signs	Serum caeruloplasmin, urinary copper, hepatic copper concentration
Cryptogenic	Female	Obesity, diabetes, parenteral exposure	Exclusion of other causes

Table II. Histological activity index (excluding fibrosis)[3]

Component	Scores
Periportal necrosis with or without bridging necrosis	0–10
Intralobular degeneration and focal necrosis	0–4
Portal inflammation	0–4

Table III. Staging for chronic hepatitis[5]

Score	Grade	Description
0	None	–
1	Mild	Portal expansion
2	Moderate	Portal–portal septa
3	Severe	Bridging with distortion
4	Cirrhosis	Cirrhosis

Clinical severity

Transaminase levels are commonly used to assess the clinical severity.

Histological grade and stage

In 1981, Knodell *et al.*[3] introduced the histological activity index (HAI), a scoring system based on three categories for necroinflammation and one for fibrosis, which has later been modified and is known as the Ishak score.[4] For grading, numbers are assigned according to the severity of the necroinflammatory features (interface hepatitis, confluent necrosis, parenchymal injury and portal inflammation), and these numbers are added to arrive at a grade that can range from 0 to 18 (Table II).

Disease stage is defined by scores between 0 and 4 for fibrosis, and may or may not be added into the Knodell score (Table III); in the Ishak score, the stage, ranging from 0 to 6, is reported separately.

CHRONIC HEPATITIS B

Virology

HBV is a member of a family of distinct viruses, known as the *Hepadnaviridae*, which infect humans and a few animal species (duck, ground squirrel and woodchuck). They are characterized by the presence of partially double-stranded DNA surrounded by an outer lipoprotein envelope and an inner core composed of nucleocapsid proteins. The virus encodes a polymerase that catalyses by reverse transcription (RT) both the generation of DNA complementary to the viral RNA template and the synthesis of positive-strand viral DNA from the negative-strand DNA template of the virus.[6]

HBV has four open reading frames (ORF) (S, P, C and X) that encode four major proteins (surface, polymerase, core and X protein, respectively). Intact

HBV virions are 42 nm in diameter and readily visualized by electron microscopy. HBsAg or S protein, which is 24 kD in size, is the major envelope protein of the virus. Two other proteins, L and M, which are 39 kD and 31 kD, respectively, are also present in the viral envelope. Both these proteins include the S protein fused to peptides of variable length at the amino terminal. The L protein, which is synthesized from an AUG initiation codon upstream from the S gene in the pre-S1 region, is believed to play a role in binding the virus to a receptor on the hepatocyte surface. The function of the M protein, which is synthesized from an AUG initiation site between the pre-S1 and S gene in the pre-S2 region, is unknown.

Within the envelope is a 27 nm structure known as the nucleocapsid core, which consists of 180 copies of the viral core protein or HBcAg surrounding the viral DNA and the virally encoded polymerase. The nucleic acid is a relaxed, circular molecule that consists of a 3.2 kB minus strand and a smaller, complementary DNA plus strand of variable length. Two short, repeat sequences, known as DR1 and DR2, which are present at the 5' ends of the plus and minus strands, are important for the initiation of DNA synthesis. The viral polymerase is bound to the 5' end of the minus strand, where it functions as both a reverse transcriptase for the synthesis of the negative DNA strand from genomic RNA and an endogenous DNA polymerase. Its function as a polymerase includes the synthesis of completely double-stranded, relaxed, circular DNA by using the 3' end of the plus strand as a primer and the 5' end of the minus strand as a template. The HBV polymerase is encoded by the P gene of the virus.

The function of the X protein has not been fully elucidated, but it appears to function as a transcriptional activator that influences the transcription of HBV genes as well as those of other viruses (e.g. HIV) by regulating the activity of transcriptional promoters.[7]

HBV encodes four major proteins: the surface, core and X proteins, and the polymerase, which is achieved by the use of overlapping ORF, so that more than one half of the nucleotides are used in a different frame for the transcription of different viral messenger RNAs (mRNAs). These mRNAs are in turn translated into more than one viral protein. For example, the S gene, which encodes HBsAg, is used in its entirety in another frame to encode part of the polymerase. Multiple related proteins are also produced by differential translation at multiple AUG translation initiation codons within the same ORF. For example, three proteins, S, pre-S1 or L, and pre-S2 or M, are synthesized from the pre-S/S gene. Two related proteins are produced by a similar mechanism from the translation of mRNAs encoded by the core gene. One of these, the core peptide, is a 21 kD protein that forms the nucleocapsid core of the virus; the translation of the second protein, HBeAg, is initiated at a start codon upstream from the core AUG codon and consists of the core peptide plus a 30-amino acid residue encoded by the precore region.

HBeAg is also a marker of active viral replication. HBeAg is translated from genomic-length mRNA transcripts, similar to those used for the synthesis of viral DNA by RT. Thus, the production of high levels of HBeAg is indicative of the synthesis of large amounts of full-length genomic mRNA, which in turn reflects active viral replication.

Much of our understanding of the mechanism of HBV replication is derived from experiments performed on ducks, woodchucks and ground squirrels. Although extremely useful, extrapolation of these results to human disease must be done with caution.

Epidemiology

Incidence and prevalence

Chronic hepatitis B is a common disease with an estimated global prevalence of over 300 million carriers, or approximately 5% of the world's population. There are wide ranges in the prevalence of HBV infection in different parts of the world. In the Far East (Southeast Asia, China, the Philippines, Indonesia), the Middle East, Africa and parts of South America, the prevalence is high, with HBsAg positivity rates ranging from 8% to 15%.[8] In regions of high seroprevalence, serological evidence of prior HBV infection (antibody to HBcAg [anti-HBc] or antibody to HBsAg [anti-HBs] positivity) is almost universal in persons without active infection.

Regions of intermediate prevalence (2%–7%) include Japan, parts of South America, Eastern and southern Europe, and parts of Central Asia. Prevalence is lowest (<2%) in the United States and Canada, northern Europe, Australia and the southern part of South America.

In India, of the 25 reports taken up for meta-analysis of HBsAg carrier rate in the general population, a range of 1.1%–12.2% was observed. The mean HBsAg carrier rate for India from these reports is 3.34%.[9] The states of India can be classified based on HBsAg carrier rates as follows:

<2%:   Jammu and Kashmir, Kerala
2%–4%: Karnataka, Maharashtra, Delhi, Haryana, Himachal Pradesh, West Bengal
>4%:   Tamil Nadu, Pondicherry, Andhra Pradesh, Madhya Pradesh, Uttar Pradesh, Arunachal Pradesh

Transmission

HBV is parenterally transmitted via blood or blood products or by sexual or perinatal exposure.

Perinatal and early childhood transmission: Infants born to HBeAg-positive mothers who have high levels of viral replication (HBV DNA level >80 pg/ml) have a 70%–90% risk of perinatal acquisition in the absence of intervention. In contrast, the risk of mother-to-infant transmission from HBeAg-negative mothers is substantially lower (10%–40%).[10] Infection occurs through occult inoculation of the infant at the time of birth or shortly thereafter. IgM anti-HBc is not detectable in cord blood, so that intrauterine infection is unlikely to have occurred. Even with active and passive immunization, 5%–10% of babies may acquire HBV infection at birth.

Children of HBsAg-positive mothers, who are not infected at birth remain at high risk of early childhood infection; 60% become infected by the age of 5 years.[11] The mechanism of this later infection, which is neither perinatal nor sexual, is unknown. Although HBsAg can be detected in breast milk, breast-feeding is not believed to be an important mode of transmission. Children living in highly endemic areas may acquire the infection from outside the family.

Sexual transmission: Sexual activity is probably the single most important mode of HBV transmission in areas where the prevalence of infection is low. Homosexuals are at particularly high risk for HBV infection.[12] Factors associated with a high risk of viral acquisition in this patient population include multiple sexual partners, anal-receptive intercourse and duration of sexual activity.[12]

Heterosexuals, including sexual partners of injecting drug users, prostitutes and clients of prostitutes, are at particularly high risk for HBV infection. In heterosexuals, factors associated with an increased risk of HBV infection include duration of sexual activity, number of sexual partners, a history of sexually transmitted diseases and positive serological results for syphilis.[12]

Sexual partners of persons infected with HBV are at risk for infection, even in the absence of high-risk behaviour. Studies of sexual and household contacts of HBV carriers have shown that 0%–3% of the spouses or sexual partners and 4%–9% of the children are HBsAg-positive. Moreover, there is a high prevalence of markers of prior HBV infection in these two groups (29%–59% of spouses or sexual contacts and 9%–12% of children). The risk of heterosexual transmission is greater when the infected person is female.

Intravenous drug use: The risk of HBV infection increases with the duration of drug use, so that serological markers of ongoing or prior HBV infection are almost universal after 5 years of drug use.

Other modes of transmission: Other risk factors for HBV infection include working in a healthcare setting, transfusion and dialysis, acupuncture, tattooing, travel abroad and residence in an institution.[8]

Epidemiology of subtypes and genotypes

Although there are a variety of serotypes and genotypes of HBV, there is remarkably little genomic variability in the virus. There are four major serological types of HBV (adw, ayw, adr and ayr), which have different geographical distributions but unclear clinical differences.

There has been an increasing interest in the clinical significance of HBV genotypes and the geographical differences in their distribution. The clinical significance of these differences appears to be related in part to the stability of the stem–loop structure of the HBV genome and the association with precore variants of HBV.

Pathogenesis

Immune pathogenesis

Clinical observations suggest that the immune response of the host is more important than viral factors in the pathogenesis of liver injury caused by HBV. Chronic HBV carriers who have normal liver enzyme levels and normal or near-normal liver histological studies, despite high levels of viral replication, have been well described; substantial liver injury would be predicted if the virus were directly cytopathic. Similarly, HBV can be grown in hepatocyte culture with no adverse effect on cell viability. Infants with immature immune systems who acquire HBV infection at birth have a high rate of chronic infection and replication yet typically have only mild liver injury. In patients with chronic HBV infection who fail to clear the virus, the number of both CD4+ and CD8+ T cells is markedly reduced. In contrast, the humoral immune response is preserved in chronic HBV infection.

Cytotoxic T lymphocytes (CTL) are responsible for the destruction of virally infected hepatocytes and viral clearance.[13] However, the number of CTL involved is generally much fewer than the number (10^{11}) of virally infected hepatocytes. Thus, secondary non-antigen-specific immune responses, such as those mediated by inflammatory cytokines, may be more important for viral clearance than the CTL-mediated mechanism. Recent data point to the importance of tumour necrosis factor (TNF)-α and interferon (IFN)-γ as prime mediators of this non-antigen-specific clearance of HBV.[14]

Viral pathogenesis

Variant viruses: Mutant forms of HBV with mutations in the precore, surface and X genes, as well as the core promoter region, have been implicated in a number of clinical syndromes. Polymerase variants that are selected by exposure to nucleoside analogues have recently been described.

Precore/core variants: Although the majority of northern European and American patients with chronic HBV infection and active viral replication are HBeAg-positive, many southern European and Asian patients have severe liver disease and active viraemia in the absence of HBeAg.[15] Sequence analysis of the precore region of HBV isolated from such patients has revealed a point mutation (G to A) at the nucleotide position 1896 that results in the production of a translational stop codon predicted to stop translation of HBeAg.[15] Such variant viruses have also been described in association with fulminant liver failure and severe chronic liver disease.[16]

Mutations in the core promoter region have also been proposed to result in the failure of HBeAg production.[17] These mutant viruses, which involve nucleotide substitutions at positions 1762 and 1764, may decrease transcription of the mRNA that encodes HBeAg. Core promoter variants have been described in association with 27% of cases of progressive chronic hepatitis.[17]

Surface gene mutants

Immune escape from neutralizing antibodies occurs in a region of HBV known as the 'a' determinant.[18] The glycine at amino acid 145 in particular is highly conserved among HBV subtypes, and a G-to-A nucleotide substitution produces amino acid changes at this position that result in major antigenic changes in the virus. Escape mutants have been described in babies who received immunoprophylaxis with polyclonal hepatitis B immune globulin (HBIG)[18] and in liver transplant recipients receiving monoclonal HBIG therapy.[19]

Low-level HBV infection

The existence of HBsAg-negative HBV infection has long been debated.[20] Low-level HBV infection is implicated or has been documented in the following clinical situations:

1. HBV infection has been transmitted by transfusion of a unit of blood from an HBsAg-negative, anti-HBc-positive blood donor;
2. HBV DNA has been detected in the serum and liver from persons lacking all serological markers of HBV infection;
3. Low-level HBV infection has been detected in patients with a variety of causes of chronic liver disease and in association with primary hepatocellular carcinoma (HCC);[21]
4. HBsAg-negative patients may become HBsAg-positive and develop overt hepatitis with cancer chemotherapy or immunosuppression following kidney transplantation.

Clinical manifestations and diagnosis

In acute HBV infection that progresses to chronicity, HBsAg, HBeAg and HBV DNA remain positive for 6 months or longer.

After the acute phase of infection, serum ALT levels fall but often remain persistently abnormal (50–200 U/L). IgM anti-HBc titres typically fall to undetectable levels after 6 months but may become detectable again during reactivation of infection. IgG anti-HBc persists indefinitely. HBV DNA is detectable by hybridization assays during the acute and chronic phases of the disease. With time, there may be a spontaneous loss of HBV DNA and HBeAg, frequently in association with a flare-up of serum ALT levels and seroconversion to anti-HBe positivity. Spontaneous loss of HBsAg is rare. Anti-HBs may be detected simultaneously with HBsAg in the serum in fewer than 10% of cases. In some cases of chronic infection, active viral replication (HBV DNA positivity) occurs in the absence of HBeAg.

The presence of anti-HBs is associated with immunity to HBV infection. Isolated anti-HBs is more likely to be acquired by vaccination than by natural infection, in which case both anti-HBs and IgG anti-HBc are typically present. Much confusion surrounds the interpretation of isolated anti-HBc positivity. The significance of this finding depends on the patient population in which it is observed. Fifty per cent of patients with chronic HBV infection are anti-HBc positive; in these patients, who have had frequent parenteral exposure, the anti-HBc positivity probably represents resolved HBV infection or low-level HBV infection of minor clinical significance. In Alaskan natives, a group with a high prevalence of HBV infection, vaccination against HBV has been used to determine whether isolated anti-HBc signifies prior exposure; those with a primary immune anti-HBs response were deemed to have a false-positive anti-HBc, whereas those with an anamnestic response were deemed to have a true-positive anti-HBc, indicative of prior or ongoing low-level HBV infection. In blood donors who have been pre-screened for parenteral risk factors, an isolated anti-HBc, particularly if it is of low optical density on EIA, most likely represents a false-positive result. Because there is no readily available 'gold standard' for the diagnosis of resolved or ongoing low-level HBV infection, the interpretation of an isolated positive anti-HBc remains problematic.

Diagnosis

The most important tests are those of viral seromarkers. Chronic HBV infection is defined by the presence of HBsAg in the serum of a given individual on two occasions at least 6 months apart. It is paramount to know the replicative status of the patient, for which the HBeAg and anti-HBe need to be determined. In the anti-HBe positive group, HBV DNA levels may be required to differentiate between a low replicative wild-type infection (low viral titres) and a precore mutant infection (high viral titres). The diagnosis of chronic hepatitis B is usually suspected on the basis of HBsAg in the serum of a patient with chronic hepatitis and confirmed by the finding of HBV DNA in the serum or HBcAg in the liver. Most patients with chronic hepatitis B also have HBeAg in the serum, reflecting high levels of viral replication. Some patients have active liver disease with HBsAg and high levels of HBV DNA but no HBeAg in the serum. These patients usually harbour a mutant HBV that replicates efficiently and is pathogenic but does not produce HBeAg.

HBV DNA quantification is generally performed by signal or target amplification tests; the liquid hybridization test (Genostics assay [Abbott Laboratories, Abbott Park, Chicago, IL, USA]) uses a liquid phase to hybridize ^{125}I-HBV DNA after the sample HBV DNA has been denatured. The lower detection limit of the assay is 1–2 pg/ml or 6×10^5 copies/ml. The RNA–DNA hybrid assay (Digene Hybrid Capture II HBV DNA Test) uses an HBV RNA probe to capture serum HBV DNA and has a sensitivity of 0.018 pg/ml or 5×10^5 copies/ml. The branched DNA assay (Bayer, Emeryville, CA, USA) is a compound nucleic hybridization assay that uses a synthetic oligonucleotide to bind single-stranded HBV DNA to a solid phase. Different oligonucleotides bind to other areas of HBV DNA (throughout the genome) and also bind amplifier oligo-nucleotides (branched DNA) that enhance the chemiluminescent signal by having multiple branches of the same sequence that bind ALP-labelled probes. The sensitivity limit is 7×10^5 DNA equivalents/ml. PCR assay is based on the amplification of viral DNA, together with an internal standard using HBV-specific complementary primers usually to the precore/core region. The PCR method can now be performed automatically in the Cobas analyser after the manual extraction of viral DNA (Cobas Amplicor HBV Monitor or Cobas-AM)[22] or using real-time fluorescent-probe PCR (TaqMan).[23] The sensitivity of the Cobas Amplicor assay is between 100 and 400 copies/ml, and that of the Taqman method is as low as 10 copies/ml; both the assays are more sensitive than the branched DNA and Genostics assays. These tests are especially less sensitive for the detection of HBV DNA in HBsAg-positive, HBeAg-negative patients (13% and 25%, respectively) but have a high specificity (100% for each assay).[24]

Extrahepatic manifestations

Polyarteritis nodosa with systemic vasculitis can occur with chronic HBV infection. This syndrome typically presents with abdominal pain resulting from arteritis of the medium-sized arteries with ischaemia of the intestine or gallbladder. Other manifestations of HBV-associated vasculitis include neuropathy (mononeuritis), renal disease, cutaneous vasculitis, arthritis and Raynaud phenomenon.[25] Chronic HBV infection has also been associated with membranoproliferative glomerulonephritis resulting from the deposition of immune complexes in the basement membrane of the glomerulus. The syndrome of type II mixed essential cryoglobulinaemia was previously believed to be caused largely by HBV infection but has been shown to be associated more frequently with chronic HCV infection. Neurological manifestations of HBV infection include the Guillain–Barré syndrome and a polyneuropathy (usually related to polyarteritis). HBV infection is rarely associated with pericarditis and pancreatitis.

Complications

Patients with chronic HBV infection are at risk of developing the long-term complications of portal hypertension and hepatic decompensation, such as variceal bleeding, ascites and the hepatorenal syndrome as well as HCC, which may ultimately result in death. The risk of developing HCC is increased 10- to 390-fold in patients with chronic HBV infection compared to those who are HBsAg-negative, and is greater in those who acquired HBV infection perinatally than in those who acquired it as adults.

Pathology

As with other chronic viral hepatitides, HBV infection is associated with a predominantly lymphocytic infiltrate that may or may not be confined to the portal tracts. The presence of ground-glass hepatocytes, in which the cytoplasm is stained pink with haematoxylin and eosin, is characteristic of chronic HBV infection, reflecting the massive overproduction of HBsAg in these chronically infected cells. A specific histological entity known as fibrosing cholestatic hepatitis has been described in liver transplant recipients with severe recurrent HBV infection in the allograft. The pathology is characterized by massive hepatocellular necrosis in the absence of a strong inflammatory response, with striking overexpression of viral proteins. Immunohistochemical and molecular methods have been developed to detect viral antigens and viral DNA, respectively, in liver tissue.

Natural history

The risk of chronicity is related to two major factors: the age at which the infection is acquired and immune status of the host. The risk of chronicity after acute HBV infection is low in immunocompetent adults.[26] The reported risk of chronic infection after acute exposure in adults ranges from <1% to 12%, but the consensus is that the risk of chronicity is <5%.

The risk of chronic infection is greatly increased in patients who have a reduced ability to recognize and clear viral infection (e.g. patients on chronic haemodialysis, those on exogenous immunosuppression following solid organ transplantation and those receiving cancer chemotherapy). Patients with concomitant HIV infection are also at significant risk of developing chronic infection (20%–30% remain HBsAg-positive after acute infection). The risk of chronicity after neonatally acquired infection is extremely high (up to 90%), presumably because neonates have an immature immune system. Children below 6 years of age have a lower but marked risk of chronic infection (approximately 30%).

The prognosis of chronic HBV infection is determined predominantly by the presence or absence of active viral replication and the degree of histological liver damage. Approximately one half of all chronic HBV carriers have evidence of active viral replication, particularly if serum aminotransferase levels are elevated.[27] Chronic HBV carriers with evidence of active viral replication are at highest risk for the development of progressive disease; cirrhosis develops in 15%–20% of them within 5 years, even if histological liver damage is initially mild. Longitudinal follow-up of such patients has shown that the spontaneous loss of HBeAg is 7%–20% per year; therefore, the prevalence of HBeAg declines with age.[28] Loss of HBeAg, which may occur spontaneously or in association with the use of antiviral therapy, is often accompanied by an exacerbation of liver disease. Loss of HBsAg occurs much less frequently, at a rate of 1%–2% per year.

In a prospective study of 379 HBV carriers, the 5-year survival rate was 97% in patients with early histological changes, including chronic persistent hepatitis (in which inflammation is limited to the portal areas), compared with 86% in patients with chronic active hepatitis (in which liver cell necrosis and inflammation extend to the hepatic parenchyma) and 55% in patients with established cirrhosis.[27]

Many patients with chronic HBV infection have normal serum amino-transferase levels, normal or near-normal liver histological findings and no symptoms. These 'healthy carriers' appear to be immunologically tolerant of the virus, and their prognosis is excellent. Liver biopsies obtained from 92 asymptomatic HBsAg-positive carriers who were identified during blood donation showed no or minimal changes in the majority. Only 5% of patients had evidence of marked histological liver damage (chronic active hepatitis), and none had histological evidence of cirrhosis. The majority of patients included in the study were HBeAg- and HBV DNA-negative. When followed up prospectively for a mean of 130 months (range 70–170 months), 12% had a sustained elevation of serum aminotransferase levels, and only 2% developed histological progression of the disease. In a minority of patients, spontaneous flares of serum aminotransferase levels were noted in association with evidence of active viral replication. With 7–11 years of follow-up, spontaneous loss of HBsAg was seen in 15% of patients.

Prevention

Three main strategies exist for the prevention of HBV infection: (i) behaviour modification to prevent disease transmission; (ii) passive immunoprophylaxis; and (iii) active immunization.

Behaviour modification

Changes in sexual practices and improved screening methods of blood products in blood banks can reduce the risk of transfusion-associated hepatitis B. Behaviour modification is unlikely to be beneficial in developing countries, where neonates and young children are at greatest risk of acquiring the infection. In these groups, immunoprophylaxis, both passive and active, is the most effective.

Passive immunoprophylaxis

Passive immunoprophylaxis is used in four situations: (i) neonates born to HBsAg-positive mothers; (ii) after needle-stick exposure; (iii) after sexual exposure; and (iv) after liver transplantation in patients who are HBsAg-positive pretransplantation.

Immunoprophylaxis is currently recommended for all infants born to HBsAg-positive mothers and should ideally be performed in combination with universal screening of all pregnant women for HBsAg; 0.13 ml/kg of HBIG immediately after or within 12 hours of delivery, in combination with the first dose of the recombinant vaccine, followed by the remainder of the vaccine series should be used. This combination results in a >90% level of protection against perinatal acquisition of HBV.[29] About 3%–15% of infants still acquire HBV infection perinatally from HBV-infected mothers.[30] Failure of passive and active immunoprophylaxis in this setting may be the result of (i) *in utero* transmission of HBV infection, (ii) perinatal transmission related to a high inoculum, or (iii) the presence of surface gene escape mutants.

After sexual or needle-stick exposure, the administration of HBIG in a dose of 0.05–0.07 ml/kg as soon after exposure as possible is recommended, preferably within 48 hours and no more than 7 days after exposure. A second dose 30 days later may decrease the risk of transmission of HBV. Active immunization should be administered concurrently.

Active immunization

Preventing primary infection by vaccination is an important strategy to decrease the risk of chronic HBV infection and its subsequent complications. Vaccination programmes targeted at high-risk groups (e.g. healthcare workers, parenteral drug users and infants of infected mothers) have failed. Universal childhood vaccination against HBV infection is recommended. The major difficulty in implementing these recommendations in developing countries is the high cost of vaccinating large populations.

Plasma-derived vaccines were the first available HBV vaccines, but concerns about the transmission of other infectious agents led to the development of recombinant vaccines. Recombinant vaccines are made by incorporating the surface gene of HBV into different expression vectors (yeast, *Escherichia coli* or mammalian cell lines). Yeast-derived recombinant vaccines are the most widely available. The standard regimen is 20 µg in adults, with the same dosing intervals (generally 0, 1 and 6 months) as used for the plasma-derived vaccine. With this schedule, the rate of induction of protective immunity is comparable to that for the plasma-derived vaccine. Current recommendations are to administer the vaccine by intramuscular injection in the deltoid muscle for adults and in the lateral aspect of the thigh in children.

The HBV vaccine is highly effective. Anti-HBs develops in over 95% of vaccine recipients; the attack rate of all HBV infections is only 3.2% in vaccine recipients compared to 25.6% in recipients of a placebo. If patients fail to develop protective antibodies in response to the standard vaccine regimen, an additional dose of either the plasma-derived or recombinant vaccine will result in an adequate response in only a small proportion of patients. Because of the high seroconversion rates in immunocompetent individuals, postvaccination testing is usually not necessary. Protective levels of the antibody persist in the majority of responders (68% at 4 years). Even if antibody levels decline to the point that anti-HBs is no longer detectable, protection is not necessarily lost. Hence, routine testing of vaccinated persons and routine booster vaccination are not recommended. In select circumstances, particularly when persons at high risk of acquiring HBV infection are vaccinated (e.g. children of HBV-infected mothers), documentation of seroconversion may be prudent. Moreover, revaccination of such high-risk persons after 5–10 years may be appropriate if anti-HBs titres have declined below 10 IU/L.

Immunocompromised patients, including those on haemodialysis, have a reduced chance of mounting a protective immune response after vaccination. Additional doses of the vaccine appear to increase the response rate. Patients over the age of 40 years also exhibit a decreased response rate. There is evidence that response to the vaccine is genetically determined.

Treatment

The primary goal of treatment is to prevent the complications of liver disease. A secondary goal is to decrease the number of chronic carriers who serve as a reservoir for HBV transmission. Because complications may take many years to develop, most treatment trials of patients with chronic HBV infection have used intermediate end-points, such as inhibition of viral replication and improvement in histological appearance of the liver, to evaluate efficacy. Loss of HBV DNA and seroconversion from HBeAg to anti-HBe are usually associated with normalization of liver enzymes and a decrease in inflammation on liver biopsy specimens.

Interferon

The usual regimen for IFN-α has been 5 million units daily or 10 million units three times a week by injection for 16 weeks. Extending the duration or administering a higher dose does not appear to increase the response rate.

The efficacy of IFN-α is variable, but a meta-analysis showed that 33% of patients receiving the drug had a loss of HBeAg compared with 12% of untreated controls; 37% of the patients had a sustained loss of HBV DNA as compared to 17% of controls.[31]

Long-term follow-up of patients treated with IFN indicates that remission is maintained in the majority of those who initially respond to therapy and additional instances of seroconversion occur after treatment is complete.[32] HBV DNA is absent in the serum of the majority of patients who clear HBeAg, and loss of HBeAg and HBV DNA in the serum is usually associated with the disappearance of replicative forms of HBV DNA in the liver.[33] Thus, patients with chronic HBV infection appear to derive long-term benefits from IFN therapy.[34]

Nucleoside analogues

Lamivudine

Lamivudine, or 3TC (the [–] enantiomer of 2'-deoxy-3'-thiacytadine), belongs to the family of nucleoside inhibitors that possess the negative 'unnatural' L-enantiomeric structure. This orally administered compound is an inactive prodrug that gains potency once it is converted intracellularly into its triphosphorylated form. The activated drug is a potent inhibitor of the HBV reverse transcriptase.[35] Lamivudine 5'-triphosphate is a competitive inhibitor of deoxycytadine (dCTP) incorporation into viral DNA, and its incorporation results in chain termination of the elongating nucleic acid strand.

Studies of the kinetics of HBV clearance during treatment with lamivudine predicted that prolonged treatment of 1–5 years' duration is required to reliably clear HBV infection.[36] However, prolonged use of lamivudine can lead to the development of viral mutations that confer resistance to this agent.[37] The most common mutation leading to lamivudine resistance is a specific point mutation in the conserved tyrosine–methionine–aspartate–aspartate (YMDD) motif of the

HBV polymerase in which a methionine residue is changed to a valine or isoleucine.[35] The emergence of YMDD mutants in the context of lamivudine therapy results in diminished therapeutic antiviral activity.[38] However, serum HBV DNA and aminotransferase levels are typically lower in the presence of the mutant virus when compared with wild-type infection. Hence, the YMDD variant appears to have diminished replicative competence and is potentially less injurious to hepatocytes than the wild-type virus.[39]

The only independent predictive factor of HBeAg seroconversion is the pretreatment aminotransferase level. HBeAg seroconversion occurred in 64%, 26% and 5% of patients with pretreatment serum ALT levels greater than five times, two to five times, and less than two times the upper limit of normal, respectively.[40] These data suggest that, as with IFN-α, a successful antiviral response to lamivudine therapy depends on an endogenous immune response to HBV.

On the basis of available data, it is clear that a 1-year course of treatment with lamivudine is insufficient to achieve a sustained antiviral response in most patients. Current recommendations are to treat with lamivudine until the loss of HBeAg, with or without acquisition of anti-HBe. Because the risk of developing lamivudine resistance is substantial in patients who receive prolonged treatment, caution is advised before instituting treatment in patients with mild histological liver disease even in the presence of active viral replication. It is unclear whether lamivudine should be continued in patients in whom evidence of resistance develops. New therapies being developed appear to be effective against resistant variants. Lamivudine therapy has also been tested in patients with precore variants of HBV. As in patients with wild-type infection, lamivudine produces a complete response in approximately two-thirds of patients, as shown by the normalization of serum ALT and loss of serum HBV DNA associated with a greater than two-point reduction in the Knodell necroinflammatory score.[41] However, the frequency of a sustained response is unknown. Preliminary data suggest that most patients relapse and a longer duration of treatment will be necessary to achieve a sustained response.

In patients with decompensated cirrhosis, treatment with lamivudine produces clinical improvement with a reduction in serum ALT and HBV DNA levels, and improvement in the Child–Turcotte–Pugh score.[42] However, on stopping lamivudine, most patients experience an increase in serum HBV DNA levels, and there is concern that relapse of the disease may be associated with a flare-up of liver disease and worsening hepatic decompensation. For this reason, it seems advisable to continue lamivudine therapy indefinitely in a patient with advanced HBV-related liver disease.

Adefovir dipivoxil

Adefovir dipivoxil is the oral prodrug of an acyclic nucleotide monophosphate analogue (9-(2-phosphonylmethoxyethyl)-adenine [PMEA]). Orally administered adefovir dipivoxil exhibits an inhibitory effect on both the HIV and HBV reverse transcriptases. Importantly, adefovir appears to be capable of inhibiting the enzymatic activity of both wild-type and YMDD-mutant variants of both these viruses.[43] Recently, adefovir has been found to be useful in the initial treatment of both HBeAg-positive and negative chronic hepatitis B.[44,45] Adefovir monotherapy and lamivudine/adefovir combination therapy trials are currently under way in previously untreated and lamivudine-resistant patients.

Combination therapy

Regimens combining IFN-α with another agent have shown controversial results compared to IFN-α alone. Specifically, the combination of lamivudine and IFN did not show superiority over lamivudine monotherapy in patients who had previously failed to respond to IFN alone. Although one trial of lamivudine plus IFN in the treatment of previously untreated patients suggested a benefit of the combination over either drug alone,[46] further investigation is required to determine the optimal timing and duration of combination therapy.

Liver transplantation

Orthotopic liver transplantation is now the standard of care for patients with decompensated HBV-induced liver disease. The risk of HBV reinfection is at least 80% without prophylaxis, and HBV-associated graft failure is the leading cause of death in patients with recurrent HBV infection. However, because of successful therapies, 2-year survival rates have improved from 70% to 80% in the most recent cohort of patients with HBV-related cirrhosis.[47] Patients treated with a combination of lamivudine and high doses of HBIG have demonstrated very low rates of recurrence (5%–10%).[47] A combination of lamivudine and HBIG is currently the standard of care in patients with decompensated HBV who undergo liver transplantation.

CHRONIC HEPATITIS C

Virology

Structure

HCV is an enveloped virus approximately 50 nm in diameter, which is visualized on electron microscopy within the cytoplasmic vesicles of lymphoblastoid cells in culture. HCV consists of a positive-strand RNA surrounded by the core (nucleocapsid), which is surrounded by two envelope proteins (E1 and E2).[48]

Genomic organization

HCV is a single-stranded, positive-sense RNA virus that belongs to the *Flaviviridae* family. The genome of HCV has approximately 9600 nucleotides and contains a single ORF capable of encoding a large viral polypeptide precursor of 3010–3033 amino acids, with regions at the 5' and 3' ends that are not translated. The cleavage of the protein by cellular and viral proteases results in a series of structural (nucleocapsid [C, p21], envelope 1 [E1, gp31], and envelope 2 [E2, gp70]) and non-structural (NS2, NS3, NS4a, NS4b, NS5a and NS5b) proteins.

Replication

Two different putative cellular receptors for HCV have been proposed: low-density lipoproteins[49] and, more recently, CD81.[50] The importance of extra-hepatic reservoirs of HCV replication (such as peripheral blood mononuclear cells) is uncertain. Studies of the kinetics of HCV in patients have shown that the turnover of the virus is rapid, with high production of the virus *in vivo* to the order of 10^{10}–10^{12} virions/day.[51]

Genotypes and quasispecies

HCV has an inherently high mutation rate that results in considerable heterogeneity throughout the genome. The RNA-dependent RNA polymerase of HCV lacks 3' to 5' exonuclease proofreading ability to remove mismatched nucleotides incorporated during replication.

The first designation used to describe genetic heterogeneity is the genotype, which refers to genetically distinct groups of HCV isolates that have arisen during the evolution of the virus.[52] Nucleotide sequencing has shown that differences of up to 34% exist between different HCV variants. The most conserved region (5' UTR) has a maximum of 9% nucleotide sequence divergence among genotypes, whereas the highly variable regions that encode the putative envelope proteins (E1 and E2) exhibit 35%–44% nucleotide sequence divergence among genotypes. There is evidence for a clustering of sequences into six major 'types' (designated by Arabic numbers), with sequence similarities of 66%–69%, and more than 50 different 'subtypes' (designated by a lower case letter) within these types, with sequence similarities of 77%–80%. The association between genotype and severity of disease is controversial.

The second component of genetic heterogeneity is known as the quasispecies.[52,53] Quasispecies are closely related yet heterogeneous sequences of the HCV genome within a single infected person that result from mutations during viral replication. The quasispecies nature of HCV may be one of the mechanisms by which the virus escapes immune responses.

Epidemiology

Incidence and prevalence

The worldwide seroprevalence of HCV infection, based on antibody to HCV (anti-HCV), is estimated to be 3%. However, marked geographical variation exists, ranging from 0.4%–1.1% in North America to 9.6%–13.6% in North Africa.[54]

Worldwide, three different epidemiological patterns of HCV infection can be identified: (i) in countries such as the United States and Australia, most HCV infections are found among persons between 30 and 49 years of age, indicating that most HCV transmission occurred in the relatively recent past, primarily among young adults infected through intravenous drug use; (ii) in areas such as Japan or southern Europe, the prevalence of HCV infection is highest in older persons, suggesting that the risk of HCV transmission was greatest in the distant past (>30 years ago). In these countries, healthcare-related procedures, particularly unsafe injection practices with reuse of contaminated glass syringes, and folk medicine practices may have played a major role in viral spread; and (iii) in countries such as Egypt, high rates of infection are observed in all age groups, suggesting that an ongoing high risk of acquiring HCV exists.

Transmission

HCV infection may be transmitted percutaneously (blood transfusion and needle-stick inoculation) and by non-percutaneous (sexual contact, perinatal exposure) routes. The latter group may represent occult percutaneous exposure.

Percutaneous transmission

Since the introduction of sensitive second-generation assays for anti-HCV, the risk of HCV-related transfusion hepatitis is estimated to be only 0.01%–0.001% per unit of blood transfused.[55] The prevalence of HCV infection in injecting drug users is 48%–90%.[54] The majority of injecting drug users become positive for anti-HCV within 6 months of initiating injecting drug use.

Chronic haemodialysis is associated with both endemic cases and, more rarely, sporadic outbreaks of HCV infection. The prevalence of anti-HCV in patients undergoing haemodialysis has been noted to be as high as 45%, although studies have more commonly found a prevalence of 10%–20%.[54] Serological assays (anti-HCV) may underestimate the prevalence of HCV infection in this relatively immunocompromised population, and virological assays (for HCV RNA by PCR amplification) may be necessary for accurate diagnosis in dialysis patients. A correlation has been found between increasing years on dialysis and anti-HCV positivity, independent of a history of blood transfusion. These data suggest that HCV might be transmitted among these patients because of incorrect implementation of infection-control procedures.

The risk of acquiring HCV infection after percutaneous exposure is as high as 10%, if PCR is used to detect infection.[56] However, healthcare professionals, including those with a high likelihood of percutaneous exposure to blood, have prevalence rates of anti-HCV similar to those described in the general population. Transmission may also occur from healthcare workers to patients.

Non-percutaneous transmission

Transmission by non-percutaneous routes is inefficient. Most seroepidemiological studies have demonstrated anti-HCV in only a small number of sexual contacts of infected persons.[54] Even in female sexual partners of male haemophiliacs, the overwhelming majority of whom are infected with HCV, anti-HCV is detected in not more than 3%.[54] Sexual partners of low-risk index subjects without liver disease and without high-risk behaviour (injecting drug use or promiscuity) have anti-HCV prevalence rates ranging from 0% to 7%.[54] In contrast, sexual partners of subjects with liver disease or with high-risk behaviour (the partners may themselves participate in high-risk behaviour) have anti-HCV prevalence rates between 11% and 27%.[54]

The efficiency of perinatal transmission of HCV is low,[54] with a risk estimated to range from 0% to 10%. Perinatal transmission occurs exclusively from mothers who are HCV RNA-positive at the time of delivery. Controversy exists regarding the role of coinfection with HIV, and vaginal as opposed to caesarean delivery. Transmission by breastfeeding is believed to be negligible.

Pathogenesis

The primary determinant of viral persistence appears to be the quasispecies nature of HCV, although other potential mechanisms may include: (i) an inadequate innate immune response; (ii) insufficient induction or maintenance of the adaptive response; (iii) viral evasion from efficient immune responses through several mechanisms, such as infection of immunologically privileged sites, viral interference with antigen processing or other immune responses, or viral suppression of the effectiveness of antiviral cytokines; and (iv) induction of immunological tolerance. Despite the development of antibodies against several viral proteins, the majority of infected patients are unable to eradicate the virus.

In general, viral infection can produce cellular injury by direct cytopathicity and indirect immune-mediated injury.

Viral mechanisms

Viral factors may be important in the pathogenesis of disease either directly, through cell injury associated with accumulation of the intact virus or viral proteins; or indirectly, through a differential immune response associated with one viral strain but not with another. HCV is directly cytopathic. Higher serum HCV RNA levels are seen in patients with greater lobular inflammatory activity than in those with minimal inflammation.

In studies from Europe, infection with genotype 1 HCV has been associated with higher levels of viral replication, and infection with HCV subtype 1b has been associated with more advanced liver disease than infection with other genotypes. In contrast, studies from the United States have shown a positive correlation between HCV genotype 2 infection and severe disease.[57]

Immune-mediated mechanisms

HCV infection elicits a specific antibody response, both circulating and liver-infiltrating virus-specific CD8+ and CD4+ T cells, and natural killer (NK) cell activity. HCV-specific CD8+ T-cell responses to HCV antigens are detectable for up to 20 years after infection in persons in whom hepatitis C resolves, but not in those with persistent HCV infection,[58] suggesting that the maintenance of HCV-specific CD8+ T cells determines a benign course of the disease.

The CD4+ T-cell response against HCV is probably impaired, because the proportion of chronic carriers able to mount an effective CD4+ T-cell response to HCV is small.[59] In turn, an early and multispecific CD4+ T-cell proliferative response seems more frequent and stronger in patients in whom acute infection resolves with clearance of HCV viraemia. In these cases, there is a predominance of Th1 CD4+ T cells in the peripheral blood.[60]

Liver-infiltrating CD8+ and CD4+ lymphocytes are detected in the portal, periportal and lobular areas of the liver in patients with chronic HCV infection. CD8+ lymphocytes predominate, suggesting that CTL are the main perpetrators of hepatocellular injury.[60] Patients with detectable intrahepatic CTL activity show lower levels of viraemia, higher ALT values and more active liver disease than those without HCV-specific CTL, suggesting a correlation between CD8+ T cell response and degree of hepatocellular injury.

The humoral response against HCV is targeted against epitopes within all viral proteins. In contrast to the cellular immune response, the antibody response to HCV antigens continues to be evident with time in patients with a chronic outcome but is lost in most recovered patients, suggesting that T cells and not antibodies effect the resolution of acute hepatitis C.[58] The most likely explanation for the ineffectiveness of the antibody response to HCV is that rapid occurrence of viral mutations within the epitopes recognized by neutralizing antibodies abrogates antibody recognition of the new variant.

Clinical manifestations and diagnosis

Approximately 85% of infected patients do not clear the virus by 6 months, and chronic hepatitis develops. Of these, the majority have elevated or fluctuating serum ALT levels, whereas one-third have persistently normal ALT values. The most common complaint of patients with chronic HCV infection is fatigue, the severity of which is not necessarily related to the severity of the underlying liver disease. Other non-specific symptoms include depression, nausea, anorexia, abdominal discomfort and difficulty in concentrating. Once cirrhosis of the liver develops, patients are at risk for complications of portal hypertension (ascites, gastrointestinal bleeding, encephalopathy, etc.). Jaundice is rarely seen in chronic HCV infection until hepatic decompensation has occurred.

Extrahepatic manifestations

Reported extrahepatic manifestations of HCV infection include membrano-proliferative glomerulonephritis, essential mixed cryoglobulinaemia, porphyria cutanea tarda, leucocytoclastic vasculitis, focal lymphocytic sialadenitis, Mooren corneal ulcers, lichen planus, rheumatoid arthritis, non-Hodgkin lymphoma and diabetes mellitus.[61] Some of these associations are more convincing than others. Extrahepatic manifestations will develop in approximately 1%–2% of HCV-infected patients. Furthermore, non-organ-specific autoantibodies are frequently expressed in patients with HCV infection (antinuclear antibodies with a titre >1:40 in 21%, ASMA with a titre >1:40 in 21%, and anti-LKM antibodies in 5%).

Anti-HCV antibodies are found in the serum in 50%–90% of patients with essential mixed cryoglobulinaemia. Furthermore, cryoglobulins are found in approximately one half of patients infected with HCV.

Diagnosis

There are several immunological and molecular assays for the detection and assessment of hepatitis C. Immunological or serological tests identify the presence of anti-HCV, which indicates exposure to the virus without differentiating among acute, chronic and resolved infection. In contrast, molecular or virological assays detect specific viral nucleic acid sequences (HCV RNA), which indicate persistence of the virus.[62] Serological assays are typically used for screening and first-line diagnosis, and virological assays are needed to confirm active infection or monitor the effects of therapy.

Serological tests

There are two types of anti-HCV assay—EIA and the recombinant immunoblot assay (RIBA). Both detect antibodies to different HCV antigens from the core and non-structural proteins, and were developed using recombinant antigens derived from cloned HCV transcripts. Serological assays are typically used for screening and first-line diagnosis. Because first-generation EIAs lacked sensitivity and specificity, confirmatory RIBAs were systematically used in samples positive by EIA. With the newer EIAs and the increased use of molecular assays, confirmatory RIBAs are needed less frequently.

Selection of serological and virological tests

A proposed algorithm for the evaluation of an anti-HCV seropositive patient is shown in Fig. 1. Initial diagnostic testing of HCV infection is currently made by detecting the specific antibody by second- or third-generation EIA tests. For low-

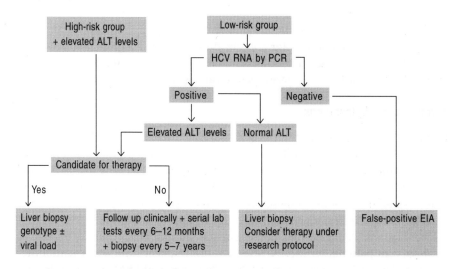

Fig. 1. Evaluation of an anti-HCV seropositive patient

risk patients, a negative EIA test result is sufficient to exclude HCV infection. In contrast, for high-risk, recently exposed, or immunocompromised patients (including HIV-infected, and chronic haemodialysis and transplant patients), further confirmatory testing is required. For years, confirmation was performed using RIBA; PCR has now supplanted RIBA as the confirmatory test of choice.

Pathology

The range of histological findings in patients with chronic HCV infection is broad—from minimal periportal lymphocytic inflammation to active hepatitis with bridging fibrosis, hepatocyte necrosis and frank cirrhosis. Steatosis, lymphoid aggregates and bile duct damage are frequent in liver biopsy specimens from patients with HCV infection. The HAI developed by Knodell *et al.*[3] can be used to quantify the degree of liver damage, but it is cumbersome. A simplified system in which inflammation is graded from 0 to 4 and fibrosis is staged from 0 to 4 has been developed by Scheuer *et al.*[63] and is gaining widespread use in clinical practice.

The role of liver biopsy in the management of HCV-infected patients has not been settled to date. The potential risks associated with a biopsy contrast with the importance of the information generated, especially in the absence of appropriate surrogate markers of hepatic fibrosis. Recent consensus conferences have stated that a liver biopsy is mandatory in patients with chronic hepatitis C and elevated serum aminotransferase levels so that correct grading and staging can be performed. This information is particularly relevant when considering antiviral therapy or when other causes of liver disease may be present. A post-treatment liver biopsy is not necessary because most trials have demonstrated that a sustained virological response is generally associated with stable or improved histological findings. In contrast, in patients with normal serum aminotransferase levels, the role of liver biopsy is less clear. Although the frequency of progression of fibrosis appears to be low in these patients, only 20% have absolutely normal histological findings on liver biopsy, and a small percentage (<15%) have considerable liver damage.[64] In patients in whom the diagnosis of cirrhosis is suggested by clinical or USG findings (ascites, splenomegaly, spider angiomata, low platelet count, prolonged PT, reduced portal flow, nodularity of the liver), histological confirmation is usually not needed.

Natural history

HCV is a less progressive disease than previously believed and only 15%–20% of HCV-infected persons eventually progress to potentially serious end-stage liver disease; the remainder will die of causes other than liver disease.[65]

Factors associated with disease progression

These include age (>40 years), male gender, immunosuppression and increased alcohol intake (>50 g daily).[66] Other less consistently documented prognostic factors include mode of transmission (higher disease progression when infection is through blood transfusion than through injecting drug use)[67] and coinfection with HBV. Conflicting results have been reported regarding the role played by genotypes or quasispecies in the severity of the disease.

Natural history of clinically compensated HCV-related cirrhosis

Even after the development of cirrhosis, the short- and medium-term natural history is fair. In the absence of clinical decompensation, actuarial survival rates are 91% at 5 years and 79% at 10 years. The survival drops to 50% at 5 years among those in whom clinical decompensation develops. The cumulative probability of an episode of decompensation is only 5% at 1 year, increasing to 30% at 10 years from the diagnosis of cirrhosis.[68–70] The risk of developing HCC is 1%–4% per year once cirrhosis is established.

Disease in patients with persistently normal aminotransferase levels

Approximately one-third of anti-HCV positive patients have normal serum ALT levels. Most of these patients have some degree of histologically proven chronic liver damage, ranging from mild chronic hepatitis to cirrhosis.[71] Strictly speaking, patients considered to be 'HCV carriers' should be those with persistently normal serum ALT levels over a period of at least 12 months, with measurement of ALT levels on several occasions at least 1 month apart and with detectable HCV RNA in the serum. Disease progression appears to be slower in these patients than in those with elevated ALT levels, and progression to cirrhosis is considered a rare event.

Prevention

General measures

Adequate sterilization of medical and surgical equipment is mandatory. Efforts should also be made to modify injection practices among persons concerned with folk medicine, rituals and cosmetic procedures. Infected patients should be instructed to avoid sharing razors and toothbrushes, and to cover any open wounds. Safe sexual practices, such as the use of latex condoms, should be encouraged in patients with multiple sexual partners. Because of the low rate of vertical transmission, pregnancy is not contraindicated in HCV-infected women; breastfeeding is also not contraindicated. Also, HCV-infected patients should be vaccinated against HAV and HBV because of the high risk of severe liver disease if superinfection with these viruses occurs.

Passive immunoprophylaxis

Immune globulin is not effective in the prevention of HCV infection.

Active immunoprophylaxis

Development of a vaccine for HCV has been difficult. Vaccination of chimpanzees with composite proteins from the envelope regions of the virus (E1/E2 fusion protein) has been demonstrated to be protective against challenge with viruses that contain homologous but not heterologous sequences.[72] Currently, development of HCV vaccines is being actively investigated.

Treatment

Goals of therapy

The primary goal of therapy for HCV infection is to eradicate the infection early in the course of the disease to prevent progression to end-stage liver disease and eventually to HCC. However, these end-points are difficult to achieve because of the long natural history of hepatitis C. Intermediate end-points that have been used to assess the success of therapy include normalization of serum aminotransferase levels, loss of serum HCV RNA measured by a variety of methods and improvement in histological findings. It is likely, although unproven, that the achievement of these end-points will translate into long-term benefit from therapy.

End-points

Normalization of serum ALT levels was the end-point of therapy in early clinical trials. After the discovery of HCV, both loss of HCV RNA and normalization of serum ALT levels have been used as treatment end-points. These responses are usually evaluated at the end of treatment (end-of-treatment response) and 6 months after the discontinuation of treatment (sustained response). Sustained biochemical and virological responses, which are often accompanied by histological improvement, are the current standard therapeutic end-points. Indeed, several studies have shown that, in patients with sustained biochemical and virological responses, the durability of the response is >95% for up to 10 years.[73]

Available drugs

IFN-α-based regimens constitute the cornerstone of current antiviral therapies. There are several types of IFN-α available, including recombinant forms (IFN-α2a and -α2b, and consensus IFN) and naturally occurring forms (lymphoblastoid IFN). IFNs are naturally occurring proteins that exert a wide array of antiviral, antiproliferative and immunomodulatory effects. New formulations of IFN, known as pegylated IFN, have been developed recently.[74] They consist of IFN bound to a molecule of polyethylene glycol of varying length, which increases the half-life of the molecule and reduces the volume of distribution, thereby allowing once-weekly dosing. These new IFNs are able to sustain more uniform plasma levels, as opposed to the fluctuations observed with every-other-day dosing, and consequently enhance viral suppression.

Ribavirin is an antiviral agent with activity against DNA and RNA viruses. It is given orally. In immunocompetent patients with chronic HCV infection, ribavirin improves serum ALT levels, but the effect is transient and no direct antiviral activity is observed.[75] Ribavirin is generally well tolerated, although marked haemolysis may be seen. Because of the potential to cause a sudden fall in haemoglobin, ribavirin is contraindicated in patients with a history of myocardial infarction or cardiac arrhythmia. As ribavirin is teratogenic, patients and partners are required to avoid pregnancy during therapy and for 6 months after the cessation of treatment. Ribavirin has a long, cumulative half-life and is excreted by the kidney so that severe side-effects, particularly haemolysis, can occur in patients with renal failure. Therefore, ribavirin cannot be removed by haemodialysis. Hence, ribavirin should not be administered to patients with a serum creatinine level >1.5 mg/dl.

Efficacy

Several recent, large, randomized controlled trials have shown that treatment with a combination of IFN-α (3 million units three times weekly) plus ribavirin (1000–1200 mg/day) results in a higher frequency of sustained biochemical and virological response than does treatment with IFN alone,[76,77] so that in the absence of contraindications to ribavirin, combination therapy is currently the standard. Overall, the success rate with combination therapy in previously untreated ('naïve') patients is 38%–42%, and is largely dependent on genotype and pretreatment viral load. Also, patients who relapse after discontinuation of IFN monotherapy show a significantly higher sustained response rate if retreated with combination therapy than with IFN monotherapy.[78] In contrast, in patients who are non-responders to IFN monotherapy, the efficacy is low either with combination therapy or a second course of IFN monotherapy in higher doses for a longer duration.

Factors predictive of a sustained response

Factors associated with a better outcome include low serum HCV RNA levels, viral genotype other than 1, absence of cirrhosis, female gender and age <40 years.[76-78] With IFN monotherapy, absence of a virological response at 12 weeks was a strong predictor of end-of-treatment non-response, and further treatment was abandoned. This may not be true for combination therapy, because approximately 10% of patients with detectable HCV RNA at 12 weeks of therapy will become sustained responders if combined treatment is continued. Recent studies suggest that response to treatment can be predicted by the degree to which the serum HCV RNA level decreases or by the quasispecies genetic divergence within the first weeks of treatment.[53]

Indications and contraindications

Theoretically, all patients with ongoing HCV infection and persistently elevated serum aminotransferase levels are potential candidates for antiviral therapy. However, patients with the lowest likelihood of progression are the ones who are most likely to respond to treatment. Paradoxically, those with the least likelihood of responding or least tolerance to side-effects are often the ones with the greatest need for treatment.

Treatment in some situations is controversial. In particular, treatment is not recommended outside clinical trials in patients with persistently normal serum ALT levels,[79] those with minimal histological abnormalities, or in those with decompensated cirrhosis.[80]

There is a strong theoretical rationale for treating patients with acute HCV infection, because the majority develop persistent infection and chronic liver disease. The few studies that have addressed this issue suggest that higher rates of disease remission are observed in patients treated with IFN at an early stage as compared with untreated controls.[81] However, these studies have included relatively few patients, and used different doses and durations of treatment. Even if early intervention is effective, identification of acute cases in the non-transfusion setting is difficult and early treatment will be limited to a small number of patients.

Treatment choices

In previously untreated patients with documented HCV infection, persistently elevated serum aminotransferase levels and moderate-to-severe necroinflammatory activity with portal or bridging fibrosis, the current standard treatment is either standard or pegylated IFN-α given subcutaneously combined with ribavirin orally. Long-acting (pegylated) IFNs as monotherapy are less effective than IFN/ribavirin combination therapy. The results of two large, prospective, randomized trials of pegylated IFN plus ribavirin compared with standard IFN plus ribavirin are shown in Table IV.

In patients who have a relapse after a course of IFN monotherapy, combination therapy is the treatment of choice. Alternatively, these patients can be retreated with a 12-month course of higher doses of IFN-α.

The treatment of choice for patients who have relapsed after an initial course of combination therapy is yet to be established.

Table IV. Results of combination treatment trials for hepatitis C virus (HCV) infection with pegylated interferon[82,83]

Pegylated (12 kD) IFN-α2b (PEG) plus ribavirin versus standard IFN-α2b plus ribavirin for chronic HCV infection

Sustained virological response	PEG 1.5 µg/kg/week plus ribavirin 800 mg/day (%)	PEG 0.5 µg/kg/week plus ribavirin 1000/1200 mg/day (%)	IFN 3 million units three times a week plus ribavirin 1000/1200 mg/day (%)
Overall	54	47	47
Genotype 1	42	34	33
Genotype non-1	82	80	79

Pegylated (40 kD) IFN-α2a plus ribavirin versus IFN-α2b plus ribavirin versus pegylated (40 kD) IFN-α2a plus placebo for chronic HCV infection

Sustained virological response	PEG 180 µg/week plus ribavirin 1000/1200 mg/day (%)	PEG 180 µg/week plus placebo	IFN 3 million units three times a week plus ribavirin 1000/1200 mg/day (%)
Overall	57	30	45
Genotype 1	46	Not available	37
Genotype non-1	76	Not available	60

There are no proven treatments for non-responders to prior treatment with IFN alone. Combination therapy administered for 12 months with either IFN-α or pegylated IFN may achieve a response in a minority of patients.[80]

Monitoring of therapy

Before starting therapy, blood tests should be done to establish the patient's baseline status, including liver biochemical tests, complete blood counts (CBC), and thyroid-stimulating hormone (TSH) level. A pregnancy test is needed before initiating ribavirin therapy in women. Genotyping and quantification of the serum viral level will help in selecting the best strategy. During the first month of therapy, a CBC should be done weekly because most side-effects, particularly haemolytic anaemia due to ribavirin, occur within this period. After the first month, serum ALT values and a CBC should be obtained monthly, and TSH values obtained every 3 months. At the end of treatment and at 6 months after the discontinuation of treatment, HCV RNA testing should be repeated to assess the patient's response. If a sustained response is achieved, it is recommended that HCV RNA testing be performed annually for at least 2 years after completion of therapy. A repeat liver biopsy after treatment is rarely necessary. In non-responders or relapsers in whom no additional treatment is considered, the follow-up should be similar to that for untreated patients, with yearly check-ups and repeated liver biopsy every 3–5 years to assess progression of the disease.

Algorithm for the treatment of patients with chronic hepatitis C

The National Institutes of Diabetes, and Digestive and Kidney Disease (NIDDK) has proposed new treatment guidelines for the use of combination therapy in patients with chronic hepatitis C (Fig. 2).[84] In the proposed algorithm, the decision to treat and duration of therapy are based mainly on the HCV genotype.

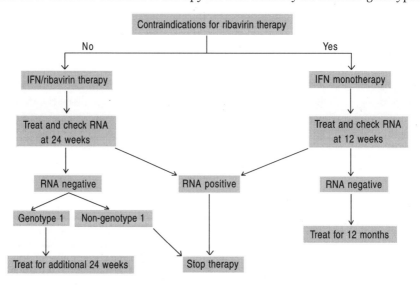

Fig. 2. Treatment algorithm for chronic hepatitis C

However, Poynard *et al.*[85] have criticized this 'simplistic approach' based on only one predictive factor and proposed an alternative approach. In an analysis of 1774 patients from the two large multicentre IFN/ribavirin studies, five independent variables were found to be associated with a sustained response: (i) genotype 2 or 3; (ii) baseline serum HCV RNA level <3.5 million copies/ml; (iii) no or minimal portal fibrosis; (iv) female gender; and (v) age <40 years. After 24 weeks of combined treatment, the authors recommend discontinuation of therapy if HCV RNA remains detectable in the serum. If HCV RNA is undetectable, the treatment should be continued until week 48 if the patient has fewer than four favourable variables. In contrast, treatment can be discontinued if four or more favourable variables are present.

AUTOIMMUNE HEPATITIS

AIH is characterized by the presence of interface hepatitis on histological examination, hypergammaglobulinaemia and autoantibodies in the serum.[86] Diagnosis requires the exclusion of other chronic liver diseases that have similar features, including Wilson disease, chronic viral hepatitis, α_1-antitrypsin deficiency, genetic haemochromatosis, drug-induced liver disease, non-alcoholic steatohepatitis and the immune cholangiopathies of PBC, primary sclerosing cholangitis (PSC) and autoimmune cholangitis.

Diagnostic criteria

An international panel codified the diagnostic criteria of AIH in 1992, and an expanded panel updated them in 1999.[87] Due to a propensity for acute, and rarely fulminant, presentation the requirement for 6 months of disease activity to establish chronicity has been waived; and lobular hepatitis is included in the histological spectrum.[87] Cholestatic histological changes, including bile duct injury and ductopenia, are incompatible features. The immunoserological tests essential for diagnosis are assays for antinuclear antibodies (ANA), anti-smooth muscle antibodies (ASMA), and antibodies to liver kidney microsome type 1 (anti-LKM1).[88] These assays are based on the indirect immunofluorescence of rodent tissues or Hep-2 cell lines or on EIA using microtitre plates with adsorbed recombinant or highly purified antigens.

Clinical criteria

The definite diagnosis of AIH requires the exclusion of other similar diseases, laboratory findings that indicate substantial immunoreactivity, and histological features of interface hepatitis (Fig. 3).[87]

A probable diagnosis is justified when findings are compatible with AIH but insufficient for a definite diagnosis.[87] Patients who lack conventional autoantibodies but are seropositive for investigational markers are classified as having probable disease.

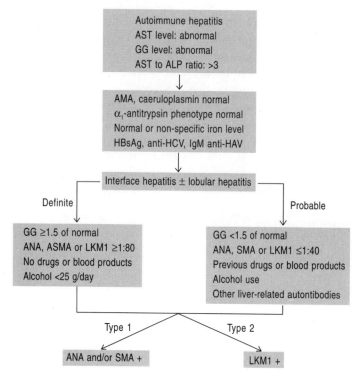

Fig. 3. Diagnostic algorithm for autoimmune hepatitis
ANA: antinuclear antibodies; LKM: liver kidney microsome; ASMA: anti-smooth muscle antibodies;
AMA: antimitochondrial antibodies; GG: gamma globulins

Scoring criteria

A scoring system proposed by the International Autoimmune Hepatitis Group accommodates the diverse manifestations of AIH and renders an aggregate score that reflects the net strength of the diagnosis before and after glucocorticoid treatment.[87] The scoring system is rarely necessary in clinical practice.

Pathogenesis

The pathogenetic mechanisms of AIH are unknown. Various interactive factors including a triggering agent, genetic predisposition and various determinants of autoantigen display; immunocyte activation and effector cell expansion are important in the pathogenesis.[89]

Multiple triggering factors have been proposed, and they include infectious agents, drugs and toxins. There can be a long lag time between exposure to the trigger and onset of the disease, and the triggering factor may not be needed for perpetuation of the disorder. Molecular mimicry of a foreign antigen and a self-antigen is the most common explanation for the loss of self-tolerance.[89]

Genetic factors influence autoantigen presentation and CD4+ helper T-cell recognition. Different ethnic groups have different susceptibility alleles, and these findings support a shared motif hypothesis of pathogenesis.[90] According to this hypothesis, the risk of disease relates to amino acid sequences in the antigen-binding groove of the class II MHC molecule, and multiple alleles encode the same or a similar sequence (shared motif).

Liver cell destruction is due to either cell-mediated cytotoxicity, antibody-dependent cell-mediated cytotoxicity or a combination of both.[86]

Subclassifications

Three types of AIH have been proposed on the basis of immunoserological markers.[86] Only two types have almost mutually exclusive autoantibodies. The International Autoimmune Hepatitis Group has not endorsed the sub-classification of AIH, and subtyping by autoantibody profile has mainly been of descriptive value.

Type 1 autoimmune hepatitis

Type 1 AIH is characterized by the presence of ASMA and/or ANA in the serum (Table V).[86] Antibodies to actin have greater specificity for the diagnosis than ASMA, but less sensitivity.[91] Perinuclear antineutrophil cytoplasmic antibodies (pANCAs), which occur in patients who have PSC and chronic ulcerative colitis,

Table V. Subclassifications of autoimmune hepatitis based on autoantibodies

Clinical features	Type 1	Type 2	Type 3
Conventional autoantibodies	Smooth muscle Nuclear	Liver kidney microsome type 1	None
Novel autoantibodies	pANCA Actin Asialoglycoprotein receptor	Liver cytosol type 1	Soluble liver antigen/ liver–pancreas
Age (years)	Bimodal (10–20 and 45–70)	Children (2–14)	Adults (30–50)
Women (%)	78	89	90
Concurrent immune diseases (%)	41	34	58
Organ-specific antibodies (%)	4	30	Uncertain
Gamma globulin elevation	Marked	Mild	Moderate
Low IgA	No	Occasional	No
HLA associations	-B8, -DR3, -DR4	-B14, -DR3, -C4A-Q0, -DR7	Uncertain
Allelic risk factors	DRB1 0301 and 0401 (White North Americans and northern Europeans)	DRB1 07 (Germans and Brazilians)	Uncertain
Glucocorticoid responsive	+++	+++	+++

pANCA: perinuclear antineutrophil cytoplasmic antibodies; HLA: human leucocyte antigen are found in up to 90% of patients who have type 1 AIH and may be surrogate markers for the disease.[92]

Type 1 AIH has a bimodal age distribution, with a female-to-male ratio of 3.6:1, with 41% of patients having concurrent extrahepatic immunological diseases. Autoimmune thyroiditis (12%), Graves disease (6%) and chronic ulcerative colitis (6%) are the most common associated immune disorders.

In 40% of patients with type 1 AIH, the onset of symptoms is acute and the disease may appear in a fulminant fashion.[93] Typically, patients who have an acute presentation have clinical (ascites, oesophageal varices, or spider angiomas), laboratory (thrombocytopenia, hypoalbuminaemia, or hypergamma-globulinaemia) and histological changes (cirrhosis) that suggest chronic liver disease. Eight per cent of patients have no features of chronicity, and the presentation of the disorder is indistinguishable from that of acute viral hepatitis. The target autoantigen of type 1 AIH is unknown, but the asialo-glycoprotein receptor (ASGPR) is a candidate.[94]

Type 2 autoimmune hepatitis

Type 2 AIH is characterized by the presence of anti-LKM1 in the serum. Children are mainly affected (2–14 years of age). An acute or fulminant presentation is possible. Type 2 AIH responds as well to glucocorticoids as type 1. The target antigen of type 2 AIH is CYP2D6.[95]

Type 3 autoimmune hepatitis

Type 3 AIH is characterized by the presence of anti-SLA (soluble liver antigen)/ LP (liver–pancreas) in the serum.[96,97] The candidate antigen is a transfer ribonucleoprotein (tRNP$^{(Ser)Sec}$) involved in the incorporation of selenocysteine into peptide chains. Patients who have anti-SLA/LP have clinical and laboratory features that are indistinguishable from those of type 1 AIH patients, and they respond well to glucocorticoids. For these reasons, anti-SLA/LP does not define a valid subgroup of AIH.

Variant forms

Such patients have autoimmune features but do not satisfy the criteria for a definite or probable diagnosis of AIH. These patients typically have manifestations of AIH and another type of chronic liver disease (overlap syndrome), or have findings that are incompatible with the diagnosis of AIH by current diagnostic criteria (outlier syndrome) (Table VI).

Prognostic indices

The prognosis of AIH relates mainly to the severity of liver inflammation at the initial medical consultation, as reflected in the laboratory indices and histological findings. HLA status influences the treatment outcome (Table VII).[98]

Table VI. Variant forms of autoimmune hepatitis (AIH)

Distinctive features	AIH+PBC	AIH+PSC	Autoimmune cholangitis	Cryptogenic chronic hepatitis
Clinical	Features of AIH	Features of AIH	ANA and/or ASMA present	Features of AIH
	AMA present	Ulcerative colitis AMA absent Abnormal cholangiogram	AMA absent No CUC Normal cholangiogram	No autoantibodies HLA-B8 or -DR3
Histological	Cholangitis Cholestasis	Cholangitis Cholestasis	Cholangitis Cholestasis	Interface hepatitis
Treatment	Empirical prednisone, if ALP ≤ twice normal; prednisone and ursodeoxycholic acid, if ALP > twice normal and/or florid duct lesions	Empirical prednisone and ursodeoxycholic acid	Empirical prednisone and/or ursodeoxycholic acid	Empirical conventional regimens for AIH

PBC: primary biliary cirrhosis; PSC: primary sclerosing cholangitis; ANA: antinuclear antibodies; AMA: antimitochondrial antibodies; SMA: smooth muscle antibodies; CUC: chronic ulcerative colitis

Table VII. Prognostic indices of autoimmune hepatitis

Prognostic indices before treatment	Outcome	Prognostic indices after treatment	Comments
AST ≥ 10-fold normal or AST ≥ 5-fold normal + gamma globulin ≥2-fold normal	50% 3-year mortality 90% 10-year mortality	HLA-B8, -DR3 or DRB1 0301	Onset at young age Severe inflammation at presentation Propensity for relapse Treatment failure common Liver transplantation
AST <10-fold normal + gamma globulin <2-fold normal	49% cirrhosis at 15 years 10% 10-year mortality	HLA-DR4 or DRB1 0401	Onset in old age Women Concurrent immunological disease Good response to glucocorticoids
Interface hepatitis	17% cirrhosis at 5 years Normal 5-year survival	C4A gene deletions	Low serum complement level Early-onset disease Associated with HLA-DR3
Bridging necrosis or multilobular necrosis	82% cirrhosis at 5 years 45% 5-year mortality	Multilobular necrosis and failure to improve on treatment; hyperbilirubinaemia after 2 weeks	High mortality rate
Cirrhosis	58% 5-year mortality	Failure to enter remission within 4 years and first sign of decompensation (ascites)	High mortality rate

Clinical manifestations

Easy fatiguability is the most common symptom (85%). Weight loss is uncommon and intense pruritus argues against the diagnosis. Hepatomegaly is the most common physical finding (78%) and jaundice is found in 69%. Splenomegaly can be present in patients with and without cirrhosis (56% and 32%, respectively), as can spider angiomas.

Hyperbilirubinaemia is present in 83% of patients, but the serum level is >3-fold normal in only 46%.[99] Similarly, the serum ALP level is commonly increased (81%), but elevations of more than two (33%) or four times (10%) normal are uncommon. The hypergammaglobulinaemia of AIH is polyclonal; the IgG fraction predominates.[99]

Concurrent immunological diseases are common and involve diverse organ systems, most frequently the thyroid. ASMA, ANA and anti-LKM1 are required for the diagnosis, but other autoantibodies may be present.

Treatment

Indications

The indications for treatment shown in Table VIII[86,100] are based on the manifestations of inflammation rather than measures of hepatic dysfunction.

Table VIII. Treatment indications for autoimmune hepatitis

Findings	Indications		
	Absolute	Relative	None
Clinical	Incapacitating symptoms Relentless clinical progression	Mild or no symptoms	Asymptomatic with mild laboratory changes Previous intolerance to prednisone and/or azathioprine
Laboratory	AST ≥ 10-fold normal AST ≥ 5-fold normal and gamma globulin ≥2-fold normal	AST 3- to 9-fold normal AST <5-fold normal and gamma globulin <2-fold normal	AST <3-fold normal Severe cytopenia
Histological	Bridging necrosis Multilobular necrosis	Interface hepatitis	Inactive cirrhosis Portal hepatitis Decompensated cirrhosis with variceal bleeding

Table IX. Preferred treatment regimens for autoimmune hepatitis

Combination therapy		Single-drug therapy
Prednisone (mg/day)	Azathioprine (mg/day)	Prednisone (mg/day)
30 mg x 1 week 20 mg x 1 week 15 mg x 2 weeks 10 mg until end-point	50 mg until end-point	60 mg x 1 week 40 mg x 1 week 30 mg x 2 weeks 20 mg until end-point

Treatment regimens

Prednisone alone or at a lower dose in combination with azathioprine is effective (Table IX).[86,100] No findings at presentation preclude a satisfactory response to therapy. The presence of ascites or hepatic encephalopathy identifies patients with a poor prognosis. These individuals, however, can still respond to glucocorticoid therapy and should be treated before a decision regarding liver transplantation is made.

Treatment end-points

Glucocorticoid therapy is continued until remission, treatment failure, incomplete response, or drug toxicity occurs (Fig. 4).[100]

Remission implies the absence of symptoms; resolution of inflammatory indices (except for a serum AST level no greater than twice normal); and

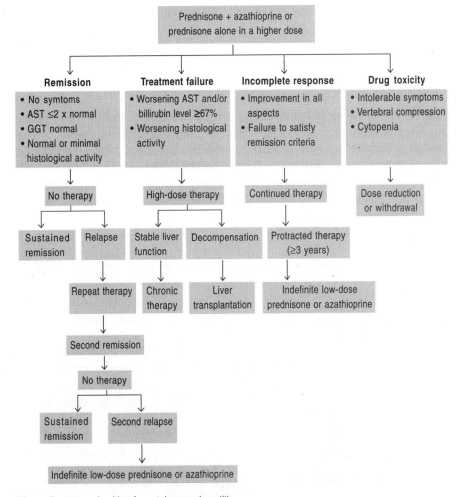

Fig. 4. Treatment algorithm for autoimmune hepatitis

histological improvement to normal or minimal activity. Histological resolution lags behind clinical and laboratory resolution by 3–6 months, and therapy must be extended accordingly. Liver biopsy examination before drug withdrawal ensures an optimal end-point. Improvement of the liver tissue to normal is associated with a frequency of relapse of only 20% after the cessation of treatment. In contrast, improvement of portal hepatitis is associated with a 50% frequency of relapse. Progression to cirrhosis or persistence of interface hepatitis is associated with a 100% frequency of relapse.

Treatment failure means deterioration during therapy,[100] evident by worsening of the serum AST or bilirubin levels by at least 67% of the previous values, progressive histological activity, or onset of ascites or encephalopathy. Conventional glucocorticoid therapy should be stopped, and a high-dose regimen instituted.

Incomplete response denotes improvement that is insufficient to satisfy the criteria for remission.[100] Failure to achieve remission within 3 years indicates that remission is unlikely and warrants the discontinuation of conventional treatment.

Drug toxicity justifies premature withdrawal of medication or a reduction in the dose.[100]

Treatment results

Prednisone alone or in combination with azathioprine induces a clinical, biochemical and histological remission in 65% of patients within 3 years.[100] The average treatment interval until remission is 22 months. Most importantly, therapy improves the survival rate; the 10-year life expectancy for treated patients with and without cirrhosis at the time of the initial presentation is 89% and 90%, respectively.[101] Patients who have histological cirrhosis respond as well as non-cirrhotic patients.

Relapse

Patients who enter remission commonly experience an exacerbation after drug withdrawal.[100] Relapse occurs in 50% of patients within 6 months, and most (70%–86%) experience exacerbation within 3 years. Reinstitution of the original treatment induces another remission, but relapse commonly recurs after termination of therapy.

Patients who have had at least two relapses require indefinite therapy with either prednisone or azathioprine. Eighty-seven per cent of patients can be managed long term on prednisone at <10 mg/day (median dose 7.5 mg/day).[102] The dose is titrated to the lowest level needed to prevent symptoms and maintain serum aminotransferase levels below 5-fold the normal value.

Continuous azathioprine therapy (2 mg/kg/day) is an alternative strategy that can be used in patients who are not severely cytopenic or pregnant.[103] Eighty-three per cent of individuals remain in remission for up to 10 years.

Mycophenolate mofetil has been found to maintain remission in patients resistant to or intolerant of azathioprine.[104]

Treatment failure

The condition of 9% of patients deteriorates during glucocorticoid therapy (treatment failure).[100] High doses of prednisone alone (60 mg/day) or prednisone (30 mg/day) in conjunction with azathioprine (150 mg/day) are the standard treatments in this group. Each schedule induces clinical and biochemical improvement in 70% of patients within 2 years. Histological resolution, however, occurs in only 20%. These patients are at risk for liver failure and serious drug toxicity. Liver transplantation must be considered at the first sign of hepatic decompensation.

Liver transplantation is effective in the decompensated patient for whom glucocorticoid therapy has failed.[105] After transplantation, the autoantibodies and hypergammaglobulinaemia disappear within 2 years, and the 5-year survival rate is 96%. Recurrent disease after transplantation is common but has been described mainly in patients with inadequate immunosuppression.[106]

Incomplete response

Thirteen per cent of patients improve during therapy but do not satisfy the criteria for remission.[100] A low-dose prednisone regimen similar to that used after relapse is reasonable. The goal of treatment is to control disease activity with the lowest possible dose of medication.

Drug toxicity

Treatment can usually be continued with the single tolerated drug (prednisone or azathioprine) in an adjusted dose. Cyclosporin, 6-mercaptopurine and cyclophosphamide have also been used following drug toxicity in isolated cases.

REFERENCES

1. Ishak KG. Pathologic features of chronic hepatitis: A review and update. *Am J Clin Pathol* 2000;**113**:40–5.
2. Goodman ZD, Ishak KG. Histopathology of hepatitis C virus infection. *Semin Liver Dis* 1995;**15**:70–81.
3. Knodell RG, Ishak KG, Black WC, *et al*. Formulation and application of a numerical system for assessing histological activity in asymptomatic chronic active hepatitis. *Hepatology* 1981;**1**:431–5.
4. Ishak KG, Baptista A, Bianchi L, *et al*. Histological grading and staging of chronic hepatitis. *J Hepatol* 1995;**22**:696–9.
5. Desmet VJ, Gerber M, Hoofnagle JH, *et al*. Classification of chronic hepatitis: Diagnosis, grading and staging. *Hepatology* 1994;**19**:1513–20.
6. Summers J, Mason WS. Replication of the genome of a hepatitis B-like virus by reverse transcription of an RNA intermediate. *Cell* 1982;**29**:403–15.
7. Rossner M. Hepatitis B virus X gene product: A promiscuous transcriptional activator. *J Med Virol* 1992;**36**:101–17.
8. Margolis H, Alter M, Hadler S. Hepatitis B: Evolving epidemiology and implications for control. *Semin Liver Dis* 1991;**11**:84–92.

9. Thyagragan SP, Jayaram S, Hari R, *et al.* Epidemiology of hepatitis B in India—a comprehensive analysis. In: Sarin SK, Okuda K (eds). *Hepatitis B and C—carrier to cancer.* New Delhi: Elsevier Science; 1999:25.

10. Alter M, Mast E. The epidemiology of viral hepatitis in the United States. *Gastroenterol Clin North Am* 1994;**23:**437–55.

11. Beasley R, Huang L. Postnatal infectivity of hepatitis B surface antigen-carrier mothers. *J Infect Dis* 1983;**147:**185–90.

12. Alter M, Hadler S, Margolis H, *et al.* The changing epidemiology of hepatitis B in the United States. Need for alternative vaccination strategies. *JAMA* 1990;**263:**1218–22.

13. Moriyama T, Guilhot S, Klopchin K, *et al.* Immunobiology and pathogenesis of hepatocellular injury in hepatitis B virus transgenic mice. *Science* 1990;**248:**361–4.

14. Guidotti LG, Ishikawa T, Hobbs MV, Matzke B, Schreiber R, Chisari FV. Intracellular inactivation of the hepatitis B virus by cytotoxic T lymphocytes. *Immunity* 1996;**4:**25–36.

15. Thomas HC, Carman WF. Envelope and precore/core variants of hepatitis B virus. *Gastroenterol Clin North Am* 1994;**23:**499–514.

16. Liang T, Hasegawa K, Rimon N, Wands J, Ben-Porath E. A hepatitis B virus mutant associated with an epidemic of fulminant hepatitis. *N Engl J Med* 1991;**324:**1705–9.

17. Laskus T, Rakela J, Nowicki MJ, Persing DH. Hepatitis B core promotor sequence analysis in fulminant and chronic hepatitis B. *Gastroenterology* 1995;**109:**1618–23.

18. Zanetti A, Tanzi E, Manzillo G, *et al.* Hepatitis B variants in Europe. *Lancet* 1988;**2:**1132–3.

19. McMahon G, Ehrlich PH, Moustafa ZA, *et al.* Genetic alterations in the gene encoding the major HBsAg: DNA and immunological analysis of recurrent HBsAg derived from monoclonal antibody-treated liver transplant patients. *Hepatology* 1992;**15:**757–66.

20. Brechot C, Thiers V, Kremsdorf D, *et al.* Persistent hepatitis B virus infection in subjects without hepatitis B surface antigen: Clinically significant or purely "occult"? *Hepatology* 2001;**34:**194–203.

21. Paterlini P, Driss F, Nalpas B, *et al.* Persistence of hepatitis B and hepatitis C viral genomes in primary liver cancers from HBsAg-negative patients: A study of a low-endemic area. *Hepatology* 1993;**17:**20–9.

22. Noborg U, Gusdal A, Pisa EK, Hedrum A, Lindh M. Automated quantitative analysis of hepatitis B virus DNA by using the Cobas Amplicor HBV monitor test. *J Clin Microbiol* 1999;**37:**2793–7.

23. Loeb K, Jerome K, Goddard J, Huang M, Cent A, Corey L. High throughput quantitative analysis of hepatitis B virus DNA in serum using the TaqMan fluorogenic detection system. *Hepatology* 2000;**32:**626–9.

24. Chan HL, Leung NW, Lau TC, Wong ML, Sung JJ. Comparison of three different sensitive assays for hepatitis B virus DNA in monitoring of responses to antiviral therapy. *J Clin Microbiol* 2000;**38:**3205–8.

25. McMahon BJ, Heyward W, Templin DW, Clement D, Lanier AP. Hepatitis B-associated polyarteritis nodosa in Alaskan eskimos: Clinical and epidemiological features and long-term follow-up. *Hepatology* 1989;**9:**97–101.

26. Hyams KC. Risks of chronicity following acute hepatitis B virus infection: A review. *Clin Infect Dis* 1995;**20:**992–1000.

27. Weissberg J, Andres L, Smith C, *et al.* Survival in chronic hepatitis B: An analysis of 379 patients. *Ann Intern Med* 1984;**101:**613–16.

28. Lok A, Lai C, Wu P, Leung E, Lam T. Spontaneous hepatitis B e antigen to antibody seroconversion and reversion in Chinese patients with chronic hepatitis B virus infection. *Gastroenterology* 1987;**92:**1839–43.

29. Stevens CE, Taylor PE, Tong MJ, *et al.* Yeast-recombinant hepatitis B vaccine: Efficacy with hepatitis B immune globulin in prevention of perinatal hepatitis B virus transmission. *JAMA* 1987;**257:**2612–16.

30. Tong MJ, Hwang SJ. Hepatitis B virus infection in Asian Americans. *Gastroenterol Clin North Am* 1994;**23**:523–36.

31. Wong DKH, Cheung AM, O'Rourke K, Naylor CD, Detsky AS, Heathcote J. Effect of alpha-interferon treatment in patients with hepatitis B e antigen-positive chronic hepatitis B: A meta-analysis. *Ann Intern Med* 1993;**119**:312–23.

32. Korenman J, Baker B, Waggoner J, Everhart J, DiBisceglie A, Hoofnagle J. Long-term remission of chronic hepatitis B after alpha-interferon therapy. *Ann Intern Med* 1991;**114**:629–34.

33. Lok A, Lai C, Lau J. Interferon alfa therapy in patients with chronic hepatitis B virus infection. Effects on hepatitis B virus DNA in the liver. *Gastroenterology* 1991;**100**:756–61.

34. Niederau C, Heinges T, Lange S, *et al.* Long-term follow-up of the HBeAg-positive patients treated with interferon alfa for chronic hepatitis B. *N Engl J Med* 1996;**334**:1422–7.

35. Ling R, Mutimer D, Ahmed M, *et al.* Selection of mutations in the hepatitis B virus polymerase during therapy of transplant recipients with lamivudine. *Hepatology* 1996;**24**:711–13.

36. Nowak M, Bonhoeffer S, Hill A, *et al.* Viral dynamics in hepatitis B virus infection. *Proc Natl Acad Sci USA* 1996;**93**:4398–402.

37. Zoulim F, Dannaoui E, Borel C, *et al.* 2',3'-dideoxy-b-L-5-fluorocytidine inhibits duck hepatitis B virus reverse transcription and suppresses viral DNA synthesis in hepatocytes, both *in vitro* and *in vivo*. *Antimicrob Agents Chemother* 1996;**40**:448–53.

38. Chayama K, Suzuki Y, Kobayashi M, *et al.* Emergence and takeover of YMDD motif mutant hepatitis B virus during long-term lamivudine therapy and re-takeover by wild type after cessation of therapy. *Hepatology* 1998;**27**:1711–16.

39. Allen M, Deslauriers, M, Andrews CW, *et al.* Identification and characterization of mutations in hepatitis B virus resistant to lamivudine. *Hepatology* 1998;**27**:1670–7.

40. Chien RN, Liaw YF, Atkins M. Pretherapy alanine transaminase level as a determinant for hepatitis B e antigen seroconversion during lamivudine therapy in patients with chronic hepatitis B. Asian Hepatitis Lamivudine Trial Group. *Hepatology* 1999;**30**:770–4.

41. Tassopoulos NC, Volpes R, Pastore G, *et al.* Efficacy of lamivudine in patients with hepatitis B e antigen-negative hepatitis B virus DNA-positive (precore mutant) chronic hepatitis B. Lamivudine Precore Mutant Study Group. *Hepatology* 1999;**29**:889–96.

42. Villeneuve J, Condreay LD, Willems B, *et al.* Lamivudine treatment for decompensated cirrhosis resulting from chronic hepatitis B. *Hepatology* 2000;**31**:207–10.

43. Xiong X, Flores C, Yang H, *et al.* Mutations in hepatitis B DNA polymerase associated with resistance to lamivudine do not confer resistance to adefovir *in vitro*. *Hepatology* 1998;**28**:1669–73.

44. Hadziyannis SJ, Tassopoulos NC, Heathcote EJ, *et al.* Adefovir dipivoxil for the treatment of hepatitis B e antigen negative chronic hepatitis B. *N Engl J Med* 2003;**348**:800–7.

45. Marcellin P, Chang TT, Lim SG, *et al.* Adefovir dipivoxil for the treatment of hepatitis B e antigen positive chronic hepatitis B. *N Engl J Med* 2003;**348**:808–16.

46. Schalm SW, Heathcote J, Cianciara J, *et al.* Lamivudine and alpha interferon combination treatment of patients with chronic hepatitis B infection: A randomised trial. *Gut* 2000;**46**:562–8.

47. Markowitz JS, Martin P, Conrad AJ, *et al.* Prophylaxis against hepatitis B recurrence following liver transplantation using combination lamivudine and hepatitis immune globulin. *Hepatology* 1998;**28**:585–9.

48. Choo Q, Richman K, Han J, *et al.* Genetic organization and diversity of the hepatitis C virus. *Proc Natl Acad Sci USA* 1991;**88**:2451–5.

49. Agnello V, Abel G, Elfahal M, Knight GB, Zhang QX. Hepatitis C virus and other *Flaviviridae* viruses enter cells via low density lipoprotein receptor. *Proc Natl Acad Sci USA* 1999;**96**:12766–71.

50. Pileri P, Uematsu Y, Campagnoli S, *et al*. Binding of hepatitis C virus to CD81. *Science* 1998;**282**:938–41.

51. Zeuzem S, Schmidt JM, Lee JH, Ruster B, Roth WK. Effect of interferon alfa on the dynamics of hepatitis C virus turnover *in vivo*. *Hepatology* 1996;**23**:366–71.

52. Bukh J, Miller R, Purcell R. Genetic heterogeneity of hepatitis C virus: Quasispecies and genotypes. *Semin Liver Dis* 1995;**15**:41–63.

53. Farci P, Purcell RH. Clinical significance of hepatitis C virus genotypes and quasispecies. *Semin Liver Dis* 2000;**20**:103.

54. Wasley A, Alter MJ. Epidemiology of hepatitis C: Geographic differences and temporal trends. *Semin Liver Dis* 2000;**20**:1–16.

55. Schreiber GB, Busch MP, Kleinman SH, *et al*. The risk of transfusion-transmitted viral infection. *N Engl J Med* 1996;**334**:1685–90.

56. Mitsui T, Iwano K, Masuko K, *et al*. Hepatitis C virus infection in medical personnel after needlestick accident. *Hepatology* 1992;**166**:1109–14.

57. Mahaney K, Tedeschi V, Maertens G, *et al*. Genotypic analysis of hepatitis C virus in American patients. *Hepatology* 1994;**20**:1405–11.

58. Gruner NH, Gerlach TJ, Jung MC, *et al*. Association of hepatitis C virus-specific CD8+ T cells with viral clearance in acute hepatitis C. *J Infect Dis* 2000;**181**:1528–36.

59. Cramp ME, Carucci P, Rossol S, *et al*. Hepatitis C virus (HCV) specific immune responses in anti-HCV positive patients without hepatitis C viraemia. *Gut* 1999;**44**:424–9.

60. Rehermann B. Interactions between the hepatitis C virus and the immune system. *Semin Liver Dis* 2000;**20**:127–41.

61. Zignego AL, Brechot C. Extrahepatic manifestations of HCV infection: Facts and controversies. *J Hepatol* 1999;**31**:369–76.

62. Morishima C, Gretch DR. Clinical use of hepatitis C virus tests for diagnosis and monitoring during therapy. *Clin Liver Dis* 1999;**3**:717–40.

63. Scheuer PJ, Standish RA, Dhillon AP. Scoring of chronic hepatitis. *Clin Liver Dis* 2002;**6**:335–47.

64. Mathurin P, Moussalli J, Cadranel JF, *et al*. Slow progression rate of fibrosis in hepatitis C virus patients with persistently normal alanine aminotransferase activity. *Hepatology* 1998;**27**:868–72.

65. Seef LB, Miller RN, Rabkin CS, *et al*. 45-year follow-up of hepatitis C virus infection in healthy young adults. *Ann Intern Med* 2000;**132**:105–11.

66. Poynard T, Bedossa P, Opolon P, for the OBSVIRC, METAVIR, CLINIVIR and DOSVIRC groups. Natural history of liver fibrosis progression in patients with chronic hepatitis C. *Lancet* 1997;**349**:825–32.

67. Gordon SC, Eloway RS, Long JC, *et al*. The pathology of hepatitis C as a function of mode of transmission. Blood transfusion vs intravenous drug use. *Hepatology* 1993;**18**:1338–43.

68. Hu K-Q, Tong MJ. The long-term outcomes of patients with compensated hepatitis C virus related cirrhosis and history of parenteral exposure in the United States. *Hepatology* 1999;**29**:1311–16.

69. Fattovitch G, Giustina G, Degos F, *et al*. Morbidity and mortality in compensated cirrhosis type C: A retrospective follow-up study of 384 patients. *Gastroenterology* 1997;**112**:463–72.

70. Serfaty L, Aumaître H, Chazouillères O, *et al*. Determinants of outcome of compensated hepatitis C virus-related cirrhosis. *Hepatology* 1998;**27**:1435–40.

71. Marcellin P. Hepatitis C: The clinical spectrum of the disease. *J Hepatol* 1999;**31** (Suppl):9–16.

72. Choo Q, Quo G, Ralston R. Vaccination of chimpanzees against infection by the hepatitis C virus. *Proc Natl Acad Sci USA* 1994;**91**:1294–8.

73. Marcellin P, Boyer N, Gervais A, *et al.* Long-term histologic improvement and loss of detectable intrahepatic HCV RNA in patients with chronic hepatitis C and sustained response to interferon-alfa therapy. *Ann Intern Med* 1997;**127**:875–81.

74. Zeuzem S, Feinman V, Rasenack J, *et al.* Peginterferon alpha-2a in patients with chronic hepatitis C. *N Engl J Med* 2000;**343**:1666–72.

75. DiBisceglie A, Conjeevaram H, Fried M, *et al.* Ribavirin as therapy for chronic hepatitis C: A randomized, double blind, placebo-controlled trial. *Ann Intern Med* 1995;**123**:897–903.

76. McHutchinson JG, Gordon SC, Schiff ER, *et al.* Interferon alfa-2b alone or in combination with ribavirin as initial treatment for chronic hepatitis C. *N Engl J Med* 1998;**339**:1485–92.

77. Poynard T, Marcellin P, Lee SS, *et al.* Randomized trial of interferon alfa-2b plus ribavirin for 48 weeks or for 24 weeks versus interferon alfa-2b plus placebo for 48 weeks for treatment of chronic infection with hepatitis C virus. *Lancet* 1998;**352**:1426–32.

78. Davis GL, Esteban-Mur R, Rustgi V, *et al.* Interferon alfa-2b alone or in combination with ribavirin for the treatment of relapse of chronic hepatitis C. *N Engl J Med* 1998;**339**:1493–9.

79. Marcellin P, Martinot M, Boyer N, Levy S. Treatment of hepatitis C patients with normal aminotransferase levels. *Clin Liver Dis* 1999;**3**:843–53.

80. Heathcote J. Antiviral therapy for patients with chronic hepatitis C. *Semin Liver Dis* 2000;**20**:185–99.

81. Orland JR, Wright TL, Cooper S. Acute hepatitis C. *Hepatology* 2001;**32**:321–7.

82. Manns MP, McHutchison JP, Gordon S, *et al.* Peginterferon alfa-2b plus ribavirin compared to interferon alfa-2b plus ribavirin for the treatment of chronic hepatitis C: 24-week treatment analysis of a multicenter multinational phase III randomized controlled trial [Abstr]. *Hepatology* 2000;**32**:297A.

83. Fried MW, Shiffman ML, Reddy RK, *et al.* Pegylated (40 kDa) interferon alfa-2a (Pegasys) in combination with ribavirin: Efficacy and safety results from a phase III, randomized, actively controlled, multicenter study [Abstr]. *Gastroenterology* 2001;**120** (Suppl):A55.

84. National Institutes of Diabetes and Digestive and Kidney Disease. Chronic hepatitis C: Current disease management. *www.niddk.nih.gov/health/digest/pubs/chrnhepc/ chrnhepc.htm* (accessed 2000).

85. Poynard T, McHutchinson J, Goodman Z, Ling M, Albrecht J. Is an 'a la carte' combination interferon α2b plus ribavirin regimen possible for the first line treatment in patients with chronic hepatitis C? *Hepatology* 2000;**31**:211–18.

86. Czaja A. Autoimmune hepatitis: Evolving concepts and treatment strategies. *Dig Dis Sci* 1995;**40**:435–56.

87. Alvarez F, Berg P, Bianchi F, *et al.* International Autoimmune Hepatitis Group report: Review of criteria for diagnosis of autoimmune hepatitis. *J Hepatol* 1999;**31**:929–38.

88. Czaja A, Homburger H. Auto-antibodies in liver disease. *Gastroenterology* 2001;**120**:239–49.

89. Czaja A. Immunopathogenesis of autoimmune-mediated liver damage. In: Moreno-Otero R, Clemente-Ricote G, Garcia-Monzon C (eds). *Immunology and the liver: Autoimmunity.* Madrid: Aran Ediciones; 2000:73–86.

90. Czaja A, Donaldson P. Genetic susceptibilities for immune expression and liver cell injury in autoimmune hepatitis. *Immunol Rev* 2000;**174**:250–9.

91. Czaja A, Cassani F, Cataleta M, *et al.* Frequency and significance of antibodies to actin in type 1 autoimmune hepatitis. *Hepatology* 1996;**24**:1068–73.

92. Targan S, Landers C, Vidrich A, et al. High-titer antineutrophil cytoplasmic antibodies in type 1 autoimmune hepatitis. Gastroenterology 1995;**108**:1159–66.
93. Nikias G, Batts K, Czaja A. The nature and prognostic implications of autoimmune hepatitis with an acute presentation. J Hepatol 1994;**21**:866–71.
94. Poralla T, Treichel U, Lohr H, et al. The asialoglycoprotein receptor as target structure in autoimmune liver diseases. Semin Liver Dis 1991;**11**:215–22.
95. Manns M, Griffin K, Sullivan K, et al. LKM-1 autoantibodies recognize a short linear sequence in P450IID6, a cytochrome P-450 monooxygenase. J Clin Invest 1991;**88**:1370–8.
96. Manns M, Gerken G, Kyriatsoulis A, et al. Characterization of a new subgroup of autoimmune chronic active hepatitis by autoantibodies against a soluble liver antigen. Lancet 1987;**1**:292–4.
97. Stechemesser E, Klein R, Berg P. Characterization and clinical relevance of liver–pancreas antibodies in autoimmune hepatitis. Hepatology 1993;**18**:1–9.
98. Czaja A. Diagnosis, prognosis, and treatment of classical autoimmune chronic active hepatitis. In: Krawitt E, Wiesner R (eds). Autoimmune liver disease. New York: Raven Press; 1991:143–56.
99. Czaja A. Natural history, clinical features, and treatment of autoimmune hepatitis. Semin Liver Dis 1984;**4**:1–12.
100. Czaja A. Drug therapy in the management of type 1 autoimmune hepatitis. Drugs 1999;**57**:49–68.
101. Roberts S, Therneau T, Czaja A. Prognosis of histologic cirrhosis in type 1 autoimmune hepatitis. Gastroenterology 1996;**110**:848–57.
102. Czaja A. Low dose corticosteroid therapy after multiple relapses of severe HBsAg-negative chronic active hepatitis. Hepatology 1990;**11**:1044–9.
103. Johnson P, McFarlane I, Williams R. Azathioprine for long-term maintenance of remission in autoimmune hepatitis. N Engl J Med 1995;**333**:958–63.
104. Richardson P, James P, Ryder S. Mycophenolate mofetil for maintenance of remission in autoimmune hepatitis patients resistant to or intolerant of azathioprine. J Hepatol 2000;**33**:371–5.
105. Sanchez-Urdazpal L, Czaja A, van Hoek B, et al. Prognostic features and role of liver transplantation in severe corticosteroid-treated autoimmune chronic active hepatitis. Hepatology 1992;**15**:215–21.
106. Ratziu V, Samuel D, Sebagh M, et al. Long-term follow-up after liver transplantation for autoimmune hepatitis: Evidence of recurrence of primary disease. J Hepatol 1999;**30**:131–41.

CHAPTER 8

Cholestasis

DINESH KUMAR SINGAL, RAKESH TANDON

Cholestasis refers to the interruption of bile flow or bile formation. This may result from a functional defect in bile formation at the hepatocyte level, or a defect in bile secretion and flow at the level of the bile ductules or ducts. Thus, cholestasis can be classified as intrahepatic when caused by hepatic disorders, or extrahepatic when caused by obstruction of the major bile ducts. The common causes of cholestasis are given in Table I. This chapter will focus on intrahepatic cholestasis.

Table I. Causes of cholestasis

Intrahepatic cholestasis	Extrahepatic cholestasis
Hepatocellular	Benign
Viral: hepatitis viruses A, B, C, E	Biliary stricture: post-cholecystectomy,
Alcohol	inflammatory, PSC
Drugs	Stone disease
Cirrhosis	Mirizzi syndrome
Chronic cholestatic disorders	Chronic pancreatitis
Primary biliary cirrhosis	Bile duct infections
Primary sclerosing cholangitis (PSC)	Malignant
Autoimmune hepatitis	Carcinoma of the gallbladder
Autoimmune cholangiopathy	Cholangiocarcinoma
Cholestasis of pregnancy	Ampullary carcinoma
Benign recurrent intrahepatic cholestasis	Carcinoma of the head of the pancreas
Progressive familial intrahepatic cholestasis	Hepatocellular carcinoma
Vanishing bile duct syndrome	
Ductopenic syndromes	
Allograft rejection	
Graft-versus-host disease	
Sepsis	
Total parenteral nutrition-associated infiltrative diseases	
Tuberculosis	
Sarcoidosis	
Lymphoma	

NORMAL BILE SECRETION AND PATHOPHYSIOLOGY OF CHOLESTASIS

Bile serves to eliminate toxic lipophilic compounds, drugs and heavy metals from the body. It helps to excrete cholesterol, as well as in the digestion and absorption of lipids and fat-soluble vitamins in the intestines. Normal bile formation is dependent on various transport systems localized on the basolateral and canalicular membranes of the hepatocytes as well as cholangiocytes. It is an osmotic secretory process driven by the concentration of bile acid-dependent and -independent components in the bile canaliculi. The bile acid-dependent component relies on the active uptake of bile acid at the basolateral membrane by the sodium taurocholate co-transporter (NTCP) and organic anion-transporting polypeptide (OATP). Once inside the hepatocytes, bile acids are transported to the canalicular membrane and secreted into the canaliculi by an ATP-dependent transport system known as the bile salt export pump (BSEP).

The bile acid-independent component results from the secretion of glutathione, glutathione conjugates and bicarbonates in the canalicular lumen mediated by the canalicular multispecific organic anion transporter (cMOAT), which is known to be the human multidrug resistance-associated protein 2 (MRP2). Other transporters that serve important functions are localized on the basolateral and canalicular membranes. Bile ductules contribute a bicarbonate-rich solution produced by the cholangiocytes to the normal bile flow. This ductular contribution is regulated by the hormone secretin. Various diseases presenting as cholestasis are associated with the decreased or absent expression of specific hepatocellular transport proteins located at the level of either the basolateral or canalicular membrane. The resultant impaired hepatocellular uptake at the basolateral membrane or reduced canalicular secretion of bile salts and other organic anions into the canaliculi leads to loss of the osmotic forces essential for bile secretion. Cholestatic disorders are also associated with an alteration in the cytoskeleton of the hepatocytes, which disrupts intrahepatic transport and increases the permeability of tight junctions. This also contributes to the loss of osmotic forces. The detailed mechanism underlying bile secretion and the pathophysiology of cholestasis are beyond the scope of this chapter and readers are referred to reviews on this subject.[1,2]

CLINICAL AND LABORATORY FEATURES

Cholestasis results in the accumulation of bile salts, bilirubin and other biliary pigments in the serum, as well as the absence/deficiency of bile salts in the intestines. These factors are responsible for the clinical features associated with cholestasis (Fig. 1). Jaundice associated with clay-coloured stools is a typical feature of cholestasis. However, not all patients with cholestasis have jaundice. Pruritus is the most debilitating symptom of cholestasis. The exact substance responsible for producing pruritus has not been established till date; however, bile acids, endogenous opioids or opiate-like substances and altered serotoninergic neurotransmission have been incriminated.[3] Fatigue is another intriguing

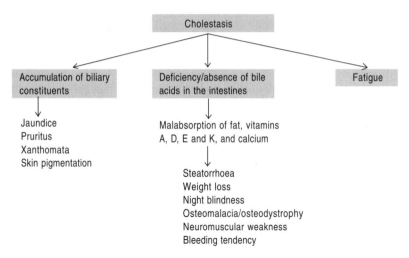

Fig. 1. Clinical features of cholestasis

symptom, which affects 20%–80% of patients with cholestatic liver disease, particularly primary biliary cirrhosis (PBC). The severity of fatigue does not correlate with the severity of the underlying liver disease. The pathogenesis of fatigue is obscure, although alterations in central neurotransmission and peripheral muscle dysfunction have been implicated.[4]

Xanthomata are usually seen around the eyes, but may also be seen in the palmar creases, below the breasts and on the neck. These occur due to the accumulation of cholesterol. Hepatic osteodystrophy constitutes both osteoporosis as well as osteopenia. This results in bone pain and fractures. The pathogenesis appears to be multifactorial and includes cholestasis-related risk factors such as vitamin D and K deficiency, and reduced calcium availability. In addition, risk factors independent of cholestasis such as ageing, female sex, reduced exposure to sunlight, reduced physical activity, low body-mass index, the menopause, steroid therapy and genetic variability may also play a role.

Biochemically, there is conjugated (direct) hyperbilirubinaemia. The serum ALP level is raised, usually to more than three times the upper limit of normal (ULN). Since the ALP level may be raised in non-hepatic disorders as well (e.g. bone disease and pregnancy), the hepatic origin of the rise in the ALP level is confirmed by an associated rise in serum GGT, 5'-nucleotidase and leucine aminopeptidase levels. The serum cholesterol level is raised and bile salts are increased. The levels of serum transaminases (AST and ALT) are usually raised only 1–2 times above the ULN, but may be higher in case of intrahepatic cholestasis. Serum protein and albumin levels are normal in acute cholestasis but, in prolonged disease, the serum albumin level falls. PT is prolonged but is usually correctable by injecting vitamin K in patients with cholestasis. Biochemically, it is difficult to distinguish between intra- and extrahepatic cholestasis.

INTRAHEPATIC VERSUS EXTRAHEPATIC CHOLESTASIS

The first step to be taken when a patient presents with cholestatic symptoms is to determine whether the condition is due to intra- or extrahepatic cholestasis. A detailed history, good clinical examination and routine biochemical investigations (Table II) provide clues to distinguish between the two. Subsequently, imaging studies will confirm the diagnosis. However, further investigations will be required to identify the underlying aetiology of cholestasis.

The presence of symptoms suggestive of cholangitis (fever with chills and rigors, right upper quadrant pain), a past history of biliary surgery, an elderly patient and a palpable mass in the right upper quadrant point towards a diagnosis of extrahepatic biliary obstruction. A history of prodromal symptoms (anorexia, malaise, nausea and arthralgia), exposure to hepatotoxins (alcohol, hepatotoxic drugs) and blood products, a family history of liver disease, the presence of stigmata of chronic liver disease (spider angiomata, gynaecomastia, parotid enlargement, testicular atrophy, Dupuytren contracture), signs of portal hypertension (ascites, splenomegaly, dilated abdominal veins and oesophageal varices) suggest an underlying intrahepatic cause. On routine biochemistry, elevation of transaminases is predominant in intrahepatic cholestasis, while in extrahepatic cholestasis, the ALP level is predominantly raised. However, these clues should be interpreted with caution as they can be misleading at times, e.g. fever and abdominal pain may be important symptoms in alcoholic and viral hepatitis as well, a patient who had undergone prior biliary surgery may develop acute viral hepatitis, a patient with chronic liver disease may have gall stones and choledocholithiasis, and a patient with acute obstruction due to choledocholithiasis may have high transaminase levels in the acute phase.

Abdominal USG examination is a good and inexpensive imaging technique that not only differentiates between extra- and intrahepatic cholestasis, but also provides additional supportive information regarding the underlying aetiology. The intrahepatic biliary ducts and/or the CBD will be dilated in the event of extrahepatic biliary obstruction. USG examination has a sensitivity of 55%–91% and specificity of 82%–95% for the diagnosis of extrahepatic biliary obstruction.

Table II. Extrahepatic versus intrahepatic cholestasis

	Extrahepatic	Intrahepatic
History	Abdominal pain Fever with rigors Past history of biliary surgery Old age	Prodromal symptoms History of exposure Family history of liver disease
Physical examination	Fever Lump in the right upper quadrant Surgical scar	Stigmata of chronic liver disease Evidence of portal hypertension (ascites, splenomegaly)
Biochemical tests	Predominant ALP rise Prolonged PT correctable with vitamin K	Predominant transaminase rise Prolonged PT not correctable with vitamin K Decreased serum albumin

It identifies the level of obstruction (hepatic ducts, hilar, CBD or ampullary) as well as the cause of obstruction (stone disease, mass lesion involving the gallbladder, CBD or pancreas). It also provides information about the hepatic parenchyma, space-occupying lesions of the liver and underlying portal hypertension (patency and diameter of the splenoportal axis, collaterals, splenomegaly and ascites). However, there are limitations associated with the use of USG; it may be difficult in obese patients and those with overlying bowel gases. The intrahepatic biliary ducts may not dilate in patients with extrahepatic biliary obstruction due to primary sclerosing cholangitis (PSC) or those with a poorly compliant hepatic parenchyma (as in underlying cirrhosis); thus, USG may be fallacious in such instances. Other imaging modalities, such as endoscopic ultrasonography (EUS), contrast-enhanced CT (CECT) scan or MRCP/ERCP are helpful in establishing the diagnosis of extrahepatic biliary obstruction in such cases.

DIFFERENTIAL DIAGNOSIS OF INTRAHEPATIC CHOLESTASIS

The various causes of intrahepatic cholestasis are enumerated in Table I. A short history with a typical prodrome followed by jaundice and markedly raised transaminase levels (10 x ULN) favours a diagnosis of acute hepatitis. Acute hepatitis A as well as E may have a prolonged course and, later in the illness, transaminase levels may become normal while cholestatic symptoms may persist along with raised ALP levels. The presence of one of the acute hepatitis markers (IgM anti-HAV, IgM anti-HEV, IgM anti-HBc) along with the absence of extrahepatic biliary obstruction on imaging will aid in the diagnosis. In case of doubt, a liver biopsy consistent with acute hepatitis will be confirmatory. In patients with negative acute hepatitis markers, drugs as a cause should be excluded on history. The presence of features of hypersensitivity (rash, arthralgia and peripheral eosinophilia) point towards drugs as a cause of cholestasis, and liver biopsy may provide a clue. Acute alcoholic hepatitis can also present with the symptoms and biochemical features of cholestasis. A history of alcohol abuse, tender hepatomegaly, spider naevi, AST>ALT and AST/ALT >2 are characteristic features. Liver histology typically reveals steatosis, ballooning degeneration, Mallory hyaline bodies, neutrophilic infiltration and pericellular fibrosis.

Chronic cholestatic diseases are prototypes of intrahepatic cholestasis. PBC typically presents with pruritus in a middle-aged female or even earlier as an asymptomatic rise in the ALP level. The presence of antimitochondrial antibodies (AMA) and characteristic liver biopsy are diagnostic. AMA-negative PBC (autoimmune cholangiopathy) is also known. PSC is associated with ulcerative colitis in 75% of cases. ERCP is usually diagnostic; it may be normal in small-duct PSC, in which case the liver biopsy is conclusive. Secondary causes of sclerosing cholangitis should also be considered and ruled out.

Many infiltrative disorders also present with cholestasis. The commonest disorders are tuberculosis and sarcoidosis. Other causes include infections such as those with *Mycobacterium avium*, leprosy, brucellosis, syphilis, fungal diseases, parasitic diseases and mononucleosis; toxins such as beryllium, quinidine, allopurinol, sulphonamides; and systemic disorders such as amyloidosis, lymphoma and Wegener granulomatosis. Most patients with these diseases present with fever and hepatosplenomegaly. Chest X-ray may reveal typical features in patients with tuberculosis and sarcoidosis. Liver biopsy is usually diagnostic.

During pregnancy, acute viral hepatitis remains the commonest cause of cholestasis and can present during any trimester. Cholestasis of pregnancy typically presents late in the second or third trimester, and is characterized by intense pruritus, absent or mild jaundice, and raised serum bile acids and transaminases. ALP levels are mildly or moderately increased, and GGT is normal or minimally increased. These patients may have experienced similar symptoms during earlier pregnancies, may give a family history of a similar disorder in their mother or sisters, and may have experienced cholestatic symptoms with oral contraceptives. Improvement occurs with delivery; those with persistent symptoms after delivery or with prolonged symptoms should be suspected of having other cholestatic disorders, particularly PBC or autoimmune hepatitis. Jaundice during pregnancy is discussed in detail in Chapter 12.

Cholestasis in neonates is due to several causes (Table III).[5] It is crucial to detect the presence of extrahepatic biliary atresia early, as surgical intervention before the eighth week of life markedly improves the prognosis (*see also* Chapter 13).

Treatment

The treatment of intrahepatic cholestasis is directed towards the underlying aetiology as well as relief of the associated symptoms of pruritus, fatigue, osteodystrophy and malabsorption. This would include symptomatic supportive treatment in acute viral hepatitis, cessation of alcohol in alcoholic hepatitis, removal of offending drugs in drug-induced cholestasis, ursodeoxycholic acid (UDCA) for cholestasis of pregnancy and PBC, steroids for

Table III. Aetiology of neonatal cholestasis at a tertiary care centre in India (n=120)[5]

Aetiology	n (%)
Neonatal hepatitis	40 (33)
Biliary atresia	47 (39)
Paucity of bile ductules (non-syndromic)	6 (5)
Choledochal cyst/Caroli disease	2 (1.6)
Sclerosing cholangitis	1 (0.8)
Galactosaemia	6 (5)
α_1-antitrypsin deficiency	3 (2.5)
Niemann–Pick disease	1 (0.8)
Giant-cell hepatitis with Coombs + haemolytic anaemia	1 (0.8)
Undetermined	13 (11)

Table IV. Antipruritic agents used in cholestatic liver disease

Agent/drug	Dosage	Adverse effects	Comments
Anion-exchange resins			
Cholestyramine	4 g before and after breakfast, and then before lunch	Bloating, constipation	First-line drug
Enzyme inducer			
Rifampicin	300 mg twice/day	Hepatotoxicity	Second-line drug
Opioid antagonist			
Naltrexone	50 mg daily	Opioid withdrawal-like syndrome	Third-line drug, efficacious in clinical trials
Serotonin antagonist			
Ondansetron	24 mg/day in divided doses	Not significant	Effective in initial trials
Bile acids			
Ursodeoxycholic acid	12–15 mg/kg/day	Not significant	Effective only in cholestasis of pregnancy and primary biliary cirrhosis

autoimmune hepatitis and antiviral agents for chronic viral hepatitis. Liver transplantation may be the only option in progressive, irreversible, end-stage liver disease. Treatment options in extrahepatic cholestasis include radiological, endoscopic or surgical interventions, and are discussed separately in Chapters 3, 4 and 19, respectively.

The management of pruritus[3] has been aimed primarily at removing or antagonizing the putative pruritogens (hydrophobic bile acids, endogenous opioids or opiate-like substances and altered serotoninergic neurotransmission) (Table IV). Antihistamine drugs are ineffective and help only by virtue of their sedative effect. Anion-exchange resins are first-line antipruritic agents that bind hydrophobic bile salts in the intestines and excrete them through the faeces, thus depleting the bile acid pool of hydrophobic bile acids. Cholestyramine is the most commonly used. It is administered in doses of 4 g before and after breakfast and then before lunch; side-effects include nausea, bloating, constipation, and reduced absorption of certain drugs and fat-soluble vitamins. It should be administered 2 hours before UDCA, if both the drugs are to be given. Colestipol is another bile salt-binding agent that is better tolerated by some patients. Colesevalem is a new bile acid-binding resin and has minimal gastrointestinal side-effects. Rifampicin is a second-line antipruritic agent. It acts by inducing enzymes of the microsomal drug-oxidizing system, and thus promotes the metabolism of endogenous pruritogens. It is administered in a dose of 300–600 mg/day. Considerable reduction in pruritus is observed within 7 days of treatment. Potential hepatotoxicity as well as the development of resistance to *M. tuberculosis* is a concern with the use of this drug. Phenobarbitone is also an enzyme inducer but has not been found to be as effective as rifampicin.

Opioid antagonists have been found effective in ameliorating pruritus in most studies. These act by antagonizing endogenous opioids. The only oral preparation available is naltrexone. Other preparations, such as nalmefene and naloxone, are for parenteral use. The use of these agents may be associated with an opioid withdrawal-like reaction in patients with cholestasis, but not in normal persons. Ondansetron, a 5-HT$_3$ serotonin receptor antagonist, has shown promising results in improving pruritus in initial studies. UDCA[6] is a hydrophilic bile acid that replaces hydrophobic hepatotoxic bile acids from the bile acid pool and becomes the predominant constituent of this pool. This is the only approved treatment in PBC; however, different studies have yielded contradictory results for the relief of pruritus in PBC with this agent. In cholestasis of pregnancy, UDCA improves maternal symptoms, including pruritus, as well as the outcome of pregnancy. Oral steroids for a duration of 3 weeks have been used for the relief of pruritus in patients with prolonged cholestatic hepatitis associated with hepatitis A infection. However, no randomized studies are available to support the belief that these are of use. In severe cases, interventions such as plasmapheresis and albumin dialysis (see MARS, pp. 314–15) have also been tried. Liver transplantation may be the only option in patients with irreversible cholestatic liver disease and severe, persistent pruritus. Finally, some simple but important measures may help, such as the application of emollients, bathing with cold water, wearing light cotton clothes, frequent cutting of nails and avoiding the urge to scratch.

No specific medical treatment is available for the fatigue associated with cholestasis. The pathogenesis of fatigue needs to be elucidated before an appropriate therapeutic intervention can be established. However, pilot trials suggest that antioxidants may be helpful.

As already noted, the osteodystrophy associated with cholestasis is multifactorial. Calcium and vitamin D should be supplemented. As a preventive measure, these patients should be encouraged to stay mobile and active, consume additional amounts of skimmed milk and have adequate exposure to sunlight. Corticosteroids worsen osteopenia and should hence be avoided. In symptomatic patients, bisphosphonates (editronate, arendronate) may be beneficial.

Steatorrhoea associated with cholestasis should be treated with a low-fat diet. The addition of medium-chain triglycerides (MCT) to the diet helps in maintaining nutrition, as MCT do not require bile acids for absorption. Commercial preparations of MCT are available; coconut oil can also be used for cooking as it provides MCT. Supplementation of calcium and the fat-soluble vitamins A, D, E and K is also required in patients with long-standing cholestasis.

DRUG-INDUCED CHOLESTASIS

Drugs are an important cause of cholestasis, although the incidence of drug-induced cholestasis has been underestimated. The diagnosis of drug-induced cholestasis is difficult and generally considered after excluding common causes of cholestasis. A high index of suspicion and a detailed drug history are required. Usually, symptoms appear within 3–6 months of starting a new drug. Occasionally, cholestasis manifests after the causative drug has already been discontinued. The presence of features of hypersensitivity (rash, lymphadeno-pathy, eosinophilia and joint pains) favours drugs as the underlying cause. Improvement after stopping the suspected drug may be a helpful clue. Often, the recurrence of symptoms after inadvertent rechallenge settles the diagnosis. Deliberate rechallenge is usually not advocated for ethical and safety reasons. Liver biopsy is useful in excluding other hepatobiliary disorders as there are no pathognomonic features of drug-induced cholestasis. Management is limited to the relief of symptoms. After withdrawal of the incriminated agent, most patients improve completely over a period of time. However, although uncommon, in severe cases the outcome may be fatal or cirrhosis may develop.

The list of drugs causing cholestasis is ever increasing and includes various herbal medicines. However, the main drug classes implicated are antimicrobials, psychotropic agents, lipid-lowering agents, and non-steroidal anti-inflammatory drugs.[7]

Based on the clinical and histological features, various syndromes associated with drug-induced cholestasis have been recognized:

1. *Pure cholestasis:* There are no associated symptoms or laboratory features of hepatitis. Histological examination of the liver shows intrahepatic cholestasis without substantial hepatic inflammation. Common drugs causing pure (bland) cholestasis are oestrogens, anabolic steroids, tamoxifen and azathioprine.
2. *Cholestatic hepatitis:* In this condition, the clinical and laboratory features of cholestasis and hepatitis overlap. In addition to cholestasis, histological examination of the liver also reveals lobular and portal inflammation. Chlorpromazine is a typical example. Other common drugs responsible are the macrolide antibiotics, phenothiazines, tricyclic antidepressants, amoxicillin–clavulanic acid, ketoconazole, enalapril and azathioprine.
3. *Cholestatic hepatitis associated with bile duct injury:* Symptoms of this condition may resemble those of acute cholangitis. Most agents causing cholestatic hepatitis can also cause bile duct injury, but typical examples are dextropropoxyphene, flucloxacillin and paraquat.
4. *Vanishing bile duct syndrome (VBDS):* When bile duct injury in patients with cholestatic hepatitis is severe, it leads to ductopenia or VBDS. The clinical features may resemble those of PBC, the only distinguishing feature being the absence of antimitochondrial antibodies. After stopping the incrimina-ting drug, complete resolution may take 2 years; however, biliary cirrhosis may develop. A number of drugs have been implicated but the commonest are chlorpromazine, flucloxacillin and erythromycin.
5. *Large bile duct strictures:* These are uncommon lesions that have a presentation similar to that of PSC. The strictures usually occur at the junction of the right and left hepatic ducts. Intra-arterial infusion of floxuridine and intralesional instillation of scolicidal agents are the commonest causes.

CHOLESTATIC DISORDERS IN INDIA

The exact incidence, prevalence and aetiology of cholestatic disorders in India are not known, as these disorders are uncommon and have not been studied systematically.

Clinical experience suggests that cholestasis associated with acute viral hepatitis due to HEV infection is the commonest cause in India; 25% of such patients have cholestatic symptoms.[8] These symptoms are transient in the majority of patients. However, an occasional patient may develop a prolonged course with predominantly cholestatic symptoms. Why some patients develop prolonged cholestatic hepatitis is not known, but all recover completely over a period of 3–6 months. Liver biopsy in these patients reveals characteristic cholangitic hepatitis.[9]

Primary biliary cirrhosis is uncommon in India and is usually mentioned only as case reports. In a tertiary care centre, only 5 patients had been diagnosed over a 5-year period.[10] The clinical presentation and course of these patients was similar to that seen in the West. A variant form of PBC without pruritus has been described in a few case reports from India.[11] A case report of the familial form of PBC has also been described.[12]

Likewise, PSC is also uncommon in India.[13] The profile of these patients as reported from a tertiary care centre in India is detailed in Table V.[14] The clinical profile and outcomes seem similar to those seen in the West. Of the total, 50% of patients had associated ulcerative colitis. The clinical profile was not different in patients with and without ulcerative colitis.

To conclude, a systematic approach helps in establishing the underlying aetiology in the majority of cases of intrahepatic cholestasis. Specific management depends on the underlying aetiology. Pruritus is the most troublesome symptom; encouraging results have been obtained with newer drugs such as rifampicin and opioid antagonists. Liver transplantation may be the only option for progressive, irreversible cholestatic liver diseases. Cholestatic disorders in the Indian context need to be studied systematically.

Table V. Characteristics at diagnosis of patients with primary sclerosing cholangitis[14]

Number of patients (n)	18
Age (years)	39±16
Male:female ratio	1.5:1
Associated ulcerative colitis (n)	9 (50)
Duration of jaundice in months (mean±SD)	12.6±16.1
Recurrent cholangitis (n)	3 (16.7)
Hepatomegaly (n)	9 (50)
Splenomegaly (n)	8 (44.8)
Bilirubin in mg/dl (mean±SD)	6.6±5.6
ALP level >2 × upper limit of normal (n)	18 (100)
Evidence of portal hypertension on sonography (n)	5 (27.8)
Varices at endoscopy (n)	2 (11.1)

Values in parentheses are percentages

REFERENCES

1. Trauner M, Boyer JL. Bile salt transporters: Molecular characterization, function and regulation. *Physiol Rev* 2003;**83**:633–70.
2. Trauner M, Peter J, Meier PJ, Boyer JL. Molecular pathogenesis of cholestasis. *N Engl J Med* 1998;**339**:1217–27.
3. Mela M, Mancuso A, Burroughs AK. Pruritus in cholestatic and other liver diseases. *Aliment Pharmacol Ther* 2003;**17**:857–70.
4. Kumar D, Tandon RK. Fatigue in cholestatic liver disease—a perplexing symptom. *Postgrad Med J* 2002;**78**:404–7.
5. Yachha SK, Mohindra S. Neonatal cholestasis syndrome: Indian scene. *Indian J Pediatr* 1999;**66** (Suppl):S94–S96.
6. Kumar D, Tandon RK. Use of ursodeoxycholic acid in liver diseases. *J Gastroenterol Hepatol* 2001;**16**:3–14.
7. Sgro C, Clinard F, Ouazir K, *et al*. Incidence of drug induced hepatic injuries: A French population-based study. *Hepatology* 2002;**36**:451–5.
8. Khuroo MS, Rustgi VK, Dawson GJ, *et al*. Spectrum of hepatitis E virus infection in India. *J Med Virol* 1994;**43**:281–6.
9. Dilawari JB, Singh K, Chawla YK, *et al*. Hepatitis E virus: Epidemiological, clinical and serological studies of north Indian epidemic. *Indian J Gastroenterol* 1994;**13**:44–8.
10. Puri AS, Kumar N, Gondal R, Lamba GS, Jain M. Primary biliary cirrhosis: An Indian experience. *Indian J Gastroenterol* 2001;**20**:28–9.
11. Sharma BC, Saraswat VA, Choudhuri G, Das A, Ghoshal UC, Pandey R. Primary biliary cirrhosis without pruritus—an Indian variant. *Trop Gastroenterol* 1996;**17**:176–7.
12. Ramakrishna B, Eapen CE, Kang G, Kurian G, Chandy GM. Familial intrahepatic cholestatic cirrhosis with positive antimitochondrial antibody: Familial primary biliary cirrhosis. *J Clin Gastroenterol* 2000;**30**:255–8.
13. Acharya SK, Vashisht S, Tandon RK. Primary sclerosing cholangitis in India. *Gastroenterol Jpn* 1989;**24**:75–9.
14. Kochhar R, Goenka MK, Das K, *et al*. Primary sclerosing cholangitis: An experience from India. *J Gastroenterol Hepatol* 1996;**11**:429–33.

CHAPTER 9

Portal hypertension and jaundice

Y.K. CHAWLA

Portal hypertension, a common complication seen in patients with cirrhosis of the liver, is characterized by an increase in the portal venous pressure. Portal hypertension promotes the development of collateral vessels through which portal blood is diverted to the systemic circulation, bypassing the liver. These portosystemic collaterals are formed by the opening and dilatation of pre-existing vascular channels connecting the portal venous system and the superior and inferior vena cavae. It is not known whether other factors such as active angiogenesis are also involved in the development of such collaterals. The most important collaterals thus formed are the gastro-oesophageal varices that drain into the azygos veins. Patients with extrahepatic portal vein obstruction (EHPVO) are known to have a high frequency of duodenal, rectal and other ectopic varices.[1]

While all known causes of portal hypertension can form varices at different sites and result in bleeding at some time during the natural history of the disease, there may be some differences in their initial clinical manifestations. Ascites is a prominent finding in posthepatic portal hypertension, as in cirrhosis and hepatic venous outflow tract obstruction, but is very rare in the prehepatic causes of portal hypertension such as EHPVO.

Jaundice in portal hypertension may occur in patients with cirrhosis either as part of the natural history or following an acute episode of viral hepatitis, reactivation of hepatitis viruses or systemic infection, and conditions that hamper the functioning of viable hepatocytes. On the other hand, patients with EHPVO invariably present with UGI bleed, have biliary changes that can be demonstrated radiologically and may occasionally present with jaundice due to choledochal varices, which give an appearance of sclerosing cholangitis. These cholangiographic appearances have been termed as pseudosclerosing cholangitis,[2] or portal biliopathy,[3] or the pseudocholangiocarcinoma sign.[4] These changes are unusual in portal hypertension due to other causes, such as cirrhosis and non-cirrhotic portal fibrosis, except when there is associated portal vein thrombosis.[5]

Jaundice in portal hypertension can broadly be classified into: (i) portal hypertension causing jaundice; and (ii) portal hypertension with jaundice.

PORTAL HYPERTENSION CAUSING JAUNDICE

Pseudosclerosing cholangitis or portal biliopathy

Biliary changes have been described in patients with portal hypertension. These are predominantly seen in patients with EHPVO, and include stricture and dilatation of both the extra- and intrahepatic bile ducts, which resemble sclerosing cholangitis on cholangiography.[1] Increased awareness of this complication along with markedly improved management of EHPVO are responsible for an increased number of patients now being recognized with this complication. The relationship between choledochal varices and jaundice was first reported in 1965.[6] Occasionally, these biliary abnormalities contribute to the development of choledocholithiasis.

Clinical presentation

Most of the patients with biliary abnormalities are asymptomatic. Patients with EHPVO and biliary symptoms are usually adults, which indicates that it is a progressive disease. A study by Condat *et al.*[7] showed a longer median time period from the diagnosis of EHPVO in patients with symptoms of biliary obstruction than in patients without such symptoms. Sezgin *et al.*[8] also studied 10 patients (mean age 36.1 years) with biliary obstruction and EHPVO. On the other hand, patients with EHPVO without biliary symptoms commonly present with haematemesis in the first and second decades of life, further supporting the fact that biliary symptoms in these patients occur later in life.

When they occur, biliary symptoms are usually in the form of obstructive jaundice, which may or may not fluctuate in intensity. Occasionally, these patients may present with abdominal pain, recurrent fever with chills and jaundice.

Meredith *et al.*[9] described a patient with cavernomatous transformation of the portal vein presenting with obstructive jaundice. In their series of 28 patients with EHPVO, Gibson *et al.*[6] observed jaundice in 5 of them. In 1979, Webb and Sherlock[10] found elevated bilirubin levels in 13 of 97 patients with portal venous obstruction, 5 of whom had persistent jaundice. In our series of 20 patients with EHPVO and biliary abnormalities, choledocholithiasis was seen in only 1 patient who presented with abdominal pain; the others were asymptomatic.[1] Sezgin *et al.*[8] reported symptoms in only 10 of 36 patients with EHPVO, 3 of whom presented with jaundice, 5 with cholangitis, 1 with pruritus and 1 with abdominal pain. In another series of EHPVO patients, only 14% had biliary symptoms.[11] Symptoms usually occur once dominant strictures or bile duct stones are formed. Condat *et al.*[7] showed that 7 of 25 patients with portal cavernoma presented with biliary symptoms, namely abdominal pain (2), acalculus cholecystitis (1), ascending cholangitis (1), pruritus (1) and obstructive jaundice (2). They also observed that biliary symptoms were more often associated with a history of variceal bleeding, larger gastro-oesophageal varices and a solid, tumour-like portal cavernoma. Biliary symptoms are more commonly seen in the idiopathic, long-standing variety of EHPVO and rarely in patients with secondary EHPVO.[12] About 60 cases of symptomatic biliary obstruction due to EHPVO have been reported in the literature to date.[8]

Pathogenesis of biliary changes

The arterial supply of the bile duct is from the branches of the gastroduodenal artery, but the veins of the bile duct are responsible for the development of abnormalities.

The exact pathogenesis of bile duct abnormalities in EHPVO remains unclear. The extrahepatic bile ducts are accompanied by two pre-formed venous systems, one being the epicholedochal venous plexus of Saint, which forms a fine reticular web on the outer surface of the CBD and hepatic duct.[13] The veins of this plexus vary in size but are normally not larger than 1 mm. Varices of this plexus alter the smooth, intraluminal surface of the CBD and cause fine intramural defects. The other venous system constitutes the pericholedochal venous plexus of Petren, which runs parallel to the CBD and is connected to the gastric veins, pancreaticoduodenal vein, portal vein and directly to the liver.[14]

Following portal venous thrombosis, several new collaterals develop, which bypass the obstruction and produce a portal cavernoma. The bile duct wall is thin and pliable, and allows protrusion of the varicose paracholedochal veins into the lumen, resulting in an appearance similar to that of oesophageal varices. The biliary strictures that develop in patients with pseudosclerosing cholangitis are possibly due to ischaemia and vascular bile duct injury, or prolonged compression of the biliary tree from portal cavernoma, as suggested by Khuroo et al.[11] They could also be due to a reaction to an infectious process that causes EHPVO.

Investigations in pseudosclerosing cholangitis

A rise in serum ALP level may be seen in 40%–80% of cases, with variable levels of serum bilirubin, depending on the symptoms.

Ultrasonography

The role of USG lies not in demonstrating choledochal varices, but in making a diagnosis of portal vein thrombosis and demonstrating gallbladder varices and, occasionally, dilatation of the bile duct. In one study, the presence of gallbladder varices seen on USG reliably predicted biliary changes detected on ERCP.[15]

Radionuclide scintigraphy

Hepatobiliary scan is not of much use in the diagnosis of pseudosclerosing cholangitis. It cannot detect minimal irregularity in calibre and angulation, but picks up dilated ductal segments as increased radiotracer activity, and strictures as decreased radiotracer activity with a partial hold-up.[16]

Choledochoscopy

This has been used for directly visualizing and diagnosing CBD varices and is useful in distinguishing between benign and malignant lesions.[17]

Endoscopic retrograde cholangiopancreaticography

Studies using ERCP have shown a prevalence of biliary tract abnormalities in 70%–100% of cases,[2,11,15,17] usually seen as irregularities in the CBD and hepatic ducts with smooth, tapering, short or long strictures that may be single or multiple. The intrahepatic ducts more commonly show strictures and dilatation on the left side. Khuroo *et al.*[11] observed portal angulation and displacement of the ducts in addition to the presence of strictures, changes in calibre and extraluminal impression on the bile duct. On the other hand, in cirrhosis and non-cirrhotic portal fibrosis, these changes are mild and are associated with pruning of the intrahepatic biliary radicles.

Magnetic resonance cholangiopancreaticography

Condat *et al.*[7] found biliary tract abnormalities in 92% of unselected patients with EHPVO. The most common abnormalities were stenosis and angulation in the suprapancreatic portion of the bile duct. All the patients had a portal cavernoma in close contact with the bile ducts. The transverse diameter of the cavernoma was larger in patients with biliary strictures compared with those without a stricture (22 mm *v.* 12 mm). Patients with biliary symptoms more often had a solid tumour-like cavernoma, as shown by a uniform mass-like structure with a solid appearance mimicking a tumour in which the venous collaterals are not clearly individualized.[7] Why these are seen in only a few patients is not known.[8]

MRCP is advantageous as it allows visualization of the bile ducts together with the adjacent blood vessels and is non-invasive as compared to ERCP.

Treatment

Asymptomatic patients do not need any treatment. At present, strategies for the management of pseudosclerosing cholangitis are directed only towards symptomatic patients. There is no consensus as to the optimal treatment of this condition as data on the various forms of therapy are inconclusive.

The treatment approach could be *direct* with endoscopic decompression or biliary digestive anastomosis, or *indirect* by portal decompression.

Surgical management of biliary obstruction in patients with EHPVO is associated with high morbidity and mortality, and is extremely difficult because of the collateral vessels around the bile ducts and in the porta hepatis.[18] In addition to the inability to carry out surgical dissection, excessive haemorrhage and death as well as restenosis decrease the success rates.[19,20]

Patients should thus undergo shunt surgery before any biliary intervention surgery is planned. Some patients improve with shunt surgery and may not require further surgical intervention. In one study, nodular defects, stenosis and irregularities of the CBD resolved in 3 out of 4 patients who underwent a transjugular intrahepatic portosystemic shunt.[5] Our own study showed partial normalization of the bile ducts after shunt surgery.[21] In patients in whom these biliary abnormalities persist, possible development of vascular neogenesis and fibrous tissue has been shown both histologically and morphologically along with paraportal collateral vessels. In these cases, cavernous transformation has spongiose, tumour-like solid features. Villazon Sahagun et al.[22] demonstrated excessive pericholedochal fibrosis and multiple congested collaterals intraoperatively. Because the biliary stenosis was induced by fibrosis in these cases, no improvement in cholestasis was obtained by the creation of a portosystemic shunt.

Hence, portal decompressive surgery should precede biliary tract surgery.[9,13] Shunt surgery may also be indicated for patients with EHPVO who have not bled but have symptomatic pseudosclerosing cholangitis.

Endoscopic therapy is the only option in patients who do not have an adequately shuntable vein. Endoscopic treatment has been undertaken in such patients with biliary obstruction. Lohr et al.[23] treated a patient with polycythaemia vera with a stent for a period of 3 years, resulting in the disappearance of cholestasis. Henne-Bruns et al.[24] successfully treated a patient by stent insertion with stent exchange every 3 months for 1 year. Mork et al.[20] treated 2 patients with the insertion of a 10 F stent.

Once stones begin to cause obstruction, they can be removed by endoscopic sphincterotomy. However, one has to be cautious while performing the sphincterotomy as venous collaterals may be present in the ampullary and juxta-ampullary area, posing a risk for bleeding during the procedure.

Sezgin et al.[8] performed biliary sphincterotomy in patients with symptomatic pseudosclerosing cholangitis. Four underwent balloon dilatation of the biliary stricture. Endoscopically, such patients may need repeated stent exchanges because of the recurrence of symptoms. The underlying stricture, however, may not improve. Endoscopic treatment could thus be considered a safe first-line treatment for patients with biliary obstruction. Tighe and Jacobson[25] reported bleeding from the bile duct during dilatation with a 6 mm balloon. Endoscopic biliary procedures were earlier considered unsafe because of the presence of choledochal varices but no major complication has been mentioned in the cases reported in the literature.

PORTAL HYPERTENSION WITH JAUNDICE

Cirrhosis with jaundice

Patients with cirrhosis of the liver may move from a compensated to a decompensated state as part of the natural history of the disease, depending on the aetiology of the cirrhosis.

HCV-decompensated cirrhosis

In such patients, the 5-year survival rate without liver transplantation is only 50%. The goals of therapy in these patients are to slow the progression of clinical disease, improve synthetic function, reverse the complications of liver disease and obviate the need for liver transplantation. Secondary goals are the eradication of HCV RNA to prevent recurrence of hepatitis C viraemia after liver transplantation, and reduce the level of HCV RNA to lessen the severity of post-transplantation liver disease.[26,27] A major concern regarding the therapy of patients with decompensated cirrhosis is the safety of administering interferon and ribavirin. These patients are at increased risk for bone marrow suppression and can suffer life-threatening infections during treatment. They are also more prone to worsening hepatic function. Unfortunately, the published literature on the treatment of hepatitis C in decompensated cirrhosis is scant.[28] Thus, the primary therapy for patients with decompensated liver disease due to hepatitis C should be a referral for liver transplantation. The 5-year survival rate after liver transplantation for hepatitis C is 60%–80%, which compares favourably with survival without transplantation.

HBV-decompensated cirrhosis

The prognosis for a patient with decompensated HBV cirrhosis is poor, with a 5-year survival rate of only 14% compared with 80% in patients with compensated cirrhosis. The causes of death in a Dutch series[29] were liver failure in 10% of patients and hepatocellular carcinoma (HCC) in 10%, while a few (6%) died of causes not related to the liver.[29]

Studies on the natural history of patients with untreated HBV cirrhosis, with active viral replication as defined by the presence of detectable serum HBV DNA using a non-PCR-based assay ($>10^5$–10^6 copies/ml) or HBeAg, show that they are at an increased risk for developing progressive liver disease and death. In the Dutch study,[29] loss of HBeAg and the development of anti-HBe during follow-up was associated with a 55% reduction in the likelihood of death. Thus, suppression of HBV replication with loss of HBeAg is an important event in the natural history of chronic HBV infection and a useful end-point of antiviral treatment.

The annual risk of HCC among HBV carriers is dependent on viral replication, severity of liver disease and demographic features. In HBV carriers with normal ALT levels, the annual risk of HCC is approximately 0.5%, whereas the risk among carriers with active viral replication and cirrhosis is up to 2%–5% per year. HBeAg-positive carriers are more likely to develop HCC.[30,31] Because the natural history of decompensated HBV cirrhosis is influenced by the level of HBV replication, it is logical to hypothesize that antiviral therapy may improve outcomes. Effective suppression of HBV replication should lead to reduced hepatic necroinflammation and potentially improve or stabilize liver function.

Interferon-alpha (IFN-α) has been shown to be safe and effective in some patients with chronic hepatitis B and selected patients with compensated HBV cirrhosis. Long-term follow-up studies have demonstrated that patients with a sustained response to IFN have improved liver histology, and a decreased risk of hepatic decompensation and development of HCC.[32] IFN is associated with life-threatening hepatitis flares and infectious complications even when used in low doses. Despite the use of a reduced dose of IFN in over 50% of patients (6–15 µg/week), 28% of patients developed bacterial infections and 50% developed hepatitis flares. Hence, IFN is contraindicated in patients with HBV-decompensated cirrhosis.[33,34]

Lamivudine, an orally administered nucleoside analogue, suppresses HBV DNA to undetectable levels by hybridization assays in 90% of patients and is associated with improved aminotransferase levels and liver histology at 1–2 months. It has no myelotoxicity and is generally well tolerated. Uncontrolled, open-labelled studies of lamivudine have shown improvement in biochemical and clinical parameters after prolonged treatment in patients with decompensated HBV cirrhosis. In a study from India, after a treatment period of 18 months, there was a significant improvement in Child–Turcotte–Pugh (CTP) scores (from 8.3 to 6.7) and serum ALT levels.[35] In another study from America, a few patients with decompensated cirrhosis after treatment with lamivudine were removed from the waiting list for liver transplantation due to clinical improvement.[36] In a study of 35 Canadian patients, there was an objective improvement in the severity of liver disease in the majority of treated patients.[37] In a study from North America, 77 HBsAg-positive candidates for liver transplantation were given lamivudine therapy that led to stabilization or improvement in the severity of liver disease.[38] Yao et al.[39] reported that candidates for liver transplantation receiving lamivudine are less likely to undergo transplantation. A greater proportion of patients treated with lamivudine showed an improvement of more than 3 points on the CTP score compared to untreated histological controls.[39]

Other co-factors associated with a more rapid progression of the disease include alcohol use, co-infection with other viruses (HAV, HCV, HDV, HEV and HIV) and the use of immunosuppressive agents.

Overall, lamivudine has been well tolerated and is safe in decompensated cirrhosis. Most studies have found that clinical improvement occurs typically in 3–6 months.

Alcoholic liver disease

Alcoholic hepatitis presents with jaundice, fever, anasarca and features of hepatic encephalopathy. It is usually present in association with cirrhosis of the liver. In fact, one-third of patients with alcoholic cirrhosis may have jaundice. They would also have features of peripheral oedema, ascites and GI haemorrhage. A combination of alcoholic hepatitis and cirrhosis has a poor prognosis, which depends on subsequent drinking behaviour, and clinical and histological severity. A poor outcome is associated with increasing age, alcohol ingestion, presence of hepatic encephalopathy, elevated serum bilirubin and creatinine levels, decreased plasma albumin, a hepatic vein pressure gradient (HVPG)

>14 mmHg and the presence of large varices.[40] In one study, the 10-year cumulative survival rate in patients with alcoholic cirrhosis was 30% in those who presented with well-compensated disease, 10% in those presenting with ascites, and 0% in those presenting with variceal haemorrhage and hepatic encephalopathy.

Cirrhosis with hepatocellular carcinoma

Patients with HBV, HCV and alcohol-related cirrhosis are prone to develop HCC. These patients may present with abdominal pain, weight loss, a palpable mass, jaundice and fever. In the presence of cirrhosis of the liver, features of hepatic decompensation are more common in patients with HCC.

Occasionally, growth of HCC into the biliary tract causes obstructive jaundice; such patients are said to have the cholestatic type of HCC. It is seen in only 1.9%–2.1% of cases.[41]

Autoimmune hepatitis and cirrhosis

Occasionally, patients with autoimmune hepatitis may present with hepatic decompensation. On investigation, they may be found to have cirrhosis of the liver. Immunosuppressive therapy is indicated only if the patient has no evidence of bleeding, infection or encephalopathy. Failure of therapy for autoimmune hepatitis is frequent if the patient has associated cirrhosis.

Drug-induced hepatitis in chronic liver disease

Patients with chronic liver disease are more prone to develop hepatotoxicity when given hepatotoxic drugs. A recent study on patients with tuberculosis and chronic liver disease divided the patients into 2 groups. Group A received INH, rifampicin and ethambutol for 2 months, and then INH and rifampicin for 7 additional months; 26% of patients developed hepatotoxicity versus 0% in the group given INH, pyrazinamide, ethambutol and ofloxacin (group B).[42]

In patients with chronic liver disease, it is now recommended that pyrazinamide be avoided as far as possible. Otherwise, a low dosage of pyrazinamide (20 µg/kg/day) should be given for a maximum of 2 months. Therapy should start with a low dose of INH (3 µg/kg/day) and then increased to the maximum dose. Additionally, hepatotoxic drugs should be avoided.[43]

REFERENCES

1. Chawla Y, Dilawari JB. Anorectal varices, their frequency in cirrhotic and noncirrhotic portal hypertension. *Gut* 1991;**32**:309–11.
2. Dilawari JB, Chawla YK. Pseudosclerosing cholangitis in extrahepatic portal venous obstruction. *Gut* 1992;**33**:272–6.
3. Sarin SK, Bhatia V, Makwane U. Portal biliopathy in extrahepatic portal vein obstruction. *Indian J Gastroenterol* 1992;**11** (Suppl):82.

4. Bayratkar Y, Balkanci F, Kayhan B, *et al.* Bile duct varices or pseudocholangiocarcinoma sign in portal hypertension due to cavernous transformation of the portal vein. *Am J Gastroenterol* 1992;**87**:1801–6.
5. Gorgul A, Kayhan B, Dogan I, *et al.* Disappearance of the pseudocholangiocarcinoma sign after TIPPS. *Am J Gastroenterol* 1996;**91**:150–4.
6. Gibson JP, Johnson GW, Fulton TT. Extrahepatic portal venous obstruction. *Br J Surg* 1965;**52**:129–39.
7. Condat B, Vilgrain V, Asselah T, *et al.* Portal cavernoma associated cholangiopathy: A clinical and MR cholangiography coupled with MR portography imaging study. *Hepatology* 2003;**37**:1302–8.
8. Sezgin O, Oguz D, Altin E, *et al.* Endoscopic management of biliary obstruction caused by cavernous transformation of the portal vein. *Gastrointest Endosc* 2003;**68**:602–8.
9. Meredith HC, Vujic I, Schabel SL. Obstructive jaundice caused by cavernous transformation of portal vein. *Br J Radiol* 1978;**51**:1011–12.
10. Webb LJ, Sherlock S. The etiology, presentation and natural history of extrahepatic portal venous obstruction. *Q J Med* 1979;**48**:627–39.
11. Khuroo MS, Yatoo GN, Zargar S, *et al.* Biliary abnormalities associated with extrahepatic portal venous obstruction. *Hepatology* 1993;**17**:807–13.
12. Chandra R, Kapoor D, Tharakan A, Chaudhary A, Sarin SK. Portal biliopathy. *J Gastroenterol Hepatol* 2001;**16**:1086–92.
13. Saint OA. The epicholedochal venous plexus and its importance as a means of identifying the common bile duct during operations on extrahepatic biliary tract. *Br J Surg* 1971; **46**:489–98.
14. Petren T. Die extrahepatischen gallenwegsveness and itioc. *Pathologisch Anat Ische Bedentum Vesh Anat Ges* 1932;**41**:139–43.
15. Malkan GH, Bhatia SJ, Bashir K, *et al.* Cholangiopathy associated with portal hypertension: Diagnostic evaluation and clinical implication. *Gastrointest Endosc* 1999;**49**:344–8.
16. Ikegami T, Matsuzaki Y, Saito Y, *et al.* Endoscopic diagnosis of common bile duct varices by percutaneous transhepatic choledochoscopy: Differential diagnosis from bile duct carcinoma. *Gastrointest Endosc* 1994;**40**:637–40.
17. Nagi B, Kochhar R, Bhasin D, *et al.* Cholangiopathy in extrahepatic portal venous obstruction. Radiological appearances. *Acta Radiol* 2000;**41**:612–15.
18. Hymes JL, Haichess BN, Schein CJ. Varices of the common bile duct as a surgical hazard. *Am Surg* 1977;**43**:667–8.
19. Chaudhary A, Dhar P, Sarin SK, *et al.* Bile duct obstruction due to portal biliopathy in extrahepatic portal hypertension: Surgical management. *Br J Surg* 1998;**85**:326–9.
20. Mork H, Weber P, Schmidt H, *et al.* Cavernous transformation of the portal vein associated with common bile duct strictures. Report of two cases. *Gastrointest Endosc* 1998;**47**:79–83.
21. Dhiman RK, Puri P, Chawla Y, *et al.* Biliary changes in extrahepatic portal venous obstruction: Compression by collaterals or ischemic? *Gastrointest Endosc* 1999;**50**:646–52.
22. Villazon Sahagun A, Yoselevitis M, Villazon Davico O, Garcia del Castillo M. [Pericholedochal varices.] *Rev Gastroenterol Mex* 1989;**54**:27–9.
23. Lohr JM, Kuchenreuter S, Grebmeier H, *et al.* Compression of the common bile duct due to portal vein thrombosis in polycythemia vera. *Hepatology* 1993;**17**:586–92.
24. Henne-Bruns D, Kremer B, Soehendra N. [Cavernous transformation of the portal vein. A rare cause of mechanical obstructive jaundice.] *Chirurg* 1989;**60**:704–6.
25. Tighe M, Jacobson I. Bleeding from bile duct varices as unexpected hazard during therapeutic ERCP. *Gastrointest Endosc* 1996;**43**:250–2.
26. Fattovich G, Giustina G, Dejos F, *et al.* Morbidity and mortality in compensated cirrhosis type C: A retrospective follow-up study of 384 patients. *Gastroenterology* 1997;**112**:463–72.
27. Charltons M, Seaber E, Wiesner R, *et al.* Predictors of patient and graft survival following liver transplantation of hepatitis C. *Hepatology* 1998;**28**:823–30.

28. Everson GT, Trouillot T, Trotter J, *et al.* Treatment of decompensated cirrhotics with a slow acceleration dose of interferon alfa 2b plus ribavarin: Safety+efficacy. *Hepatology* 2000;**32**:308-A.

29. De Jongh FE, Janssen HL, De Man RA, *et al.* Survival and prognostic indications in hepatitis B surface antigen positive cirrhosis of liver. *Gastroenterology* 1992;**103**:1630–5.

30. Beasely RP. Hepatitis B virus. The major etiology of hepatocellular carcinoma. *Cancer* 1988;**61**:1942–56.

31. Yang HI, Lu SN, Liaw YF, *et al.* Hepatitis B e antigen and the risk of hepatocellular carcinoma. *N Engl J Med* 2002;**347**:168–74.

32. Niederau C, Heinteges T, Lange S, *et al.* Long term follow up of HBeAg positive patients treated with interferon alfa for chronic hepatitis B. *N Engl J Med* 1996;**334**:1422–7.

33. Lin SM, Sheen IS, Chien RN, *et al.* Long term beneficial effect of interferon therapy in patients with chronic hepatitis B virus infection. *Hepatology* 1999;**29**:971–5.

34. Hoofnagle JH, DiBisceglie AM, Waggoner JG, Park Y. Interferon alfa for patients with clinically apparent cirrhosis due to chronic hepatitis B. *Gastroenterology* 1993;**104**:1116–21.

35. Kapoor D, Guptan RC, Wakil SM. Beneficial effects of lamivudine in hepatitis B-related decompensated cirrhosis. *J Hepatol* 2000;**33**:308–12.

36. Yao FY, Ban NM. Lamivudine treatment in patients with severely decompensated cirrhosis due to replicating hepatitis B infection. *J Hepatol* 2000;**33**:301–7.

37. Villeneuve J, Candreay CD, Willems B. Lamivudine treatment for decompensated cirrhosis resulting from chronic hepatitis B. *Hepatology* 2000;**31**:207–10.

38. Perrillo RP, Wright T, Rakela J, *et al.* A multicentre US Canadian trial to assess lamivudine monotherapy before and after liver transplantation for chronic hepatitis B. *Hepatology* 2001;**33**:424–32.

39. Yao FY, Tersault NA, Fresc C, *et al.* Lamivudine treatment is beneficial in patients with severely decompensated cirrhosis and actively replicating hepatitis B infection awaiting liver transplantation, a comparative study using a matched untreated cohort. *Hepatology* 2001;**34**:411–16.

40. Bircher J, Benhamou JP, McIntyre N, Rizetto M, Rodes J (eds). *Oxford textbook of clinical hepatology.* 2nd ed. Oxford: Oxford University Press; 1999:671.

41. Saunders JB, Wallent JRF, Davies P, *et al.* A 20-year prospective study of cirrhosis. *Br J Med* 1981;**282**:263–6.

42. Saigal S, Agrawal SR, Sarin SK, *et al.* Safety of an ofloxacin based antituberculosis treatment of tuberculosis in patients with underlying chronic liver disease. A preliminary report. *J Gastroenterol Hepatol* 2001;**16**:1028–32.

43. Kimmoun E, Samuel D. Antituberculosis drugs in patients with chronic liver disease. *J Gastroenterol Hepatol* 2002;**17**:S408–S412.

CHAPTER 10

Jaundice and infections

RUPA BANERJEE

Infectious diseases due to viral, bacterial, fungal and rickettsial organisms, either primary or part of a multisystemic disorder, can cause jaundice. The classical 'viral hepatitis' (hepatitis A, B, C, D and E) forms the commonest group and has been discussed in Chapters 6 and 7. Non-viral hepatic infections are the primary focus of this chapter. The liver serves as the initial site for the filtration of absorbed luminal contents and is particularly susceptible to contact with microbial antigens. A variety of infectious agents affect the liver, either as the result of direct hepatocellular or biliary invasion, or through the production of toxins. Systemic infectious processes can also cause jaundice, and non-specific liver function abnormalities are a well recognized complication of severe bacterial infections.[1]

Jaundice associated with bacterial pneumonia, appendicitis, bacteraemia in infants and other extrahepatic infections has long been recognized.[2] The possibility must be considered when encountering unusual cases of hepatitis with a cholestatic biochemical profile.[3] The newer immunofluorescence and PCR techniques have facilitated the early diagnosis of non-viral hepatic infections in contrast to the retrospective serological diagnoses in the past. However, a high degree of clinical suspicion is often necessary for diagnosis. This is especially important since early institution of appropriate therapy can avert serious or fatal complications, and save lives. Non-viral hepatic infections that cause jaundice are shown in Table I.

BACTERIAL SEPSIS AND JAUNDICE

In patients with sepsis, the liver plays two opposing roles: it is a source of inflammatory mediators as well as a target organ for the effects of the same.[4] Thus, the liver is pivotal in modulating the systemic response to severe infection. It contains the largest mass of macrophages (Kupffer cells) in the body, which can clear the endotoxins as well as the bacteria that initiate the inflammatory response.

Table I. Non-viral hepatic infections

Bacterial	Fungal
General	Histoplasmosis
Gram-negative/Gram-positive bacteraemia	Candidiasis
Sepsis syndrome	Actinomycosis
Toxic shock syndrome	Coccidioidomycosis
Specific	Paracoccidioidomycosis
Salmonella hepatitis	*Rickettsial*
Tuberculosis	Q fever
Legionnaires disease	Ehrlichosis
Brucellosis	Rocky Mountain spotted fever
Tularaemia	*Others*
Listeriosis	*Neisseria*
Melioidosis	*Chlamydia*
Spirochaetal	*Campylobacter*
Leptospirosis	Cat-scratch disease
Syphilis	
Lyme disease	

The mechanism by which bacterial infection causes cholestasis and jaundice is not clear but endotoxaemia appears to be the likely cause. Endotoxaemia can occur in the absence of documented sepsis.[5] In fact, endotoxin-mediated cytokine release, particularly tumour necrosis factor (TNF)-α, inhibits the transport of bile acids and other organic anions across the hepatic sinusoidal and bile canalicular membranes leading to intrahepatic cholestasis.[6]

The jaundice associated with sepsis was historically described as occurring in paediatric patients but a marked elevation in direct and total serum bilirubin levels has been reported in bacteraemic adults.[7,8] Antecedent liver disease, particularly that due to chronic alcohol consumption, is an important factor in the development of jaundice.

Classically, Gram-negative organisms have been implicated in hepatic dysfunction due to bacteraemia. However, numerous reports have also indicted Gram-positive organisms, especially *Staphylococcus aureus*.[9] Interestingly, infections of the lung and urinary tract are more prone to LFT abnormalities, with or without septicaemia, compared to infections at other sites.

The sepsis syndrome

The syndrome of septic jaundice is highly variable and may range from non-specific biochemical cholestasis to deep jaundice. Jaundice usually develops within a few days of the onset of bacteraemia. However, hyperbilirubinaemia may be detected much before the initial positive blood culture. Manifestations of the underlying infection usually dominate the clinical picture. Hepatomegaly is found in approximately 50% of cases and the serum bilirubin level varies from 5 to 10 mg/dl.

The magnitude or duration of jaundice does not correlate with the mortality and complications, which include acute renal failure, adult respiratory distress syndrome (ARDS) and disseminated intravascular coagulation (DIC). These complications are the same as those seen in non-jaundiced patients with severe sepsis.[9] Frank hepatic failure is usually not apparent. Jaundice, however, reflects the severity of the underlying infection. Altered LFT with no jaundice is associated with a better prognosis.[10]

Blood culture and samples from likely sources of infection must be taken before starting empirical antibiotic therapy. The results of culture of liver biopsy specimens are usually negative. When sepsis is treated with appropriate antibiotics, the LFT return to normal. Mortality rates ranging from 10% to 50% have been reported.

Though ursodeoxycholic acid (UDCA) has been used in many cholestatic liver disorders to replace toxic hydrophobic bile salts in the serum, liver and bile, so far it plays no accepted role in the cholestasis of sepsis. Treatment with recombinant human interleukin-1 receptor antagonist (rh IL-1ra),[11] and its safety and efficacy are currently under evaluation.

Toxic shock syndrome (TSS)

This is a severe, multisystem disorder occurring in patients infected with a strain of *Staph. aureus* producing a specific toxin, TSST-1. It was originally described in association with the use of tampons in women (menstrual TSS), but is now more commonly seen in surgical wounds and abscesses (non-menstrual TSS).

TSST-1 is a superantigen with high-potency lymphocyte-transforming activity.[12] The mechanism of toxicity of TSST-1 appears to be related to the release of cytokines, particularly IL-1, and TNF. Histological examination shows evidence of vasculitis and microvesicular steatosis. Liver biopsy findings include microabscesses and granulomas.

The disease is clinically characterized by high fever, a scarlatiniform rash, vomiting, diarrhoea and hypotension. Hepatic involvement is common and marked by deep jaundice with high aminotransferase levels. The diagnosis is confirmed by culture of toxigenic *Staph. aureus* from the wound, blood or other body sites. An overall mortality rate of 8%–10% has been reported.

Treatment is primarily supportive, with removal of the infected foreign bodies, drainage of infected sites and maintenance of haemodynamic stability. The early use of antistaphylococcal antibiotics may help in halting the progress of the disease.[13]

Salmonella hepatitis

Both *Salmonella typhi* and *S. paratyphi* cause enteric fever, an acute systemic disease. It is estimated that approximately 16 million cases occur every year with at least 600 000 deaths.[14] The disease affects all ages, and persons with immune deficiency are particularly at risk. Among HIV-infected people, the most commonly isolated serotypes are *S. enteritidis* and *S. typhimurium*.[14] Alcoholism has been identified as a predisposing factor in severe forms of disease due to *S. enteriditis*.[15]

Liver involvement is present in almost all cases,[16] though clinical hepatitis is not that common. Some patients may present with an acute hepatitis-like picture characterized by fever and tender hepatomegaly. The mechanism by which the organism causes hepatitis has not been established but it appears that bacterial endotoxins are the major mediators of damage. Immune mechanisms may play a role. The liver histology of *Salmonella* hepatitis is non-specific with focal necrosis, periportal mononuclear infiltration and Kupffer cell hyperplasia. The changes appear similar to those seen in Gram-negative sepsis. Lobular aggregates of Kupffer cells, known as typhoid nodules,[17] have also been described.

The manifestations are similar to those seen in other forms of acute hepatitis. Certain features, including high fever with bradycardia, may indicate infection with *Salmonella*. Patients with jaundice have more severe disease, and complications such as glomerulonephritis, liver abscess, cholangitis, neuropsychiatric disorders, encephalitis, disseminated intravascular coagulation (DIC) and even rhabdomyolysis have been reported.[18]

The biochemical profile is an important aid in diagnosis. Patients with *Salmonella* infection have a disproportionately increased serum ALP level while the aminotransferase levels are far lower than those seen in acute viral hepatitis (AVH). The ALT to LDH ratio is usually less than 4 in *Salmonella* hepatitis. A ratio >5 is seen in AVH whereas values <1.5 occur in central zonal injury, including hepatic ischaemia or acetaminophen injury.[19]

Prompt diagnosis and early intervention with proper antibiotics ensure a good prognosis. Blood culture and sensitivity proves extremely useful in view of the high incidence of resistance to chloramphenicol, amoxycillin and trimethoprim–sulphamethoxazole. Ceftriaxone and fluoroquinolones are the preferred drugs.

The organism may enter the bile and reside in the gallbladder, shedding for long periods and causing a carrier state. Long-term fluoroquinolone therapy may help eradicate the carrier state.

NON-VIRAL GRANULOMATOUS DISEASE

Many infectious organisms cause hepatic granulomatosis: proliferative inflammatory reactions resulting in granular, circumscribed lesions. The classic granuloma is a focal accumulation of modified macrophages usually surrounded and infiltrated by lymphocytes. Liver involvement is always a part of the generalized disease process.

Tuberculosis remains the commonest cause of hepatic granulomas. There is renewed interest in tuberculous infection of the liver because of the increasing incidence of extrapulmonary tuberculosis related to AIDS.[20]

An unusual but increasingly reported variant of hepatobiliary tuberculosis is obstructive jaundice[21] caused by involvement of the bile duct, pancreas and gallbladder. Compression of the biliary tree by the involved lymph nodes, or possibly by direct involvement of the biliary epithelium, or rupture of a caseating granuloma into the lumen of the bile duct may cause jaundice and biochemical cholestasis.

Bile duct tuberculosis may manifest as bile duct dilatation and common hepatic duct stricture.[22] Biliary cytological findings at ERCP may yield the diagnosis. Such patients have painless jaundice and weight loss that mimic malignant disease of the pancreas. Biliary stenting has been tried but reports are variable. Isolated pancreatic tuberculosis may also manifest as a tumour. Similarly, gallbladder tuberculosis may manifest as biliary colic with acute cholecystitis.

JAUNDICE IN PATIENTS WITH AIDS

Patients with AIDS frequently develop hepatic dysfunction. Kupffer cells are the major hepatic target cell population for HIV-1.[23] Deficits in cell-mediated immunity in AIDS may cause hepatic complications such as granulomas, CMV hepatitis, multimicrobial AIDS cholangiopathy, Kaposi sarcoma and lymphoma. Hepatic injury may also result indirectly from malnutrition, hypotension, administered medications, sepsis or other conditions.

Mycobacterium avium intracellulare typically occurs in severely immuno-compromised patients with systemic symptoms due to widely disseminated infection. CMV infection may produce acute hepatitis. CMV and cryptosporidial infections have been implicated in acalculus cholecystitis and secondary sclerosing cholangitis. About 10%–20% of patients with AIDS have chronic hepatitis B infection. These patients tend to develop minimal hepatic inflammation and necrosis. The clinical findings in patients with hepatic cryptococcal infection are usually due to concomitant extrahepatic infection.[24]

Patients with liver dysfunction and HIV-related disease should undergo a sonographic or CT examination of the liver. Patients with dilated bile ducts should undergo ERCP because opportunistic infection may produce biliary obstruction. Patients with a focal hepatic lesion should be considered for a guided liver biopsy. Liver biopsy will demonstrate considerable disease involving the liver in about 50% of patients with AIDS. The clinical impact of a diagnostic biopsy is blunted by the lack of efficacious therapy for many opportunistic infections.

LEPTOSPIROSIS

Leptospirosis has a worldwide distribution. It results from direct or indirect exposure to the urine of infected animals, usually rodents. The severity of the disease varies with the serotype, the most common of which are *Leptospira icterohaemorrhagica, canicola, autumnalis, hebdomdis, australis* and *pomona*. The organism enters the body through skin wounds or intact mucous membranes. The risk of exposure is highest among sewer workers, slaughter-house workers, miners or laboratory personnel; however, cases have been reported following recreational activity such as swimming.

The clinical picture of leptospirosis is not classical and cases may be missed if a high index of clinical suspicion is absent. The initial anicteric phase presents with high-grade fever and an influenza-like illness, often with abdominal pain, cough, chest pain, headache and myalgia. In fact, the pain may present as a biliary colic or even cholecystitis.[25] After about a week, the icteric phase begins with milder symptoms. Severe leptospirosis with deep jaundice, renal failure and haemorrhagic diathesis may develop in some patients; it is labelled Weil disease.[26]

Doxycycline may be an effective prophylaxis for Weil disease. Doxycycline or penicillin is also effective when administered in the initial stages of the disease. Hence, early diagnosis is extremely important. During the early phase, *Leptospira* can be isolated from the CSF, blood or urine. PCR assay is now available and allows rapid detection in the first 10 days of illness. Serological tests, including the IgM-specific dot ELISA technique, help to make a rapid diagnosis in the second phase of the illness.

FUNGAL INFECTIONS

The extensive use of immunosuppressive therapies, the spread of AIDS and improvement in the management of bacterial infections affecting debilitated patients have led to an increase in opportunistic fungal infections. Non-opportunistic fungal diseases in immunocompetent hosts may affect the liver. These include diseases due to dimorphic fungi such as histoplasmosis, coccidioidomycosis, paracoccidioidomycosis, blastomycosis and sporotrichosis.

In the majority, the liver is involved in cases of disseminated disease. In such a scenario, the infection may travel from the lungs to involve other organs. Hepatic involvement may manifest as fever of unknown origin. It may also manifest as unexplained biochemical cholestasis with fatigue and weight loss mimicking neoplasia or cholangitis.[27] Hepatic lesions may include diffuse granulomas distributed throughout the liver or parenchymal infiltration. The macrophages are filled with fungal elements that can be demonstrated with fungal staining.[27] Early diagnosis may be life-saving.

Management for all disseminated fungal infection is usually with intravenous amphotericin B. Disseminated candidiasis, though rare, deserves special mention because of the tendency to relapse on inadequate treatment. Further-more, radiological findings may disappear transiently during neutropenia leading to confusion about the duration of treatment.[28]

REFERENCES

1. Miller DJ, Irvine RW. Jaundice in acute appendicitis. *Lancet* 1969;**1**:321–3.
2. Neale G, Caughey DE, Mollin DL, *et al.* Effects of intrahepatic and extrahepatic infection on liver function. *BMJ* 1996;**1**:382–7
3. Elton NW. Icterus index in lobar pneumonia. *N Engl J Med* 1929;**201**:611–17.
4. Szabo G, Romics L Jr, Frendl G. Liver in sepsis and systemic inflammatory response syndrome. *Clin Liver Dis* 2002;**6**:1045–6.
5. Nolan JP. Intestinal endotoxins as mediators of hepatic injury: An idea whose time has come again. *Hepatology* 1989;**10**:887–91.

6. Moseley RH. Sepsis and cholestasis. *Clin Liver Dis* 1999;**3**:465–75.

7. Moseley RH. Sepsis associated cholestasis. *Gastroenterology* 1997;**112**:302–6.

8. Zimmerman HJ, Fang M, Utili R, *et al.* Jaundice due to bacterial infection. *Gastroenterology* 1979;**77**:362–3.

9. Franson TR, LaBrecque DR, Buggy BP, *et al.* Serial bilirubin determinations as a prognostic marker in clinical infections. *Am J Med Sci* 1989;**297**:149–50.

10. Goldman IS, Farber BF, Brandborg LL. Bacterial and miscellaneous infections of the liver. In: Zakim D, Boyer TD (eds). *Hepatology: A textbook of liver disease*. Philadelphia: WB Saunders; 1996:1232–41.

11. Fisher CJ Jr, Dhainaut JF, Opal SM, *et al.* Recombinant human interleukin 1 receptor antagonist in the treatment of patients with sepsis syndrome. *JAMA* 1994;**271**:1836–43.

12. Alouf JE, Muller-Alouf H. Staphylococcal and streptococcal superantigens: Molecular, biological and clinical aspects. *Int J Med Microbiol* 2003;**292**:429–40.

13. Herzer CM. Toxic shock syndrome: Broadening the differential diagnosis. *J Am Board Fam Pract* 2001;**14**:131–6.

14. Pramoolsinsap C, Viranuvatti V. *Salmonella* hepatitis. *J Gastroenterol Hepatol* 1998; **13**:745–50.

15. Bassa A, Parras F, Reina J, *et al.* Non typhi *Salmonella* bacteremia. *Infection* 1989; **17**:290–3.

16. Morgenstern R, Hayes PC. The liver in typhoid fever: Always affected, not just a complication. *Am J Gastroenterol* 1991;**86**:1235–9.

17. Khosla SN, Singh R, Singh JP, *et al.* The spectrum of hepatic injury in enteric fever. *Am J Gastroenterol* 1988;**83**:413–16.

18. Khan M, Coovadia Y, Sturm AW. Typhoid fever complicated by acute renal failure and hepatitis: Case reports and review. *Am J Gastroenterol* 1998;**93**:1001–3.

19. El Newihi HM, Alma ME, Reynolds TB. *Salmonella* hepatitis: Analysis of 27 cases and comparison with acute viral hepatitis. *Hepatology* 1996;**24**:516–19.

20. Alvarez SZ. Hepatobiliary tuberculosis. *J Gastroenterol Hepatol* 1998;**13**:833–9.

21. Abascal J, Martin F, Abreu L, *et al.* Atypical hepatic tuberculosis presenting as obstructive jaundice. *Am J Gastroenterol* 1988;**83**:1183–6.

22. Kok KYY, Yapp SKS. Tuberculosis of the bile duct: A rare cause of obstructive jaundice. *J Clin Gastroenterol* 1999;**29**:161–4.

23. Lefkowitch JH. The liver in AIDS. *Semin Liver Dis* 1997;**7**:335–44.

24. Capell MS. Hepatobiliary manifestations of the acquired immune deficiency syndrome. *Am J Gastroenterol* 1991;**86**:1–15.

25. Guarner J, Shieh WJ, Morgan J, *et al.* Leptospirosis mimicking acute cholecystitis among athletes participating in a triathlon. *Hum Pathol* 2001;**32**:750–2.

26. Scribe JS. The liver in enteric fever and leptospirosis. *Indian J Gastroenterol* 2001;**20**:c44–c46.

27. Lamps LW, Molina CP, West AB, *et al.* The pathologic spectrum of gastrointestinal and hepatic histoplasmosis. *Am J Clin Pathol* 2000;**113**:64–72.

28. Pestalozzi BC, Krestin GP, Schanz U, *et al.* Hepatic lesions of chronic disseminated candidiasis may become invisible during neutropenia. *Blood* 1997;**90**:3858–64.

CHAPTER 11

Jaundice in alcoholics

SANJEEV SACHDEVA, VIVEK A. SARASWAT

Alcohol has been known to mankind since the beginning of recorded history and has been linked to liver disease for centuries.[1] The word 'alcohol' is attributed to Paracelsus (c.1530 AD), and is derived from the Arabic word *al-kuhl* meaning 'the finest part'. It is probably the most easily available and widely used mood-altering substance worldwide, and is a hepatotoxin that has achieved social acceptance. Most people drink in moderation without any problem, but some indulge in alcohol abuse; that is, overindulgence resulting in physical damage. Alcohol addiction may follow and is defined by the presence of physical and/or psychological dependence on alcohol. Alcoholism is well described by the acronym TyPICAL (Tolerance, Physical dependence, Impaired Control or craving for ALcohol). Alcoholic liver disease (ALD) is the commonest cause of cirrhosis in the western world[2] and, with improving socioeconomic standards of living, it has also become an important cause of liver injury in a number of developing countries.

Alcohol intake (g/day) may be calculated by the formula $0.79 \times \%$ alcohol content of the beverage $\times$ intake in ml/day. For beer, wine and whisky, 10 g alcohol equivalents are 250 ml, 100 ml and 30 ml, respectively. The severity of ALD is related not only to the quantity of alcohol consumed; several other factors also play an important role in its pathogenesis.

FACTORS ASSOCIATED WITH THE FREQUENCY AND SEVERITY OF ALD

The risk of developing ALD begins at an intake level of 30 g/day and becomes substantial beyond 80 g/day.[3,4] Liver disease is 2–4 times more likely to develop in women who drink excessively than in men.[5] If consumed regularly for over 5–10 years, the threshold for alcohol-induced hepatic injury is 60 g/day for men and 30 g/day for women. However, not all who ingest large amounts of alcohol (>60 g/day) develop ALD; serious liver disease develops only in approximately 1 in 10 individuals.[3] Apart from gender, dose and duration of alcohol consumption, other factors that influence the frequency and severity of ALD include heredity (certain human leucocyte antigen [HLA] haplotypes, mutations in the tumour necrosis factor [TNF] promotor region, genetic isomorphisms for different enzymes responsible for alcohol metabolism), coexistent liver diseases (chronic hepatitis C or B, others), concurrent exposure to hepatotoxins (acetaminophen), immunological response, body iron stores, malnutrition[6] and obesity.[7]

ALCOHOL AS A PROBLEM IN INDIA

In a survey of the general population of Mumbai, the prevalence of alcoholism was found to be about 18% in men >45 years of age.[8] A drinking problem was present in 23.3% of patients admitted to a general hospital in Bangalore.[9] However, alcohol was considered to be the cause in only 1.7% of 175 patients with chronic liver disease in West Bengal.[10] A cumulative alcohol dose of >2000 ml-years was found to be a reliable cut-off for association with liver disease.[11]

JAUNDICE IN ALCOHOL USERS

As in any individual, jaundice may occur in alcohol users due to hepatic and extrahepatic causes. Hepatic causes are the commonest.

Hepatic causes

Due to or influenced by alcohol abuse
Alcoholic liver disease (fatty liver, hepatitis, cirrhosis)
Alcohol-related iron overload
Altered hepatic drug metabolism
Interaction with other chronic hepatitis agents (HCV, HBV)
Hepatocellular carcinoma (HCC)
Porphyria cutanea tarda (PCT)

Concomitant liver diseases unrelated to alcohol abuse
Acute viral hepatitis
Drug-induced liver disease
Infiltrative disorders, e.g. tuberculosis
Space-occupying lesions of the liver, e.g. amoebic liver abscess
Hepatic venous outflow tract obstruction

Extrahepatic (haematological) causes

Megaloblastosis with ineffective erythropoiesis
Haemolytic anaemia (burr cell, spur cell, Zieve syndrome, hypersplenism)

Extrahepatic (non-haematological) causes

Cardiac: Alcohol-related cardiomyopathy, congestive cardiac failure, cardiac cirrhosis

Extrahepatic biliary obstruction: Gall stone disease, pancreatic carcinoma, acute or chronic pancreatitis.

METABOLISM OF ALCOHOL

Alcohol is predominantly metabolized in the liver, though other parts of the gastrointestinal tract such as the stomach also play a role.

Gastric metabolism

The activity of gastric alcohol dehydrogenase (ADH), the first enzyme to process alcohol in the body, is lesser in women than in men.[12]

Hepatic metabolism

Three enzyme systems (ADH, cytochrome P450 2E1 [CYP2E1] and catalase) are involved in the metabolism of alcohol in the liver. ADH is the main enzyme that metabolizes alcohol at low blood levels (<50 mg/dl), while at higher levels CYP2E1 becomes more important and produces oxyradicals. Catalase plays a minor role. Alcohol is converted to a potentially toxic metabolite, acetaldehyde, by ADH/CYP2E1. Acetaldehyde is converted to acetate by aldehyde dehydro-genase (ALDH) at low acetaldehyde concentrations, while the aldehyde/xanthine oxidase pathway is activated at higher concentrations, and also results in the formation of oxyradicals.

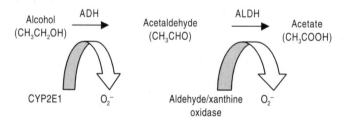

PATHOGENESIS OF ALCOHOLIC LIVER INJURY

Alcohol-induced liver injury occurs due to three pathogenetic mechanisms: (i) toxic and metabolic; (ii) immunological and inflammatory; and (iii) mechanisms leading to liver fibrosis (Table 1). Damage induced by alcohol may be direct (Fig. 1) or indirect (Fig. 2), wherein endotoxin activation and release of cytokines play a key role.

Table I. Mechanisms involved in the pathogenesis of alcoholic liver disease

Toxic and metabolic mechanisms
• Oxidant stress
• Redox alteration
• Effects of hypoxia
• Toxicity due to acetaldehyde

Immunological and inflammatory mechanisms
• Neoantigens. Adducts between hydroxyethyl radicals/acetaldehyde and hepatocellular proteins
• Kupffer cell activation with release of inflammatory cytokines such as transforming growth factor (TGF)-β, tumour necrosis factor (TNF), interleukin-1,-6, -8, nuclear factor kappa B (NF-κB), superoxide, monocyte chemoattractant protein-1 (MCP-1), etc.

Mechanisms leading to fibrosis
• Activation of hepatic stellate cells stimulated by TGF-β, oxyradicals, acetaldehyde–protein adducts

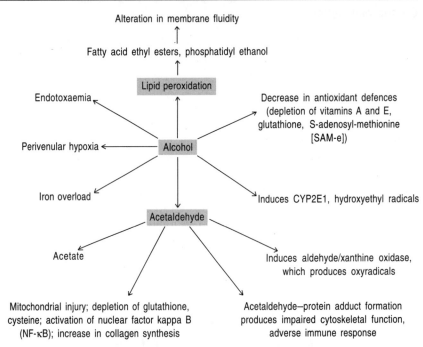

Fig. 1. Direct pathway of alcohol-induced liver injury

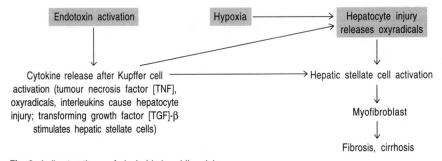

Fig. 2. Indirect pathway of alcohol-induced liver injury

SPECTRUM AND NATURAL HISTORY OF LIVER INJURY

The spectrum of liver damage due to alcohol ranges from fatty change to malignant transformation. The spectrum of liver lesions includes:

- Alcoholic fatty liver (classic and alcoholic foamy degeneration)
- Alcoholic hepatitis (fulminant, chronic aggressive, chronic persistent, 'pseudotumour')
- Alcoholic cirrhosis (with/without concomitant hepatitis)
- HCC

Classically, the disease progresses through phases of fatty change, inflammation, fibrosis and cirrhosis, with or without evident portal hypertension. Only a minority (5%–15%) develop HCC. With sustained abstinence, the liver lesions may regress; however, this is not possible if advanced fibrosis or cirrhosis has set in (Fig. 3).

Alcoholic foamy degeneration

This is a variant of fatty liver and is a rare entity seen in <10% of all cases of fatty liver. It was described for the first time by Uchida in 1983.[13] The characteristic histological feature is the accumulation of finely dispersed perivenular microvesicular lipid (Fig. 4). Other histological features include cholestasis, megamitochondria, focal liver cell necrosis, and macrovesicular steatosis in other zones, occasional perivenular fibrosis, negligible inflammation and no Mallory bodies. Cholestasis is possibly due to compression of the intrahepatic biliary radicles and/or increased permeability of the bile ductules.

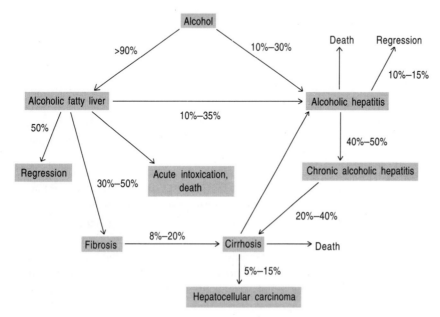

Fig. 3. Natural history of alcoholic liver disease

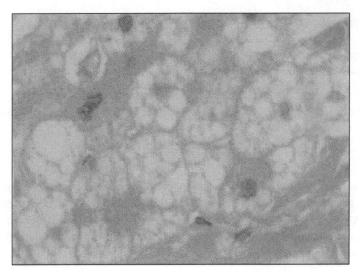

Fig. 4. Alcoholic foamy degeneration (H&E)

Clinically, it may present as a first episode of hepatic decompensation in the absence of encephalopathy or portal hypertension. Jaundice is generally marked with features of cholestasis and hepatomegaly but, in contrast to alcoholic hepatitis, there is no pyrexia or peripheral blood leucocytosis.

Laboratory evaluation reveals persistent marked elevation of serum ALP and cholesterol levels. In most cases, the condition resolves following cessation of alcohol.

Alcohol-related cholestasis

Cholestasis is a not infrequent problem and is seen in about 20% of all patients with ALD (range 10%–86%).[14-17] It may be intrahepatic or extrahepatic.

Intrahepatic cholestasis may be due to hepatocellular disease (fatty liver, alcoholic hepatitis, alcoholic cirrhosis) or a space-occupying lesion in the liver. The AST/ALT ratio is generally >1.4.

Extrahepatic cholestasis may be due to a CBD stone, stenosis at the lower end of the CBD due to alcohol-related chronic pancreatitis, or pancreatic carcinoma. The AST/ALT ratio is generally <1.4.

Diagnosis is based on the laboratory findings (elevated serum bilirubin, serum ALP, serum bile acids, hypercholesterolaemia) and liver histology (characterized by intracellular, canalicular, and/or bile ductular cholestasis, frequently forming bile plugs). Levels of serum bilirubin and serum ALP (generally >4 times the upper limit of normal) are more strikingly elevated than those of AST or ALT (generally <200 U/L). USG reliably differentiates intrahepatic from extrahepatic causes of cholestasis. Cholangiography (MRCP/ERCP) may be required in case there is a strong suspicion of extrahepatic cholestasis that is not confirmed by sonography.

A variety of mechanisms contribute to intrahepatic cholestasis. These include disturbances in basolateral uptake, intracellular transport and metabolism of bile acids and bile salts, microscopic cholangitis, idiosyncratic immunologically mediated response with release of cytokines (e.g. IL-1, TNF-α) and hepatic steatosis. Steatosis alone can cause cholestasis, presumably by compressing the biliary radicles or impairing ductular permeability.

A severe cholestatic syndrome may be observed in patients with alcoholic fatty liver, mimicking the clinical picture of extrahepatic biliary obstruction. Severe forms may progress to acute liver failure.[18] Nissenbaum *et al.*[14] found a significant correlation between cholestasis and malnutrition, PT, AST, serum ALP, serum bilirubin, serum albumin, serum cholylglycine levels and histological severity score. They found cholestasis to be a highly significant prognostic indicator of outcome in alcoholic hepatitis.

Therapy depends on whether cholestasis is intrahepatic or extrahepatic. For extrahepatic causes, surgery is the mainstay of therapy. For intrahepatic causes, abstinence from alcohol, improved nutrition, and administration of ursodeoxycholic acid and corticosteroids are known to be of help.

Alcohol and chronic hepatitis B virus infection

The prevalence of serum HBV markers in alcoholics is 2–4-fold higher than that in control populations and ranges between 30% and 50%. This is mainly due to the increased prevalence of markers of past infection such as anti-HBc and anti-HBs, alone or in combination. Whereas HBsAg is found in only about 5%, indicating that while exposure to HBV may be commoner than in the general population, the risk of chronicity is not increased among alcoholics.

Ethanol impairs host defence by decreasing the inflammatory response, altering cytokine production and inducing generation of abnormal reactive oxygen intermediates. Ethanol inhibits the antiviral response to IFN-α and promotes viral replication. HBV sensitizes the hepatocytes to TNF-α or ethanol-induced apoptosis by a caspase-3 dependent mechanism. Ethanol potentiates HBV-mediated activation of nuclear factor kappa B (NF-κB) in the liver.

The adverse effects of chronic HBV infection in an alcoholic include accelerated progression of liver injury, increased risk for cirrhosis[19,20] and HCC.[21]

Management of HBV infection in an alcoholic requires sobriety before the initiation of IFN treatment and continued sobriety during the course of therapy.

Alcohol and chronic hepatitis C virus infection

The frequency of chronic HCV infection may be as high as 45% in alcoholics, being higher in those with ALD. The prevalence of fatty liver, hepatitis and cirrhosis is 20%, 21% and 43%, respectively.[22]

The coexistence of alcohol abuse and chronic HCV infection amplifies the severity of liver injury due to interaction at various levels. Alcohol impairs host defences by decreasing inflammatory response, altering cytokine production and inducing abnormal reactive oxygen intermediates, and may compromise the host immune response to HCV infection, resulting in chronicity. Alcohol also enhances HCV replication resulting in greater HCV viraemia and direct cytopathic damage. Alcohol-induced liver injury synergistically aggravates histological damage due to HCV infection, resulting in faster progression. A higher content of hepatic iron associated with ALD may increase the replication of HCV.

Clinical implications

In the presence of chronic HCV infection, alcohol consumption has important effects on the natural history of liver disease. The threshold dose that induces liver injury is reduced; intake >30 g/day of alcohol is considered harmful. There is a 34% increased risk of progression of fibrosis in alcoholics consuming >50 g/day compared to non-drinkers,[23] and the risk of cirrhosis is increased 4-fold in those who consume >80 g/day of alcohol.[24] Viral replication is enhanced, with higher HCV RNA levels and more HCV quasispecies.[25,26]

The histopathological picture is generally that of chronic HCV infection and not ALD. In HCV-infected patients, alcohol has been found to increase the histological activity as well as fibrosis indices[27,28] and results in higher aminotransferase levels.[29] The risk for HCC is increased almost 4-fold[30,31] and the risk of death is increased 10-fold.[32] The response to antiviral therapy is poorer in moderate and heavy alcohol drinkers, with sustained virological response seen in 20% and 9%, respectively.[33] Abstinence is essential before and during antiviral treatment. Most researchers suggest that antiviral therapy should be offered only after 1–2 years of sobriety.

Alcohol and hepatocellular carcinoma

Hepatocellular carcinoma arises in 5%–15% of patients with alcoholic cirrhosis,[34] and is 2–6 times more frequent than in cirrhosis due to other causes. Development of HCC accounts for one-third of all deaths due to ALD.[35] The risk increases once the intake exceeds 65 g/day for more than 5 years.[30] The relationship between alcohol and HCC is attributed primarily to cirrhosis, the key precursor lesion, but studies show that even without cirrhosis, the incidence of HCC is increased,[36,37] which may be partly related to chronic HCV or HBV infection.[38,39] In alcoholic cirrhosis, the 10-year cumulative risk of developing HCC is 81% in patients with chronic HCV infection as compared to 19% in alcoholics without HCV infection.

Alcoholic beverages may contain carcinogens such as nitrosamines, polycyclic hydrocarbons and asbestos fibres. Secondary iron overload may contribute as well. The possibility that alcohol may have carcinogenic potential *per se* has been raised because of reports of HCC arising in non-cirrhotic alcoholic patients.[40]

Alcohol may act as a co-factor or indirect tumour promotor by virtue of its effects on hepatocellular metabolism such as:

- changes in membrane properties with respect to cellular absorption of carcinogens;

- increased biotransformation of carcinogens by mixed function oxidases and activation of the microsomal ethanol oxidizing system by ethanol intake;
- altered immune surveillance (suppression of natural killer cell activity and numbers via TGF-β1);
- general hypomethylation of oncogenes (c-*myc*, c-n-*ras*) in association with areas of regional hypermethylation of tumour suppressor genes (p53);[41]
- toxicity of its metabolite acetaldehyde;
- decrease in retinoic acid levels; and
- acetaldehyde–protein adducts that act as neo-antigens, and have mutagenic and antigenic properties.

Apart from ensuring abstinence, the management of HCC in this situation is similar to that in any other setting.

Altered hepatic drug metabolism

The mechanisms of drug toxicity in alcoholics include the following:

- selective induction of specific types of cytochrome P450 enzymes;
- depletion of hepatic glutathione reserves;
- competitive inhibition of certain CYP2E1 enzymes;
- selective induction of glucuronosyltransferases;
- decreased production of uridine diphosphate (UDP)–glucuronic acid; and
- stimulation of acetylation by increasing the hepatic concentration of acetyl-CoA.

Alcohol and porphyria

Alcohol intake can provoke clinical expression of hepatic porphyria.[44] This is true for PCT as well as both the acute and latent phases of chronic hepatic

Drugs/toxins that induce hepatoxicity in alcoholics	
Acetaminophen	Methotrexate
Non-steroidal anti-inflammatory drugs	Halothane
Vitamin A[42]	Cocaine
Beta-carotenoids[43]	Carbon tetrachloride
Antitubercular drugs	Aflatoxins
Herbal drugs (e.g. germander, chapperal)	Industrial solvents

porphyria, and the acute form. Over 50% of cases of PCT are associated with excess consumption of alcohol.[45]

The mechanisms of induction of hepatic porphyria include: (i) inhibition of uroporphyrin decarboxylase; (ii) induction of delta-amino-laevulinic acid synthetase; and (iii) increase in iron absorption, thereby accelerating the development of PCT. Management includes avoiding not only sunlight but also alcohol.

Alcohol and iron overload

Alcohol ingestion leads to secondary iron overload.[46] Hepatic iron stores are increased in 40%–60% of alcoholics[47] but the increase is usually mild to moderate. Clinically, it may present as cirrhosis associated with diabetes mellitus, hypogonadism and skin pigmentation.

The mechanisms of iron overload in alcoholics include the following:

- increased intake and intestinal absorption of iron;
- stimulation of production of desialylated transferrin, which promotes hepatic iron uptake;
- impaired utilization of iron due to impaired erythropoiesis as a result of folate deficiency and myelotoxicity of alcohol;
- repeated episodes of haemolysis;
- enhanced hepatic iron deposition due to liver damage; and
- portosystemic shunting, which may provoke iron deposition in the liver.

Alcohol-associated iron overload may be differentiated from primary haemochromatosis by *HFE* gene mutation analysis, and a liver biopsy with hepatic iron index.

The degree of iron deposition is lesser in alcohol-associated iron overload than in primary haemochromatosis (Fig. 5). The site of excess iron deposition is primarily the Kupffer cell and not the hepatocyte, as occurs in primary haemochromatosis. The hepatic iron index is below 2.

The clinical implications of alcohol-associated iron overload are that iron may contribute to alcohol-induced liver disease by increased peroxidation and increased susceptibility of the liver to other damaging agents. It may contribute to liver fibrosis

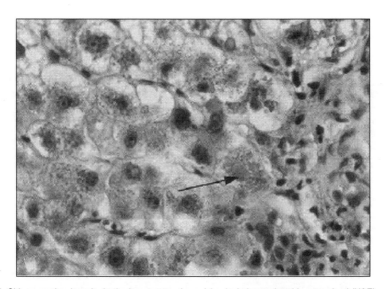

Fig. 5. Siderogranular deposits in the hepatocytes (arrow) in alcohol-associated iron overload (H&E)

and there is a higher incidence of HCC. In other respects, the prognosis of iron overload associated with ALD seems to be that of the underlying ALD.

Alcohol and macrocytic anaemia with ineffective erythropoiesis

The mean corpuscular volume of RBCs is increased in up to 90% of heavy alcoholics.[48] Macrocytosis in alcoholics may occur as a result of vitamin deficiency in the malnourished alcoholic. Folic acid deficiency occurs in 6%–80% of cases,[49,50] and deficiency of vitamins B_1, B_2, B_6 and B_{12} is common. The metabolism of vitamin B_{12} and folic acid is also impaired.

Other causes of macrocytosis in alcoholic patients include: (i) reticulocytosis associated with haemolysis and/or bleeding; (ii) direct effect of alcohol on the bone marrow through primitive erythroid precursor cell vacuolization and antagonism of the effect of folic acid on haemopoiesis;[51] and (iii) increase in the cholesterol and phospholipid content of the RBC membrane.

Management

A full work-up including complete haemogram and peripheral smear examination, bone marrow aspiration and biopsy is desirable. Therapy includes abstinence and adequate supplementation of vitamins.

ALCOHOL AND HAEMOLYSIS

Haemolysis in alcoholics may be due to extracorpuscular or intracorpuscular factors. These may cause morphological abnormalities in the RBCs which can lead to haemolysis.

The pathophysiological basis of defects in the RBC membrane includes: (i) changes in the lipid composition of the RBC membrane; (ii) changes in plasma lipoproteins secondary to alcohol consumption resulting in reduced membrane fluidity; and (iii) hypophosphataemia that may cause low levels of RBC adenosine triphosphate (ATP).

Morphological abnormalities of RBCs in ALD	Important causes of haemolysis in ALD
• Spherocytes (in Zieve syndrome) • Schistocytes (burr cell anaemia) • Acanthocytes (spur cell anaemia) • Macrocytes • Stomatocytes (tear-drop poikilocytes) • Target cells • Triangulocytes • Knizocytes	• Hypersplenism • Spur cell anaemia • Burr cell anaemia • Zieve syndrome • Hypophosphataemia

Burr cell anaemia

This is related to reversible, saturable binding of abnormal high-density lipoprotein (HDL) by the RBC surface and is characterized by spiculated RBCs or echinocytes seen well on electron microscopy in peripheral blood smears. The anaemia is generally mild. The pathophysiological significance is unknown.

Spur cell anaemia

This condition was first described by Smith *et al*.[52] Mechanisms involved in the development of spur cell anaemia in alcoholics include increase in the ratio of free cholesterol to phospholipid in the erythrocyte membrane, resulting in a decrease in membrane fluidity,[53] and hypophosphataemia, resulting in ATP deficiency in severely malnourished alcoholics. Abnormal lipids contained in the membrane of erythrocytes make them susceptible to damage from oxidant stress, leading to their deformation. Cooper *et al*.[53] suggested a two-stage hypothesis. The first stage is dependent on abnormal serum lipoprotein composition. This results in erythrocytes passively accumulating excess cholesterol, thereby acquiring an increased surface area and being transformed into cells with scalloped contours. The second stage is characterized by loss of cell surface area as the cells pass through the spleen, resulting in their transformation to cells with spiculated contours, and lysis by the splenic macrophages.

Spur cell anaemia is characterized by the presence of acanthocytes (spur cells—erythrocytes with irregular, spiny projections of the cell membrane). The resulting anaemia is generally marked, and usually occurs in the presence of alcoholic cirrhosis and severe underlying disease. Jaundice, ascites, encephalopathy and/or GI bleeding usually precede or follow the development of haemolysis. Although patients may survive for many months with acanthocytosis, the prognosis of the underlying liver disease is generally poor. There is no effective treatment other than liver transplantation.[54] Combination therapy with flunarizine, pentoxyfylline and cholestyramine may help.[55]

Zieve syndrome

In 1958, Zieve[56] described a syndrome consisting of a triad of hyperlipidaemia, jaundice and haemolytic anaemia in the presence of liver disease. He suggested that this was a distinct syndrome, with haemolysis being caused by the hyperlipoproteinaemia. The syndrome appears to be distinctly uncommon, in spite of the fact that alcohol abuse is so common.

Pathogenesis

The exact cause of the transient haemolysis remains obscure. Erythrocytes have been shown to have a low ATP content, high 2,3 diphosphoglycerate (DPG) and decreased glucose utilization. The enzyme erythrocyte pyruvate kinase shows marked thermal instability and an altered *Km*; it is probably inhibited by acetaldehyde, the highly reactive metabolite of ethanol. Acetaldehyde also binds to the RBC membrane and produces stomatocytes that affect the RBC ion flux.[57] These red cell defects predispose to autohaemolysis by a circulating, non-corpuscular haemolysin, possibly lysolecithin or lysocephalin.[58] Goebel *et al.*[59] proposed that low levels of vitamin E in the RBCs cause an increase in glutathione oxidation, thus causing pyruvate kinase instability which triggers haemolytic anaemia. Hence, Zieve syndrome represents a peculiar reaction to alcohol in predisposed individuals, perhaps due to an enzyme deficiency that prevents adequate detoxification of alcohol or its metabolites in the RBCs.

Diagnosis

Jaundice, abdominal pain, nausea, vomiting, diarrhoea and fever are the usual presenting symptoms[60] generally following an alcoholic binge, and may mimic an acute abdomen. Zieve syndrome almost always affects men in their forties, though it may occur in all forms of ALD.

A history of alcohol abuse, an elevated autohaemolysis test result, and RBC pyruvate kinase heat instability should establish the diagnosis as the hyperlipid-aemia is transitory and not always present when the diagnosis is made. The hyperlipidaemia generally involves all the lipid fractions. Rapidly developing anaemia results in reticulocytosis, and is at the same time responsible for increased erythropoiesis; this boosts the lipid-storing reticular cells (so-called foam cells) in the bone marrow.

Treatment

The condition usually reverses within a few weeks of abstinence.

ALCOHOL AND THE HEART

The association between alcohol intake and congestive cardiomyopathy was reported more than a century ago. Previously this was attributed to nutritional deficiencies or toxic additives rather than the alcohol itself. Several recent studies excluding alcoholics with malnutrition have established a direct relationship between alcohol consumption and cardiac damage.[61] Alcohol consumption >60 g/day for 10 years or more is required for the development of cardiac decompen-sation. Up to 30%–50% of heavy alcoholics may have echocardiographic abnormalities suggestive of congestive cardiomyopathy.

Clinical features

The onset is generally insidious with non-specific fatigue, chest discomfort, palpitations or an isolated episode of atrial fibrillation.[62] As the condition progresses, manifestations of overt right heart failure (elevated right atrial pressure with distension of the jugular veins and peripheral oedema); and left heart failure (orthopnoea and paroxysmal nocturnal dyspnoea) become apparent.

Mild jaundice can occur as a result of congestion and later as a result of cardiac cirrhosis, in case the disease persists for a long period. Continued alcohol abuse after decompensation of cardiac function can result in death in 2–4 years from cardiac failure; sudden cardiac death from ventricular arrhythmias may also occur.

Laboratory, electrocardiographic and echocardiographic abnormalities are similar to those of congestive cardiomyopathy due to any other cause. Management includes strict abstinence from alcohol combined with supportive therapy for associated heart failure and arrhythmias.

ALCOHOL AND GALL STONES

There are conflicting reports in the literature regarding the relationship between alcohol consumption and the formation of gall stones.

Alcohol consumption might protect against the development of cholesterol gall stones by lowering bile cholesterol saturation. However, the development of cirrhosis predisposes to pigment stone formation and alcohol is one of the commonest causes of cirrhosis worldwide. There is increased haemolysis as a result of megaloblastosis and the resultant ineffective erythropoiesis. RBC membrane defects as in Zieve syndrome, and burr and spur cell anaemias increase haemolysis. Hypersplenism as a result of chronic liver disease also aggravates haemolysis.

Schwesinger et al.[63] proposed that both liver cirrhosis and alcohol abuse predispose to the formation of pigment gall stones, and that the effects of alcohol may occur independent of cirrhosis. In cirrhotics, 80% of gall stones are pigment stones as compared to subjects without chronic liver disease in whom 80% are cholesterol stones.

Buchner and Sonnenberg[64] in their large study involving 38 459 patients and 69 336 controls, found a 5.2% prevalence of gall stones in the general population, 7.5% in patients with liver disease, 9.5% in those with alcoholic cirrhosis, and 9.1% in patients with alcoholic fatty liver.

Cholelithiasis may be associated with choledocholithiasis which, in turn, may cause episodes of jaundice if untreated.

ALCOHOL AND THE PANCREAS

Chronic ethanol abuse is the commonest cause of acute and chronic pancreatitis in western countries. Heavy intake (>80 g/day) on a regular basis for >15 years predisposes to this complication. The mean age at onset is 35–50 years; 72% are men.[65]

Three main pathogenetic hypotheses have been proposed.

1. *Big duct hypothesis* implicates the premature activation of pancreatic enzymes by the entry of bile or duodenal contents through the common channel, i.e. biliopancreatic and duodenopancreatic reflux, and sphincter of Oddi spasm;

2. *Small duct hypothesis* invokes ductal obstruction by protein plugs due to increased viscosity or hypersecretion of proteins, increased lactoferrin and decreased lithostathine;
3. *Initial acinar cell injury hypothesis* postulates that free radical injury, hyperstimulation of leucocytes, lysosomal hyperreactivity and cholinergic hyperactivity initiate the necrosis–fibrosis sequence causing pancreatic damage.

Natural history and clinical course

The clinical course is characterized initially by recurrent attacks of acute pancreatitis precipitated by alcohol abuse. This is followed by chronic, persistent, or intermittent abdominal pain (chronic pancreatitis) with or without attacks of acute pancreatitis and the development of pancreatic calcification (median 9 years), steatorrhoea (median 13 years), and diabetes mellitus (median 20 years).[65] In addition, local pancreatic or extrapancreatic complications (e.g. pseudocyst formation, strictures of the adjacent organs, haemorrhages) may occur during the second decade of symptomatic disease. One-third of the patients with recurrent acute alcoholic pancreatitis do not progress to chronic pancreatitis, which develops in about 5%–15% of alcoholic patients.

Although the incidence of cirrhosis in patients with alcoholic chronic pancreatitis is 0%–30.7%, the presence of pancreatic damage does not seem to be related to the severity of ALD.[66,67] In some cases, however, the clinical course is insidious and the illness progresses to pancreatic insufficiency without acute inflammatory episodes.[68]

Carcinoma of the pancreas may occur more frequently in alcoholic patients. The majority of patients with pancreatic cancer also have lesions of chronic pancreatitis. The reported incidence of pancreatic carcinoma in alcoholic chronic pancreatitis is 2.8%[69] and the reported increased cumulative risk of developing carcinoma in chronic pancreatitis is 2% per decade.[70]

The diagnosis of chronic pancreatitis is made on the basis of imaging studies (USG and CT scan of the abdomen, MRCP/ERCP) and pancreatic function tests.

Common bile duct stenosis in chronic pancreatitis

This was first reported in 1900 by Mayo Robson[71] and is seen in about 10% of patients. Its prevalence varies from 5% to 46%.[72,73]

Clinical features

It may manifest as an incidental finding on MRCP/ERCP, an isolated elevation of serum ALP, or may present with pain and jaundice with or without cholangitis. The risk of developing secondary biliary cirrhosis has been stressed in some studies,[74,75] but questioned by others.[76,77] The natural history of this condition is influenced by numerous factors including pancreatic oedema,

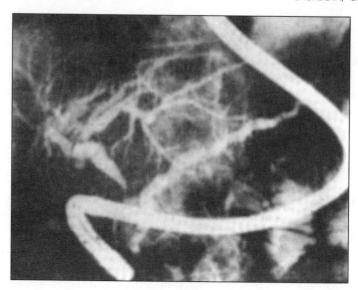

Fig. 6. Alcoholic chronic pancreatitis. ERCP shows dilatation and irregularity of the pancreatic duct, and narrowing of the common bile duct (stricture) at the lower end.

pseudocyst formation or pancreatic abscess during acute relapses that may reverse or resolve, and progressive, irreversible pancreatic fibrosis and calcification during the end stage of the disease. Pancreatic carcinoma is another cause of CBD stenosis in the background of chronic pancreatitis, but narrowing of the distal CBD is usually due to fibrosis (stricture) in the majority. This may or may not be associated with choledocholithiasis. Jaundice is present in about 50% of cases where CBD stenosis is due to fibrosis, while its incidence is about 20% when it is due to reversible factors such as local oedema.[78]

Diagnosis

This is made by estimation of the serum bilirubin, serum ALP, USG of the abdomen to look for evidence of extrahepatic biliary obstruction and cholangiography (MRCP/ERCP) (Fig. 6). Persistent elevation of serum ALP (equal to or more than twice the upper limit of normal) can be used as a reliable screening test for the detection of CBD stenosis. Normal levels of serum transaminases and a normal serum aminotransferase ratio (AST/ALT≤1.4) may help to differentiate extrahepatic cholestasis as in CBD stricture from intrahepatic cholestasis due to ALD.[78] Liver biopsy may be necessary to rule out ALD with intrahepatic cholestasis and to evaluate the long-term effect of CBD stricture on the liver (early or advanced secondary biliary cirrhosis).

Treatment

The treatment is primarily surgical. While conservative management may be appropriate in asymptomatic patients with a normal or minimally raised serum ALP level, a bilioenteric anastomosis is indicated in those with persistent elevation of serum ALP or jaundice not associated with ALD and persistent

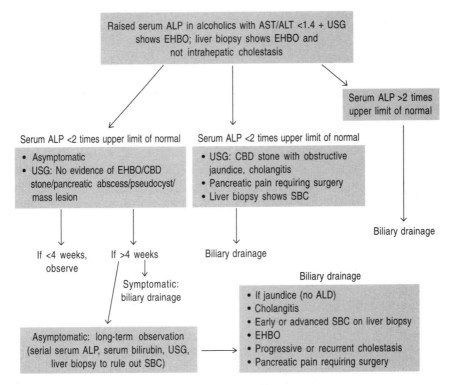

Fig. 7. Management of biliary obstruction in chronic pancreatitis
EHBO: extrahepatic biliary obstruction; SBC: secondary biliary cirrhosis; ALD: alcoholic liver disease

biliary obstruction (>4 weeks) on imaging because of the risk of cholangitis and secondary biliary cirrhosis.[79,80] Biliary drainage is also indicated in the presence of choledocholithiasis, cholangitis and in patients undergoing pancreatic surgery for pain relief (combined biliopancreatic decompression).

Choledochoduodenostomy is preferable to choledochojejunostomy unless a Roux loop is required to drain a pseudocyst or when a pancreatic duct drainage procedure is needed.[81] Careful, long-term observation of patients treated without biliary drainage should include serial estimations of serum ALP and bilirubin, USG of the abdomen, MRCP/ERCP and radionuclide biliary scintigraphy, and perhaps liver biopsy (Fig. 7).[82] The presence of secondary biliary cirrhosis (SBC) constitutes an indication for biliary drainage. Several series of patients have been reported in which comparable long-term results have been obtained after endoscopic biliary drainage and repeated biliary stenting.

CONCLUSION

Jaundice in an alcoholic individual may be as varied and multifactorial as in a person not taking alcohol. Close attention to the clinical history and investigations are required to determine the likely cause or combination of causes of jaundice in the given patient and the best management strategy. Some entities that are peculiar to alcohol abusers need particular consideration such as foamy degeneration and alcohol-related intrahepatic cholestasis. The numerous drug interactions due to induction of the hepatic microsomal enzyme systems in the alcoholic also need to be borne in mind. The management of jaundice in the alcoholic individual is often rewarding, since correctable, reversible factors are not uncommon and much may be achieved by abstinence from alcohol, relief of biliary obstruction, and treatment of concomitant hepatitis virus infections.

REFERENCES

1. Ravi Varma LA. Alcoholism in Ayurveda. *Q J Stud Alc* 1950;**11**:484–91.
2. Leiber CS. Alcoholic liver disease: A public health issue in need of a public health approach. *Semin Liver Dis* 1993;**13**:105–7.
3. Kerr WC, Fillmore KM, Marvy P. Beverage-specific alcohol consumption and cirrhosis mortality in a group of English-speaking beer-drinking countries [Comments]. *Addiction* 2000;**95**:339–46.
4. Lelbach WK. Cirrhosis in the alcoholic and its relation to the volume of alcohol abuse. *Ann N Y Acad Sci* 1975;**252**:85–105.
5. Tuyns AJ, Pequignot G. Greater risk of ascitic cirrhosis in females in relation to alcohol consumption. *Int J Epidemiol* 1984;**13**:53–7.
6. Mendenhall CL, Tosch T, Weesner RE, *et al.* VA Cooperative Study on alcoholic hepatitis, II. Prognostic significance of protein–calorie malnutrition. *Am J Clin Nutr* 1986;**43**:213–18.
7. Bellantani S, Saccoccio G, Masutti F, *et al.* Prevalence of and risk factors for hepatic steatosis in northern Italy. *Ann Intern Med* 2000;**132**:112–17.
8. Gupta PC, Saxena S, Pednekar MS, *et al.* Alcohol consumption among middle-aged and elderly men: A community study from Western India. *Alcohol Alcohol* 2003;**38**:327–31.
9. Sri EV, Raguram R, Srivastava M. Alcohol problems in a general hospital—A prevalence study. *J Indian Med Assoc* 1997;**95**:505–6.
10. De U, Ghoshal UC, Deb AC, *et al.* Aetiological spectrum of chronic liver disease in eastern India. *Trop Gastroenterol* 2000;**21**:60–2.
11. Narawane NM, Bhatia S, Abraham P, Sanghani S, Sawant SS. Consumption of 'country liquor' and its relation to alcoholic liver disease in Mumbai. *J Assoc Physicians India* 1998;**46**:510–13.
12. Frezza M, di Padova C, Pozzato G, *et al.* High blood alcohol levels in women: The role of decreased gastric alcohol dehydrogenase activity and first-pass metabolism. *N Engl J Med* 1990;**322**:95–9.
13. Uchida T, Kao H, Quispe-Sjogren M, Peters RL. Alcoholic foamy degeneration—A pattern of acute alcoholic injury of the liver. *Gastroenterology* 1983;**84**:683–92.
14. Nissenbaum M, Chedid A, Mendenhall C, Gartside P, and the VA Cooperative Study Group. Prognostic significance of cholestatic alcoholic hepatitis. *Dig Dis Sci* 1990;**35**:891–6.
15. Glover SC, McPhie JL, Brunt PW. Cholestasis in acute alcoholic liver disease. *Lancet* 1977;**2**:1305–7.
16. Harinasuta U, Chomet B, Ishak K, Zimmerman HJ. Steatonecrosis—Mallory body type. *Medicine* 1967;**46**:141–62.
17. Perrillo RP, Griffin R, DeSchryver-Keeskemeti K, Lander JJ, Zuckerman GR. Alcoholic liver disease presenting with marked elevation of serum alkaline phosphatase: A combined clinical and pathological study. *Am J Dig Dis* 1978;**23**:1061–6.
18. Ballard H, Bernstein M, Farrar JT. Fatty liver presenting as obstructive jaundice. *Am J Med* 1961;**30**:196–201.

19. Kondili LA, Tosti ME, Szklo M, *et al.* The relationships of chronic hepatitis and cirrhosis to alcohol intake, hepatitis B and C, and delta virus infection: A case–control study in Albania. *Epidemiol Infect* 1998;**121**:391–5.

20. Shiomi S, Kuroki T, Minamitani S, *et al.* Effect of drinking on the outcome of cirrhosis in patients with hepatitis B or C. *J Gastroenterol Hepatol* 1992;**7**:274–6.

21. Ohnishi K, Iida S, Iwama S, *et al.* The effect of chronic habitual alcohol intake on development of liver cirrhosis and hepatocellular carcinoma: Relation to hepatitis B surface antigen carriage. *Cancer* 1982;**49**:672–7.

22. Kim WH, Hong F, Jaruga B, *et al.* Additive activation of hepatic NF-kappa B by ethanol and hepatitis B protein X (HBX) or HCV core protein: Involvement of TNF-alpha receptor 1-independent and dependent mechanisms. *FASEB J* 2001;**15**:2551–3.

23. Poynard T, Bedossa P, Opolon P. Natural history of liver fibrosis progression in patients with chronic hepatitis C: The OBSVIRC, METAVIR, CLINIVIR, and DOSVIRC groups. *Lancet* 1997;**349**:825–32.

24. Harris DR, Gonin R, Alter HJ, *et al.* The relationship of acute transfusion-associated hepatitis to the development of cirrhosis in the presence of alcohol abuse. *Ann Intern Med* 2001;**134**:120–24.

25. Romero-Gomez M, Grande L, Nogales MC, Fernandez M, Chaver M, Castro M. Intrahepatic hepatitis C virus replication is increased in patients with regular alcohol consumption. *Dig Liver Dis* 2001;**33**:698–702.

26. Sherman KE, Rouster SD, Mendenhall C, Thee D. Hepatitis C RNA quasispecies complexity in patients with alcoholic liver disease. *Hepatology* 1999;**30**:265–70.

27. Cromie SL, Jenkins PJ, Bowden DS, Dudley FJ. Chronic hepatitis C: Effect of alcohol on hepatitic activity and viral titre. *J Hepatol* 1996;**25**:821–5.

28. Roudot-Thoraval F, Bastie A, Pawlotsky JM, *et al.* Epidemiological factors affecting the severity of hepatitis C virus-related liver disease: A French survey of 6,664 patients, The Study Group for the Prevalence and Epidemiology of Hepatitis C Virus. *Hepatology* 1997;**26**:485–90.

29. Pessione F, Degos F, Marcellin P, *et al.* Effect of alcohol consumption on serum hepatitis C virus RNA and histological lesions in chronic hepatitis C. *Hepatology* 1998;**27**:1717–22.

30. Donato F, Tagger A, Gelatti U, *et al.* Alcohol and hepatocellular carcinoma: The effect of lifetime intake and hepatitis virus infections in men and women. *Am J Epidemiol* 2002;**155**:323–31.

31. Yamauchi M, Nakahara M, Maezawa Y, *et al.* Prevalence of hepatocellular carcinoma in patients with alcoholic cirrhosis and prior exposure to hepatitis C. *Am J Gastroenterol* 1993;**88**:39–43.

32. DiMartino V, Rufat P, Boyer N, *et al.* The influence of human immunodeficiency virus coinfection on chronic hepatitis C in injection drug users: A long-term retrospective cohort study. *Hepatology* 2001;**34**:1193–9.

33. Tabone M, Sidoli L, Laudi C, *et al.* Alcohol abstinence does not offset the strong negative effect of lifetime alcohol consumption on the outcome of interferon therapy. *J Viral Hepat* 2002;**9**:288–94.

34. Lee FI. Cirrhosis and hepatoma in alcoholics. *Gut* 1966;**7**:77–85.

35. Morgan MY, Sherlock S. Sex-related differences among 100 patients with alcoholic liver disease. *Br Med J* 1977;**1**:939–41.

36. Adami HO, Hsing AW, McLaughlin JK, *et al.* Alcoholism and liver cirrhosis in the etiology of primary liver cancer. *Int J Cancer* 1992;**51**:898–902.

37. Fisher RL, Schewer PJ, Sherlock S. Primary liver cell carcinoma: Alcohol and chronic liver disease. *Gut* 1974;**15**:343–4.

38. Smith PG, Tel LGB, Geoh GCT. Appearance of oval cells in the liver of rats after long term exposure to ethanol. *Hepatology* 1996;**23**:145–54.

39. Miyakawa H, Sato C, Izumi N, *et al.* Hepatitis C virus infection in alcoholic liver cirrhosis in Japan: Its contribution to the development of hepatocellular carcinoma. *Alcohol Alcohol* 1993;**28**:85–90.

40. Bassendine MF. Alcohol and hepatocellular carcinoma. *J Hepatol* 1985;**2**:513–19.

41. Stickel F, Schuppan D, Hahn EG, HK Seitz. Cocarcinogenic effects of alcohol in hepato-carcinogenesis. *Gut* 2002;**51**:132–9.

42. Worner TM, Gordon G, Leo MA, Lieber CS. Vitamin A treatment of sexual dysfunction in male alcoholics. *Am J Clin Nutr* 1988;**48**:1431–5.

43. Leo MA , Kim CI, Lowe N, Lieber CS. Interaction of ethanol with β-carotene: Delayed blood clearance and enhanced hepatotoxicity. *Hepatology* 1992;**15**:883–91.

44. Hines JD. Effects of alcohol in inborn errors of metabolism: Porphyria cutanea tarda and hemochromatosis. *Semin Hematol* 1980;**17**:113–18.

45. Lefkowitch JH, Grossman ME. Hepatic pathology in porphyria cutanea tarda. *Liver* 1983;**3**:19–29.

46. Powel LW. The role of alcoholism in hepatic iron storage disease. *Ann N Y Acad Sci* 1975;**252**:124–7.

47. Ludwig J, Hashimoto E, Porayko MK, Moyer TP, Baldus WP. Hemosiderosis in cirrhosis: A study of 447 native livers. *Gastroenterology* 1997;**112**:882–8.

48. Morgan MY, Camilo ME, Luck W, Sherlock S, Hoffbrand AV. Macrocytosis in alcohol related disease: Its value for screening. *Clin Lab Haemat* 1981;**3**:35–44.

49. Herbert V. Folate deficiency in alcoholics. *Ann Intern Med* 1963;**58**:977–88.

50. Jandl JH. Macrocytic anaemia in alcoholics. *Ann Intern Med* 1956;**45**:1027–44.

51. Sullivan LW, Herbert V. Suppression of hematopoiesis by ethanol. *J Clin Invest* 1964;**43**:2048–62.

52. Smith JA, Lonergan ET, Sterling K. Spur cell anemia: Hemolytic anemia with red cell resembling acanthocyte in alcoholic cirrhosis. *N Engl J Med* 1964;**271**:396–8.

53. Cooper RA, Kimball DB, Durocher JR. Role of the spleen in membrane conditioning and hemolysis of spur cells in liver disease. *N Engl J Med* 1974;**290**:1279–84.

54. Thompson A, Kerlin P, Clouston A, Cobcroft R. Spur cell anaemia resolves after orthotopic liver transplantation. *Aust N Z J Med* 1997;**27**:198–9.

55. Aihara K, Azuma H, Ikeda Y, *et al.* Successful combination therapy—flunarizine, pentoxifylline, and cholestyramine—for spur cell anemia. *Int J Haematol* 2001;**73**:351–5.

56. Zieve L. Jaundice, hyperlipidemia and hemolytic anaemia: A heretofore unrecognized syndrome associated with alcoholic fatty liver and cirrhosis. *Ann Intern Med* 1958;**48**:471–96.

57. Green RJ, Baron DN. The acute *in vitro* effect of ethanol, its metabolites and other toxic alcohols in ion flux in isolated human leucocytes and erythrocytes. *Biochem Pharmacol* 1986;**35**:3457–64.

58. Kunz F, Stummvoll W. The significance of plasma phospholipids in Zieve syndrome. *Blut* 1970;**21**:210–26.

59. Goebel KM, Goebel FD, Schubotz R, Schneidner J. Red cell metabolic features in haemo-lytic anaemia of alcoholic liver disease (Zieve's syndrome). *Br J Haematol* 1977;**35**:573–85.

60. Melrose WD, Bell PA, Jupe DML, Baikie MJ. Alcohol-associated haemolysis in Zieve's syndrome: A clinical and laboratory study of five cases. *Clin Lab Haematol* 1990;**12**:159–67.

61. Dancy M, Bland JM, Leech G, Gaitonde MK, Maxwell JD. Preclinical left ventricular abnormalities in alcoholics are independent of nutritional status and cigarette smoking. *Lancet* 1985;**1**:1122–5.

62. Steinberg J, Hayden MT. Prevalence of clinically occult cardiomyopathy in chronic alcoholism. *Am Heart J* 1981;**101**:461–4.

63. Schwesinger WH, Kurtin WE, Levine BA, Page CP. Cirrhosis and alcoholism as patho-genetic factors in pigment gallstone formation. *Ann Surg* 1985;**201**:319–22.

64. Buchner AM, Sonnenberg A. Factors influencing the prevalence of gallstones in liver disease: The beneficial and harmful influences of alcohol. *Am J Gastroenterol* 2002; **97**:905–9.
65. Sarles H. Alcoholic pancreatitis. In: Burns GP, Banks S (eds). *Disorders of the pancreas: Controversies in diagnosis and management.* New York: McGraw Hill; 1992:273.
66. Greiner VL, Schubert E, Franken FH. Koinzidenz von chronisacher pancreatitis und leberzirrhose bei alkoholabusus. Eine rontgen-und histomorphologische studie. *Z Gastroenterologie* 1983;**21**:526–32.
67. Angelini G, Merigo F, Degani G, *et al.* Association of chronic alcoholic liver disease and pancreatic disease: A prospective study. *Am J Gastroenterol* 1985;**80**:998–1003.
68. Ammann RW, Buehler H, Bruehlmann W, Kehl O, Muench R, Stamm B. Acute (non-progressive) alcoholic pancreatitis: Prospective longitudinal study of 144 patients with recurrent alcoholic pancreatitis. *Pancreas* 1986;**1**:195–203.
69. Layer P, Yamamoto H, Kalthoff L, *et al.* The different courses of early- and late-onset idiopathic and alcoholic pancreatitis. *Gastroenterology* 1994;**107**:1481–7.
70. Lowenfels AB, Maisonneuve P, Cavallini G, *et al.* Pancreatitis and the risk of pancreatic cancer. *N Engl J Med* 1993;**328**:1433–7.
71. Mayo Robson AW. On pancreatitis with special reference to chronic pancreatitis, its simulation of carcinoma of the pancreas and its treatment by operation with illustrative cases. *Lancet* 1900;**2**:235–40.
72. Littenberg G, Afroudakis A, Kaplowitz N. Common bile duct stenosis from chronic pancreatitis: A clinical and pathologic spectrum. *Medicine* 1979;**58**:385–412.
73. Siegel JH, Sable RA, Ho R, Balthazar EJ, Rosenthal WS. Abnormalities of the bile duct associated with chronic pancreatitis. *Am J Gastroenterol* 1979;**72**:259–66.
74. Afroudakis A, Kaplowitz N. Liver histopathology in common bile duct stenosis due to chronic alcoholic pancreatitis. *Hepatology* 1981;**1**:65–71.
75. Schutte WJ, LaPorta AJ, Condon RE, *et al.* Chronic pancreatitis: A cause of biliary stricture. *Surgery* 1977;**82**:303–9.
76. Sarles H, Sahel J. Cholestasis and lesions of the biliary tract in chronic pancreatitis. *Gut* 1978;**19**:851–7.
77. Segal I, Lawson HH, Rabinowitz B, Hamilton DG. Chronic pancreatitis and the hepato-biliary system. *Am J Gastroenterol* 1982;**77**:867–74.
78. Buchler H, Muench R, Schmid M, Ammann R. Cholestasis in alcoholic chronic pancreatitis. Diagnostic value of the transaminase ratio for differentiation between extra- and intra-hepatic cholestasis. *Scand J Gastroenterol* 1985;**20**:851–6.
79. Warshaw AL, Schapiro RH, Ferrucci JT Jr, Galdabini JJ. Persistent obstructive jaundice, cholangitis, and biliary cirrhosis due to common bile duct stenosis in chronic pancreatitis. *Gastroenterology* 1976;**70**:562–7.
80. Gregg JA, Carr-Locke DL, Gallagher MM. Importance of common bile duct stricture associated with chronic pancreatitis: Diagnosis by endoscopic retrograde cholangio-pancreatography. *Am J Surg* 1981;**141**:199–203.
81. Newton BB, Rittenbury MS, Anderson MC. Extrahepatic biliary obstruction associated with pancreatitis. *Ann Surg* 1983;**197**:645–52.
82. Kalvaria I, Bornman PC, Cochrane L, *et al.* ^{99m}Tc-DISIDA cholescintigraphy of biliary strictures due to chronic pancreatitis [Abstr]. *S Afr Med J* 1985;**68**:520.

CHAPTER 12

Jaundice in pregnancy

ANIL ARORA, SANJAY JAIN

Liver diseases that occur during pregnancy have varied aetiologies. It is customary to classify liver diseases occurring during pregnancy into those coincidental to pregnancy, those specifically related to pregnancy, and chronic liver disease that antedates pregnancy. Most disorders complicating pregnancy are coincidental, e.g. acute viral hepatitis or drug-induced hepatitis. Some diseases are induced by pregnancy and hence resolve following delivery. These include intrahepatic cholestasis of pregnancy, pre-eclampsia, acute fatty liver of pregnancy and hepatic dysfunction due to hyperemesis gravidarum. Finally, pregnancy may be superimposed on pre-existing chronic liver disease.

HEPATIC PHYSIOLOGY

Pregnancy normally results in appreciable physiological alterations, modifying some of the biochemical tests that are usually employed to assess liver function (Table I).

LIVER DISEASE RELATING TO PREGNANCY

Hyperemesis gravidarum

This condition affects 0.5–10/1000 pregnancies, and is characterized by persistent nausea and vomiting. The liver may be involved and biopsy findings are either normal or show fatty changes. There may be mild hyperbilirubinaemia and hypertransaminasaemia in 25%–40% of patients with hyperemesis. Serum enzyme (ALT/AST) levels seldom exceed 200 U/L.

Intrahepatic cholestasis of pregnancy

Intrahepatic cholestasis of pregnancy is also known as recurrent jaundice of pregnancy or icterus gravidarum. Its incidence is 1 in 500–1000 pregnancies. It

Table I. Results of some liver function tests done during pregnancy

Test	Effect of pregnancy
Enzymes	
Alkaline phosphatase	Markedly elevated
Aminotransferases	Unchanged
Lactic acid dehydrogenase	Unchanged
Bilirubin	Unchanged
Proteins	
Albumin	Decreased by 1 g/dl
Globulin	Slightly elevated
Hormone-binding proteins	Elevated
Transferrin	Elevated
Lipids	
Triglyceride	Elevated
Cholesterol	Elevated
Clotting factors	
Fibrinogen	Elevated
Factors VII, VIII, X	Elevated
Clotting time	Unchanged

is characterized clinically by pruritus, icterus or both, and usually occurs in the third trimester of gestation. Jaundice develops in a minority of patients. Laboratory tests confirm the presence of cholestasis. The level of ALP is modestly elevated but the GGT level is normal or only minimally elevated, an unexpected finding that is atypical of other forms of cholestatic liver injury. The cause for this is unknown, and it is believed to be due to the high oestrogen concentrations in suspectible persons. However, Leslie *et al.*[1] recently reported that maternal plasma oestrogen levels are decreased in affected women compared with matched controls. Reyes and Sjovall[2] have postulated that there is a defect in the secretion of sulphated progesterone metabolites. Amelioration of symptoms and improvement in laboratory tests begin with delivery, and are usually prompt and complete. Patients who have cholestasis of pregnancy have no hepatic sequelae but are at an increased risk for gall stone formation. The disease may recur in 60%–70% of the affected women in subsequent pregnancies.

Acute fatty liver of pregnancy

This condition is also known as acute fatty metamorphosis or acute yellow atrophy. It is an uncommon complication (about 1 in 10 000 pregnancies), and may prove fatal for both the mother and the foetus. It is a form of true hepatic failure, with coagulopathy and often encephalopathy. The diagnostic criteria include a prolonged PT with a low serum fibrinogen level in a woman who is in her second half of gestation. Characteristic abnormalities on histological exmination are swollen hepatocytes with microvesicular fatty changes and minimal hepatocellular necrosis. Current evidence regarding the aetiopathogenesis suggests that this is a recessively inherited mitochondrial abnormality of fatty acid oxidation; however, if the foetus is homozygous, the mother manifests liver failure. Sims *et al.*[3] described a familial deficiency of long-chain 3-hydroxyacyl CoA dehydrogenase (LCHAD) caused by mutation of a single codon. Affected homozygous children had Reye-like syndromes, and some of these heterozygous women suffered fatty liver of pregnancy.

Acute fatty liver usually manifests late in pregnancy (between 34 and 37 weeks of gestation), although Monga and Katz[4] described a typical case that manifested at 22 weeks. It begins with nausea, vomiting and abdominal pain, and is more common in primigravidae. Many patients have pregnancy-related problems, such as premature labour, vaginal bleeding or a decrease in foetal movement. In half the patients, hypertension, proteinuria and pedal oedema suggestive of pre-eclampsia are present. Pruritus may be an initial symptom. Abnormal test results include leucocytosis, a prolonged PT, decreased level of serum fibrinogen, hyperbilirubinaemia (usually <10 mg/dl) and serum transaminase levels of 300–500 U/L. In patients with altered sensorium, hypoglycaemia or hyperammonaemia should be ruled out.

A diagnosis of acute fatty liver is made by the typical clinical features in females in a late stage of gestation and compatible laboratory parameters. The histological hallmark is microvesicular fatty infiltration which mainly affects zone 3 (centrizonal) hepatocytes. The differential diagnosis includes viral hepatitis, drug-induced hepatotoxicity and other forms of liver disease associated with pregnancy, including the haemolysis, elevated liver enzymes and low platelets (HELLP) syndrome, and hepatic infarct or rupture.

Because spontaneous resolution usually follows delivery, many clinicians assume that delivery is essential for cure. This should be followed by maximal supportive care till the liver recovers. This support may include infusion of blood products, mechanical ventilation, dialysis, administration of antibiotics and an antihepatic coma regimen. Patients with liver failure may require liver transplantation and maximal supportive care. A maternal survival rate to the tune of 100% has been reported, whereas perinatal mortality rates have been reported to be 6%–7%. Recurrence of acute fatty liver is rare in subsequent pregnancies.

Pre-eclampsia and eclampsia

This condition is also known as toxaemia of pregnancy and complicates 3%–5% of all pregnancies. It is more common in primiparae and those with multiple gestation. It is a multisystem disorder which begins in the second trimester. The diagnostic criteria are a blood pressure of 140/90 mmHg or higher in a woman known previously to be normotensive, with proteinuria of 500 mg/L or more on 24-hour urine analysis. The liver disease usually takes the form of the HELLP syndrome. It is also presumed to underlie hepatic haematoma and rupture in pregnancy.

The HELLP syndrome

The HELLP syndrome is a complication seen in about 20% of patients with pre-eclampsia. The patient presents with abdominal pain, nausea, vomiting, headache and blurred vision. About 5% of patients present with jaundice. The haemolysis is usually modest. Serum aminotransferase levels may be modestly or substantially elevated. Liver biopsy demonstrates periportal haemorrhage, fibrin deposition and hepatocyte disruption of varying severity, especially in zone 1. The clinical course of the HELLP syndrome is marked by the prompt return of all the abnormal features to normal after delivery. In a few patients, the disease continues to worsen, resulting in multiple organ failure, sepsis, disseminated intravascular coagulation, hepatic failure and even death.

Hepatic haematoma and rupture

Haemorrhage from hepatic and subcapsular haematomas are two feared complications of liver involvement due to pre-eclampsia. The incidence of haemorrhage varies from 1 in 15 000 to 45 000 pregnancies. In typical cases, the haematoma develops on the diaphragmatic surface of the right lobe. The patient presents with right upper quadrant pain and tenderness. The diagnosis can be confirmed by a CT scan. If the haematoma is intrahepatic and intact, close observation is reasonable. In some cases, liver rupture stimulates further bleeding and may lead to haemorrhagic shock that requires prompt surgical intervention. Maternal mortality is high with overt rupture in up to 60% of patients.

LIVER DISEASE NOT RELATED TO PREGNANCY

Viral hepatitis

Hepatitis is the most common serious liver disease encountered in pregnant women. In most cases, acute viral hepatitis due to hepatitis virus A, B or C does not affect the natural course of the pregnancy. However, viral hepatitis E and acute herpes simplex infection during pregnancy, particularly during the third trimester, may lead to acute liver failure.

Hepatitis A

Previously called infectious hepatitis, this infection is caused by a 27 nm RNA picorna virus transmitted by the faeco-oral route. In developed countries, the effects of hepatitis A on pregnancy are not dramatic. However, in some under-privileged populations, hepatitis A causes a substantial increase in both perinatal and maternal deaths. Treatment consists of supportive care, including a balanced diet and restricted activity. There is no evidence that the hepatitis A virus is teratogenic. The risk of transmission to the foetus is negligible, though the risk of pre-term birth appears to be increased.

Hepatitis B

Once referred to as serum hepatitis, this infection is endemic in Asia and Africa. Hepatitis B is a DNA hepadnavirus transmitted by the parenteral route. Neither the prevalence nor the clinical course of hepatitis B infection in the mother, including fulminant hepatitis, is altered by pregnancy. Treatment is supportive and, as with hepatitis A, there is an increased likelihood of pre-term delivery.

Hepatitis C

The hepatitis C virus (HCV) is a single-stranded RNA virus of the *Flaviviridae* group. The mode of transmission of hepatitis C infection appears to be identical to that of hepatitis B. The course of hepatitis C is not different in pregnant women as compared to the general population. However, hepatitis C infection is transmitted vertically, the rate varying between 3% and 6%.

Hepatitis D

Also called the delta virus, this is a defective RNA virus that is a hybrid particle with a hepatitis B surface antigen coat and a delta core. The virus must be infected with hepatitis B. The mode of transmission is similar to that of hepatitis B. Neonatal transmission has been reported but hepatitis B vaccination usually prevents delta hepatitis.

Hepatitis E

This water-borne RNA virus is transmitted enterically. Acute infection during the third trimester of pregnancy carries a high risk of acute liver failure with a maternal mortality rate of up to 20%. Hepatitis E has also been associated with intrauterine death and increased risk of abortion. Maternal–foetal transmission of hepatitis E resulting in neonatal symptomatic hepatitis has been reported.

CHRONIC LIVER DISEASE ANTEDATING PREGNANCY

Chronic hepatitis

Most cases of chronic viral hepatitis are caused by the hepatitis B, C or D virus. Early recognition of these disorders is the key to prevent vertical transmission. Most young women who have chronic hepatitis B infection are healthy carriers and have a low risk of developing hepatic failure or decompensation during gestation or parturition. Chronic hepatitis B infection has little effect on the course of pregnancy and the reverse also holds true. Maternal–foetal transmission of hepatitis B virus is responsible for most cases of the chronic carrier state in endemic areas.[5] Infants born to mothers who are HBsAg-positive should receive hepatitis B immunoglobulin at birth as well as hepatitis B vaccine on day 1, and at months 1 and 6 after birth.[6]

Chronic hepatitis C infection does not appear to affect the outcome of pregnancy. One report suggested that pregnancy[7] may worsen the histopathological liver injury associated with hepatitis C.[8] Currently available data suggest that patients maintain normal serum aminotransferase levels during pegnancy. Perinatal transmission of hepatitis C virus seems to be uncommon.[9] Hepatitis D virus infection requires the presence of hepatitis B virus infection. There is no evidence that pregnancy has any impact on the natural course of acute or chronic hepatitis D. Vertical transmission of hepatitis D is prevented by vaccination against hepatitis B.

Autoimmune liver disease

Autoimmune diseases are commoner in women than in men. Immunosuppression for autoimmune hepatitis should be continued during pregnancy. The low doses of azathioprine used in standard treatment regimens are not known to be teratogenic. Occasionally, autoimmune hepatitis may flare up after delivery when the relative immunosuppression of pregnancy resolves. Therefore, patients with autoimmune hepatitis should undergo frequent measurement of liver enzyme levels for up to 6 months after delivery. Primary biliary cirrhosis is more common in women past the childbearing age than younger women. During pregnancy, there may be exacerbation of pruritus in patients with primary biliary cirrhosis.

Budd–Chiari syndrome

Pregnancy is a relatively hypercoagulable state, particularly during the peripartum period; and the Budd–Chiari syndrome, which causes thrombosis of the hepatic veins, can complicate it.[10] The Budd–Chiari syndrome has been associated with the HELLP syndrome and with eclampsia or pre-eclampsia.[11]

Wilson disease

Wilson disease is associated with amenorrhoea and infertility in women of childbearing age. Successful treatment of this disease with copper chelation therapy may result in the resumption of ovulatory cycles and subsequent pregnancy. Chelation with D-penicillamine or trientine has been proved to be safe in pregnancy, but the use of zinc sulphate for pregnant patients remains controversial.[12,13]

Hepatic neoplasia

Benign neoplasms of the liver include adenoma, focal nodular hyperplasia and haemangioma. Hepatic adenoma is associated with the use of oral contraceptives. Adenomas may enlarge during pregnancy and serial USG is indicated to measure the size of the tumour or detect haemorrhage. During pregnancy, hepatocellular carcinoma may be suggested by the detection of high alpha-fetoprotein levels during screening but other causes of its elevation, such as neural tube defects, hydatidiform mole and Down syndrome, should be ruled out.

REFERENCES

1. Leslie KK, Reznikov L, Simon FR, Fennessey PV, Reyes H, Ribalta J. Estrogens in intra-hepatic cholestasis of pregnancy. *Obstet Gynecol* 2000;**95**:372–6.
2. Reyes H, Sjovall J. Bile acids and progesterone metabolites in intrahepatic cholestasis of pregnancy. *Ann Med* 2000;**32**:94–106.
3. Sims HF, Brackett JC, Powell CK, *et al*. The molecular basis of pediatric long chain 3-hydroxyacyl-CoA dehydrogenase deficiency associated with maternal acute fatty liver of pregnancy. *Proc Natl Acad Sci U S A* 1995;**92**:841–5.
4. Monga M, Katz AR. Acute fatty liver in second trimester. *Obstet Gynecol* 1999;**93**:811–13.
5. Lok A. Natural history and control of perinatally acquired hepatitis B virus infection. *Dig Dis* 1992;**10**:46–52.
6. American Academy of Pediatrics Committee on Infectious Disease. Universal hepatitis B immunization. *Pediatrics* 1989;**89**:795–800.
7. Silverman N, Jenken B, Wi C, *et al*. Hepatitis C virus in pregnancy: Seroprevalence and risk factors for infection. *Am J Obstet Gynecol* 1993;**169**:583–7.
8. Fontaine H, Nalpas B, Carnot F, *et al*. Effect of pregnancy on chronic hepatitis C: A case–control study. *Lancet* 2000;**356**:1328–9.
9. La Torre A, Biadaioli R, Capobianco T, *et al*. Vertical transmission of HCV. *Acta Obstet Gynecol Scand* 1998;**77**:889–92.
10. Gordon S, Polson D, Shirkhoda A. Budd–Chiari syndrome complicating preeclampsia: Diagnosis by magnetic resonance imaging. *J Clin Gastroenterol* 1991;**13**:460–2.
11. Segal S, Shenhave S, Segal O, *et al*. Budd–Chiari syndrome complicating severe pre-eclampsia in a parturient with primary antiphospholipid syndrome. *Eur J Obstet Gynecol Report Biol* 1996;**68**:227–9.
12. Walshe J. The management of pregnancy in Wilson's disease treated with trientine. *Q J Med* 1986;**58**:81–7.
13. Brewer G, Johnson V, Dick R, *et al*. Treatment of Wilson disease with zinc XVIII. Treatment during pregnancy. *Hepatology* 2000;**31**:531–2.

CHAPTER 13

Neonatal cholestasis syndrome

MALATHI SATHIYASEKARAN

Neonatal cholestasis is not a rarity and occurs due to a variety of causes. The neonatal cholestasis syndrome (NCS) has recently received more attention, probably due to an increased awareness among paediatricians. NCS comprises two major groups: extrahepatic and intrahepatic. Biliary atresia (BA) is the most important cause of extrahepatic NCS. Idiopathic neonatal hepatitis (INH) and intrauterine infections constitute nearly 50% of the intrahepatic subset, commonly termed as neonatal hepatitis (NNH).

Prompt and accurate distinction between NNH and BA is crucial for management.[1] Postoperative restoration of bile flow occurs in up to 80% of infants with BA who had surgery before 8 weeks of age, but in only 20% if intervention is delayed beyond 12 weeks.[2] Identification of the underlying aetiology in the intrahepatic group is essential because some subgroups are treatable or preventable.

Progress in the management of NCS, particularly successful surgical correction and liver transplantation, has focused on the need for prompt referral and early intervention. However, most cases present late, probably because of the complacent attitude of both caregivers and the medical fraternity towards jaundice, as they consider it to be 'normal' or 'prolonged' physiological jaundice.

DEFINITION

NCS is a heterogeneous group of hepatobiliary disorders resulting in cholestasis. It occurs in the neonatal period and early infancy. It is characterized by jaundice, high-coloured urine, pale stools, direct serum bilirubin level >1.5 mg/dl or more than 20% of the total in an infant above 14 days of age. Since some of the affected infants are not strictly neonates, a better term would be 'prolonged cholestasis of infancy'.

INCIDENCE

Infantile cholestasis occurs in 1 in 2700 live-births, with NNH seen in 1 in 5000–10 000 and BA in 1 in 5000–15 000 live-births. In India, NCS comprises 30% of the hepatobiliary disorders seen in children.[3]

CLASSIFICATION

Based on the primary site of involvement, NCS may be intrahepatic or extrahepatic. In the intrahepatic group, an important subset is NNH, of which the idiopathic type is the most common, whereas in the extrahepatic group, BA is an important cause.

Causes of intrahepatic neonatal cholestasis syndrome

These may be:

1. Idiopathic
2. *Infections:* intrauterine, toxoplasma, rubella, CMV, herpes simplex virus, syphilis, human herpesvirus-6, herpes zoster, Coxsackie, HBV, HCV, HIV, parvovirus B19, paramyxovirus, echovirus, rotavirus and reovirus type 3
3. *Neonatal hepatobiliary infections:* generalized bacterial sepsis, syphilis, tuberculosis, malaria, urinary tract infection (UTI) and hepatitis B
4. *Genetic/chromosomal:* trisomy 18 and 21, cat-eye syndrome, Donahue syndrome and Turner syndrome
5. *Endocrine:* hypopituitarism (septo-optic dysplasia) and hypothyroidism
6. *Ductal paucity syndromes:* syndromic (Alagille syndrome) and non-syndromic ductal paucity
7. *Metabolic:* α_1-antitrypsin (AT) deficiency, cystic fibrosis, galactosaemia, tyrosinaemia, hereditary fructosaemia, glycogen storage disease type IV, Niemann–Pick disease types A and C, Wolman disease, primary disorders of bile acid synthesis, progressive familial intrahepatic cholestasis (PFIC) 1, 2 and 3, and the Zellweger syndrome
8. *Immune:* neonatal lupus erythematosus and neonatal hepatitis with autoimmune haemolytic anaemia
9. *Toxic/drug-related:* total parenteral nutrition (TPN), sepsis with endotox-aemia and drugs
10. *Anatomical:* congenital hepatic fibrosis, Caroli disease
11. *Miscellaneous:* shock, histiocytosis X, intestinal obstruction and the Dubin–Johnson syndrome.

Causes of extrahepatic neonatal cholestasis syndrome

These include extrahepatic BA, choledochal cyst, neonatal sclerosing cholangitis, hair-like bile duct syndrome, spontaneous perforation of the CBD, inspissated bile duct syndrome and cholelithiasis.

INTRAHEPATIC NEONATAL CHOLESTASIS SYNDROME

Some of the major causes of intrahepatic NCS are discussed below.

Idiopathic neonatal hepatitis[4]

A majority of infants (up to 30%) with NCS of the intrahepatic type belong to this subgroup in which no aetiology is identified. If cholestasis is severe, differentiation from BA is difficult albeit important. Infants with INH are more likely to be premature or small for their gestational age. Liver biopsy shows extensive giant-cell transformation of the hepatocytes with inflammation. The prognosis is generally good, and predictors of poor prognosis include prolonged jaundice beyond 6 months of age, pale stools, familial occurrence, persistent hepatomegaly and findings of severe inflammation on biopsy. If the infants survive the first year of life with no evidence of chronic liver disease, the outcome is very good.

Intrauterine infections

Several intrauterine infections have been implicated in the aetiology of NCS, the most common being the TORCH group of infections. This group often has similar clinical features such as hepatosplenomegaly, jaundice, pneumonitis, petechial or purpuric rash, and a tendency to prematurity or intrauterine growth retardation (IUGR). Conventional TORCH titres are not the preferred method of diagnosis, and identification of the viral infection by measuring the specific IgM antibody is necessary.

Toxoplasmosis

Congenital toxoplasmosis is relatively rare. Involvement of the central nervous system, presenting as chorioretinitis, hydrocephaly or microcephaly, intracranial calcifications, convulsions and nystagmus, forms a predominant feature along with NNH. Specific therapy with spiramycin may prevent progression of the disease in the central nervous system and liver.

Rubella

Congenital rubella infection has been reported less frequently since the introduction of immunization. The characteristic features seen in this syndrome are IUGR, anaemia, thrombocytopenia, hepatosplenomegaly, congenital heart disease (patent ductus arteriosus or pulmonary artery stenosis), cataracts, chorioretinitis, mental retardation and deafness. Liver disease in the congenital rubella syndrome may be self-limiting or progress to cirrhosis.

Cytomegalovirus infection

CMV is a common intrauterine infection causing NNH. The clinical findings include hepatosplenomegaly, jaundice and petechiae (60%–80%). CMV usually involves the central nervous system, resulting in microcephaly, intracranial calcification, chorioretinitis and sensorineural deafness. Liver biopsy demonstrates a giant-cell hepatitis. Infection with CMV may be associated with extrahepatic BA. The diagnosis of CMV requires documentation of rising titres of antibodies, high CMV DNA levels or the isolation of CMV inclusion bodies on liver biopsy. The presence of isolated IgM positivity cannot be considered to be an indicator of CMV infection as this infection is very common in India. Ganciclovir is the drug of choice for CMV hepatitis.

Parvovirus B19 infection

Infection with parvovirus B19 can cause severe anaemia, leading to hydrops foetalis. The infant can present with neonatal cholestasis, hepatomegaly, severe coagulopathy and dermal erythropoiesis ('blueberry muffin' rash). The serum aminotransferase levels are low or near normal. The diagnosis is made by detecting parvovirus B19 by PCR.

Hepatotropic viruses A, E, B and C

Though infections due to these viruses are usually not a cause of neonatal cholestasis, they may be an important cause of maternal jaundice. Rarely, infants may present with acute liver failure or severe hepatitis.

Other viral infections

Infection with human herpesvirus-6 can present with acute liver failure. Paramyxovirus infections can cause a severe liver disease known as syncytial giant-cell hepatitis. In neonates, the presentation can take the form of severe hepatitis that progresses to chronic cholestasis and cirrhosis over a period of 6–12 months. Liver biopsy shows the characteristic syncytial type of giant cell, which differs from the giant cells of NNH by the presence of 'smudged' borders between the cells.

Enteroviruses such as the echovirus, Coxsackie virus and adenovirus can cause systemic viral infection in neonates resulting in severe hepatitis and acute liver failure. This form of enteric viral sepsis occurs between 1 and 5 weeks after birth and presents with jaundice, high transaminase levels, coagulopathy and meningitis.

Bacterial infections

Intrahepatic NCS can also occur with sepsis, UTI, and streptococcal and staphylococcal infections. Infants with galactosaemia may present for the first time with sepsis.

Chromosomal disorders

Several chromosomal disorders, such as trisomy 18 and 21, and the cat-eye syndrome have been associated with intrahepatic NCS. The characteristic features of the chromosomal disorder help in identifying the aetiology. In trisomy 21, the association between neonatal cholestasis and BA is not well substantiated.

Ductal paucity syndrome

The bile duct paucity syndrome is of two types: syndromic and non-syndromic. The Alagille syndrome, the syndromic form of ductal paucity, is identified by the characteristic facies, butterfly vertebra, peripheral pulmonary artery stenosis and failure to thrive. Non-syndromic ductal paucity can be due to prematurity, infections, and metabolic or genetic causes.

Endocrine disorders

The two important endocrine causes of intrahepatic NCS are hypothyroidism and hypopituitarism. In the absence of trophic hormones that moderate or stimulate bile canalicular development and bile acid synthesis, cholestasis may occur. In septo-optic dysplasia, the characteristic midline facial abnormalities, wandering nystagmus and microgenitalia may be present.

Metabolic disorders

Several metabolic disorders have been associated with cholestasis, the common ones being α_1-AT deficiency, galactosaemia and tyrosinaemia. α_1-AT deficiency is probably the most common metabolic liver disease seen in the West. The deficiency is due to a mutation in the Pi (protease inhibitor) locus on chromosome 14. The most common deficiency variant is Z. The liver is frequently involved in the PiZZ phenotype due to the accumulation of abnormal α_1-AT in the endoplasmic reticulum. These infants present with IUGR, severe cholestasis and hepatomegaly. Spenomegaly is unusual unless there is marked hepatic fibrosis. The diagnosis is made by the demonstration of periodic acid Schiff-positive, diastase-resistant granules in the hepatocytes and demonstration of low serum α_1-AT levels (normal >1.0 g/L).

Galactosaemia

This autosomal recessive disorder can present with neonatal cholestasis, hypoglycaemia, cataracts, intraocular haemorrhage and retinal detachment. There is a high incidence of Gram-negative sepsis in infants with galactosaemia. Urinary screening for reducing substances and estimating erythrocyte galactose-1-phosphate uridyl transferase may be helpful. Dietary management with absolute elimination of galactose is mandatory.

Tyrosinaemia

This autosomal recessive disorder can present with NCS, and the clinical features include coagulopathy, encephalopathy and ascites. In addition, failure to thrive and rickets may be seen in older infants. The presence of grossly elevated alpha-fetoprotein levels (40 000–70 000 µg/L), increased plasma tyrosine, significant urinary succinyl acetone in addition to findings of renal involvement, such as proximal tubular dysfunction and radiological evidence of rickets, help in the diagnosis. The formation of toxic metabolites is prevented by 2-(2-nitro-trifluoromethylbenzoyl)-1,3-cyclohexenedione (NTBC), which forms a part of the management protocol.

Progressive familial intrahepatic cholestasis

The recent characterization of hepatobiliary transporters has helped in elucidating the mechanism of bile formation. Patients with PFIC 1 (Byler disease) and 2 have low or normal GGT levels.

Toxic and drug-related cholestasis

Total parenteral nutrition-related cholestasis

Total parenteral nutrition (TPN)-related cholestasis is a well recognized entity seen in neonates dependent on TPN. The mechanism of TPN-related cholestasis could be specific deficiencies of undelivered nutrients. Enteral starvation and deprivation of intraluminal nutrients may exacerbate the cholestasis. A high concentration of amino acids may be toxic to the hepatocytes. Recovery is slow unless parenteral nutrition is discontinued.

EXTRAHEPATIC NEONATAL CHOLESTASIS SYNDROME

The important causes of extrahepatic NCS are BA, choledochal cysts and spontaneous perforation of the bile duct. The latter two conditions are identified on USG and require surgery.

Biliary atresia

BA is a progressive, idiopathic, necroinflammatory process initially involving a segment of or the entire extrahepatic biliary tree. It is a dynamic disease and, as it progresses, the lumen of the extrahepatic bile ducts is obliterated and bile flow obstructed, resulting in cholestasis and chronic liver damage.[5]

The aetiology of BA remains obscure. Apart from the hypothesis of Landing[6] (*see below*), several others have been implicated, namely:

1. viral infections such as those with reovirus type 3 and rotavirus;
2. a catastrophe of blood supply;
3. abnormal bile acid metabolism;

4. pancreaticobiliary malformation;
5. genetic influences;
6. developmental anomalies; and
7. immune-mediated.

The developmental theory has been proposed to explain the 10%–15% of cases associated with multiple congenital anomalies such as the polysplenia syndrome. BA may be the result of a 'two-hit phenomenon' dependent on genetic vulnerability to environmental precipitating factors. A significant increase in the frequency of human leucocyte antigen (HLA)-B12 among patients with BA has also been reported.[7]

BA is of 2 types—the foetal type (15%) and the more common postnatal type (70%–85%). The foetal type is a result of a true defective embryogenesis, and is associated with multiple congenital anomalies and a high mortality. Infants with BA usually have normal birth weight, high-coloured urine and persistent pale stools. The liver is usually firm and splenomegaly is a late sign. BA has been classified into 3 different categories by the Japanese Association of Paediatric Surgeons.

Type I: Atresia at the site of the CBD—correctable (10%)

Type II: Atresia at the site of the hepatic duct (5%)

Type III: Atresia up to the porta hepatis—non-correctable (85%)

RELATIONSHIP BETWEEN NEONATAL HEPATITIS AND BILIARY ATRESIA

The 'infantile obstructive cholangiopathy' hypothesis, as proposed by Landing,[6] suggests that a single process results in the spectrum of BA, choledochal cysts and NNH. Depending on the dominant injury, NNH or extrahepatic BA occurs. The triggering event could be an infection, immune mechanism or ischaemic process.

PATHOGENESIS OF CHOLESTASIS

Unlike in adults, several conditions can cause cholestasis in infants. The factors predisposing to physiological cholestasis, such as decreased size of the bile acid pool, decreased canalicular excretion of bile acids, decreased intraluminal bile acid concentration, defective ileal transport of bile acids, decreased conjugation, sulphation and glucuronidation of bile acids, increased bilirubin load and altered bile acid synthesis, could play a role in perpetuating cholestasis in the vulnerable liver.

CONSEQUENCES OF CHOLESTASIS

The three major consequences of cholestasis are as follows: (i) bile does not enter the duodenum at all or only partially; (ii) substances normally excreted in the bile are retained in the circulation; and (iii) bile stasis occurs in the canaliculi

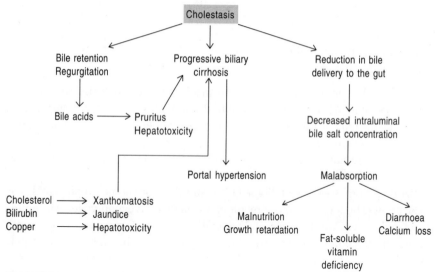

Fig. 1. The consequences of cholestasis in neonates[8]

and hepatocytes. The excretion of conjugated bilirubin and bile salts is responsible for the dark-coloured urine that stains the diaper. The decreased excretion of bile into the biliary tree results in decreased bile in the intestine, causing pale stools.

The actual mechanism of pruritus is not clear. Retention of bile acids is probably only one of the mechanisms responsible for pruritus. Endogenous opioid peptides may be responsible by increasing central opioidergic neurotransmission. Other neurotransmitters, such as serotonin (5HT-3), may also play a role. Pruritus is prominent after the age of 6 months and may become relentless. Retention of bile acids also results in injury to various biological membranes of the body, resulting in biliary cirrhosis and portal hypertension, haemolytic anaemia, bronchospasm and epistaxis.

Hyperlipidaemia is characteristic of cholestasis. Much of the plasma cholesterol is in the form of lipoprotein (x) (Lp[x]). This type of packaging of cholesterol in Lp(x) prevents the damage to the vascular endothelium normally expected with hypercholesterolaemia. Deposition of cholesterol in the skin leads to the formation of xanthomas.

A major clinical effect of neonatal cholestasis is poor growth. This is due to malabsorption, poor nutrient utilization, hormonal disturbances and secondary tissue injury. Malabsorption is due to the lack of bile in the small bowel, resulting in the inefficient absorption of fats and fat-soluble vitamins. Simultaneously, there is loss of calcium due to Ca^{++} soap formation with fats, which are also lost in the stools. Vitamin D deficiency leads to the development of vitamin E deficiency, which may present as neuropathy and haemolysis. Vitamin A deficiency leads to blindness and hyperkeratotic skin. Vitamin K deficiency is responsible for the coagulopathy and bleeding (Fig. 1).

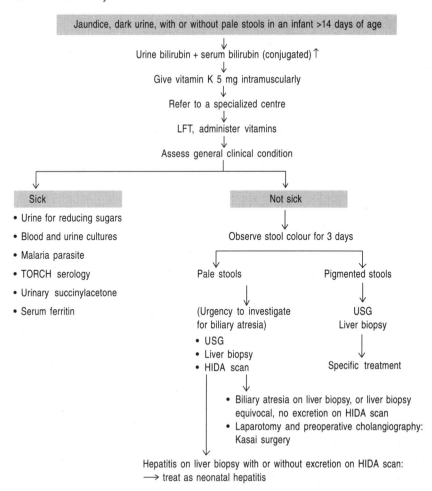

Fig. 2. Approach to the management of an infant with the neonatal cholestasis syndrome[10]
HIDA: hepatobiliary scan with an iminodiacetic acid derivative

APPROACH TO THE NEONATAL CHOLESTASIS SYNDROME

In NCS, it is mandatory to differentiate between NNH and BA. However, there is no gold standard test that can differentiate between the two.[9] A combination of clinical findings, stool examination, USG, liver biopsy wherever possible, and hepatobiliary scan with an iminodiacetic acid (HIDA) derivative, if readily available, may help in arriving at a reasonable diagnosis. Whenever there is a suspicion of BA, it may be advisable to plan a laparotomy and an intraoperative cholangiogram with a liver biopsy, which will increase the specificity of the diagnosis (Fig. 2).

Clinical examination

A simple, cheap and fairly reliable test is macroscopic examination of the stools

Table I. Differentiation between neonatal hepatitis (NNH) and biliary atresia (BA)

Clinical finding	NNH	BA
Intrauterine growth retardation/small for gestational age	++	–
Sepsis/sick, failure to thrive	++	–
Bleeding tendency	++	+ (corrected by vitamin K)
Facies	Dysmorphic	–
Eyes	Cataract, chorioretinitis	
Skin: erythropoiesis	++ (blueberry muffin rash)	–
Hepatomegaly	++	++
Splenomegaly	Early	Usually later

for three days. If the stool is golden-yellow in colour, a diagnosis of BA is unlikely. On the other hand, if the stool is white in colour, then it is highly suggestive of BA, and if pale yellow, then either NNH or extrahepatic BA could be present (Table I).

Babies with extrahepatic BA are usually born at term with normal weight; 20% of these babies may have associated congenital malformations. Babies with NNH may have IUGR, dysmorphic facies and ophthalmic findings such as cataract, chorioretinitis, coloboma, etc.

Biochemical tests

Biochemical tests may not help in differentiating between BA and NNH. Serum ALP and GGT may be very high in BA compared to NNH. Liver enzymes, such as ALT and AST, are near normal in BA but are always raised in NNH. In severe cholestasis, there may be an overlap. The GGT level is usually high in cholestasis but may be normal or low in PFIC 1 and 2, and inborn errors of bile acid metabolism.

Prothrombin time

In BA, prolonged PT usually responds to vitamin K administration, whereas in NNH, fresh frozen plasma (FFP) may be required, and the prolonged PT is not correctable with vitamin K.

Duodenal intubation

Duodenal intubation, 24-hour collection and visual examination of the duodenal fluid for the presence of bilirubin pigment has been described as an easy, inexpensive and non-invasive method for determining complete biliary obstruction with a high sensitivity and specificity. The string test involves detection of the radioactivity of a string placed in the duodenum during scintigraphy.

Ultrasonography

USG is useful in identifying choledochal cysts, spontaneous perforation of the bile duct, Caroli disease and cholelithiasis. A contracted gallbladder on a milk-free diet, non-visualization of the gallbladder and the triangular cord sign are suggestive of BA. Visualization of a normal gallbladder, which contracts normally on feeding following a 4-hour fast, is more suggestive of NNH.

Upper gastrointestinal endoscopy

Visualization of the ampulla and the presence of bile in the duodenum are suggestive of intrahepatic cholestasis and exclude BA. However, if bile is not seen, it could be either severe cholestasis or BA.

Scintigraphy

HIDA scan is a radionuclide study of the hepatobiliary system using imino-diacetic (IDA) derivatives. The radionuclide commonly used is ^{99m}Tc mebrofenin. A normal study will demonstrate a good uptake by the liver in 10 min, followed by excretion into the duodenum in 30 min and complete excretion by 5 hours. The test is done after priming with phenobarbitone for 3–5 days. This study is undertaken to evaluate both hepatic uptake and excretion. In NNH, there is poor uptake and delayed excretion even up to 22 hours. In BA, no intestinal activity is seen even at the end of 22 hours. In severe forms of NNH also there may be no evidence of intestinal activity. This test has a high rate of false-positivity.

Endoscopic retrograde cholangiopancreaticography

This is a valuable tool in expert hands and helps in the diagnosis of BA, choledochal cyst and Caroli disease. It is useful in selecting patients before subjecting them to laparotomy. Difficulty in cannulation may yield a false-positive result in BA.

Magnetic resonance cholangiopancreaticography

MRCP is a useful diagnostic technique but has problems similar to those seen with USG. The false-positivity rate is very high but wherever visualization of the biliary tree, including the gallbladder, is reported, BA can be ruled out. The cost and duration of the procedure restrict its use.

Liver biopsy

A liver biopsy, which should be interpreted by an experienced pathologist, is mandatory. BA is characterized by the presence of interlobular duct proliferation, bile lakes and fibrosis. The liver parenchyma may be normal; however, it may show intrahepatocytic or canalicular cholestasis. In advanced cases, there may be full-fledged changes of secondary cirrhosis. If the biopsy is done early, between 4 and 6 weeks of life, the classical changes of BA may be less prominent.

In NNH, the characteristic changes are the presence of giant cells, hepato-cellular necrosis and cholestasis. Certain specific findings, such as inclusion bodies in CMV hepatitis and PAS-positive diastase-resistant granules in α_1-AT deficiency, may be seen. Ductopenia is diagnosed by counting the number of bile ducts in the portal triad. If the ratio of the bile ducts to the portal triad is less than 0.4, it is confirmative of ductopenia.

Other investigations

When NNH is suspected, urinary screening for metabolic disorders, TORCH, blood and urine culture should be done. When BA is suspected, the child should be referred to a competent paediatric surgeon, and a laparotomy followed by an intraoperative cholangiogram and liver biopsy done. If intraoperative cholangiography is suggestive of BA, the surgeon proceeds with Kasai surgery in the same sitting.

MANAGEMENT OF THE NEONATAL CHOLESTASIS SYNDROME

Management depends on whether the child has NNH, a metabolic disorder or an extrahepatic cause of NCS. All extrahepatic causes of NCS should be referred to the paediatric surgeon.

Biliary atresia[11]

Infants diagnosed to have BA should undergo surgery within 60 days. The results of surgery depend on the age of the child, status of the liver, nutritional status and type of BA. Even when subjected to early surgery, 30% of these infants may have features of cirrhosis and require liver transplantation.

Neonatal hepatitis

Specific treatment is given for the treatable causes of NNH, such as sepsis, UTI and malaria. Metabolic disorders such as galactosaemia and hereditary fructose intolerance are treated by avoiding the offending agent. Endocrine disorders such as hypothyroidism can be managed with replacement therapy.

Supportive management of the neonatal cholestasis syndrome[12,13]

Nutritional support

It is essential that the child be given good nutritional support with 200 cal/kg and 1–2 g protein/day. If the child is not on breast milk, dietary fat should be modified to contain more medium-chain triglycerides.

Water-soluble vitamins

Twice the recommended daily allowance is given.

Fat-soluble vitamins

Regular and correct replacement of vitamins A, D, E and K should be done to help the child grow normally and prevent problems related to fat-soluble vitamin deficiency.

Vitamin A

Vitamin A should be given in a dose of 2500–5000 IU/day. If the levels of vitamin A can be monitored, the blood level can be maintained at 30 μg/dl. For practical purposes, an aqueous solution of vitamin A is given intramuscularly with a first dose of 50 000 IU and then at doses of 30 000–50 000 IU at 3-month intervals till cholestasis resolves. Precaution is taken to prevent the development of hypervitaminosis A.

Vitamin D

Vitamin D is recommended in a daily dose of 400–1200 IU; 25,hydroxy-cholecalciferol 5–7 μg/kg can be given daily. An injection of 300 000 units of vitamin D_3 is given once in 5 months or earlier, depending on the biochemical values and radiological findings.

Vitamin E

Vitamin E deficiency should be recognized. The recommended dosage of vitamin E is 15–200 mg daily. Serum monitoring is mandatory. If serum levels are low, then a higher dose may be required. Six-monthly neurological and yearly eye examinations are necessary.

Vitamin K

In case of prolonged cholestasis, vitamin K 5 mg monthly should be given intramuscularly.

Minerals and trace elements

Regular replacement of calcium, zinc and iron are also essential in the management of NCS. Oral calcium is given in a dose of 50–100 mg/kg/day, oral phosphorus 25–50 mg/kg/day, zinc 1 mg/kg/day, magnesium 1–2 mg/kg/day and elemental iron 5–6 mg/kg/day.

Choleretic therapy

Choleretics stimulate either the bile salt-dependent or -independent mechanisms of bile flow. Ursodeoxycholic acid in a dose of 15–20 mg/kg/day and phenobarbitone in a dose of 5–10 mg/kg/day are effective in both these mechanisms. Steroids also help to some extent, and are preferred by surgeons in the pre- and postoperative periods.

Antipruritic therapy

Since the cause of pruritus is not known, treatment also comprises a combination of various drugs acting at different levels. Choleretics may not be sufficient to treat pruritus and the child may in addition require cholestyramine, rifampicin, ondansetron, naloxone, terfenadine, propofol, ultraviolet B light, plasmapheresis and, at times, even surgery.

PROGNOSIS

Neonatal hepatitis

Of the total, 60% of patients with INH recover with no residual sequelae, 10% may present with bleeding and fulminant hepatic failure, and 10%–30% may progress to chronic liver disease. If the child continues to be icteric even after the age of 1 year, a poor prognosis is indicated.

Biliary atresia

If the infant is operated on within 60 days, the results of surgery are good, with 30% living to adulthood, 30% up to 15 years of age and 30% requiring liver transplantation. On the other hand, if the child does not undergo surgery, mortality is 100% within 2 years of age. The timing of surgery and the 10-year survival as reported by Ohi[14] is 68% when the patient is operated on within 60 days of birth, 39% between 61 and 70 days, 33% between 71 and 90 days, and 15% when the infant is more than 91 days old.

Liver transplantation

A proportion of children with either extrahepatic BA or intrahepatic causes of NCS such as metabolic disorders would eventually require a liver transplant. The results of transplantation are encouraging, and the procedure will definitely play a substantial role in the future.

CONCLUSION

NCS is a common hepatobiliary disease of infancy. To improve survival, it is essential that an early diagnosis of BA be made. Supportive management of NNH is also beneficial in a large number of children.

REFERENCES

1. Balistreri WF. Neonatal cholastasis—medical progress. *J Pediatr* 1985;**106:**171–84.
2. Ohi R, Haamatsu M, Mochizuki I, *et al.* Progress in treatment of biliary atresia. *World J Surg* 1985;**9:**285–93.
3. Bhave SA, Bavdekar AR, Pandit AN. Neonatal cholestasis syndrome in India—a diagnostic and therapeutic challenge. *Indian Pediatr* 1996;**33:**753–62.
4. Roberts EA. The jaundiced baby. In: Kelly DA (ed). *Diseases of the liver and biliary system in children.* 1st ed. Oxford: Blackwell Science; 1999:11–45.
5. Haber BA, Russo P. Biliary atresia. *Gastroenterol Clin North Am* 2003;**32:**891–911.
6. Landing BH. Considerations of the pathogenesis of neonatal hepatitis, biliary atresia and choledochal cyst—the concept of infantile obstructive cholangiopathy. *Prog Pediatr Surg* 1974;**6:**113–39.
7. Silveira TR, Salzano FM, Donaldson PT, *et al.* Association between HLA and extrahepatic biliary atresia. *J Pediatr Gastroenterol Nutr* 1993;**16:**114–17.
8. Whitington PI. Chronic cholestasis of infancy. *Pediatr Clin North Am* 1996;**43:**1–26.
9. Lai MW, Chang MH, Hsu SC, *et al.* Differential diagnosis of extraphepatic biliary atresia from neonatal hepatitis: A prospective study. *J Pediatr Gastroenterol Nutr* 1994;**18:**121–7.
10. Yachha SK. Consensus report on neonatal cholestasis syndrome. *Indian Pediatr* 2000;**37:**845–51.
11. Kasai M, Kimura S, Asakura S. Surgical treatment of biliary atresia. *J Pediatr Surg* 1968;**3:**665–8.
12. Thapa BR. Cholestasis of infancy: Definition, practical approach and management. *Gasroenterol Today* 2001;**1:**29–36.
13. Shah HA, Spivak W. Neonatal cholestasis. New approaches to diagnostic evaluation and therapy. *Pediatr Clin North Am* 1994;**41:**943–66.
14. Ohi R. Surgery for biliary atresia. *Liver* 2001;**21:**175–82.

CHAPTER 14

Drug-induced hepatitis

R.R. RAI, S. NIJHAWAN, N. AGARWAL

Hepatotoxicity is defined as liver injury caused by drugs and other chemicals. In a community, drug-induced liver diseases (DILD) constitute less than 5% of cases of jaundice and even fewer cases of chronic liver disease.[1] Drug-induced liver damage has been an important cause of mortality associated with liver disease. An abnormality in the LFT, i.e. an increase in liver enzymes by more than two-fold, usually suggests liver injury. Hepatotoxicity may vary from minor asymptomatic derangements of LFT to structural damage in the form of fulminant hepatic failure, acute hepatitis, chronic hepatitis, cirrhosis and neoplasia. Hepatotoxicity is also an important cause of the severe form of liver damage and liver disease seen in the elderly.

EPIDEMIOLOGY

The incidence of this condition is very difficult to determine. Moreover, it is not appropriate because the frequency of DILD is not linearly related to the duration of exposure, and non-recognition of the condition adds to the difficulty. The incidence of most types of DILD is about 1 per 10 000–100 000 persons exposed.[2–4]

TYPES OF DRUG REACTIONS

Two types of drug reactions take place—idiosyncratic and dose-dependent.

Idiosyncratic reactions

These occur at the therapeutic level and are seen in 1 in every 1000–100 000 patients, with the pattern being consistent for each drug and its class. The reaction can occur between 5 and 90 days from the day of ingestion of the drug and may continue thereafter, and could be fatal. Rechallenge is usually associated with a much more severe reaction; an exception is isoniazid, which produces drug injury and mild hepatotoxicity that disappears with continued use.

Direct toxic liver injury

This is caused by highly reactive liver metabolites, for example, carbon-based radicals, nitroradicals, oxyradicals and reduced oxygen species formed by cytochrome-mediated oxidation of drugs that cause cell injury by peroxidative damage of the lipid moiety of the biological membrane, and direct covalent binding with proteins or DNA. Covalent binding of the reactive metabolites with macromolecules may produce injury by inactivating key enzymes or forming protein–drug adducts, which are a potential target for immune-mediated injury.

RISK FACTORS

Although drug-induced hepatitis can develop even in an apparently normal person, a few drugs are more prone to cause drug-induced hepatitis in certain risk groups. The risk factors can be classified into 2 categories: (i) host factors and (ii) drug-related factors (Table I).

Table I. Risk factors for drug-induced liver disease

Factors	Description	Common examples
Host factors		
Age[5]	Elderly people are at ↑ risk	Isonicotinic acid hydrazide (INH), nitrofurantoin, halothane
	Children are at ↑ risk	Valproic acid, salicylates
Sex	Men at ↑ risk	Amoxi/clavulanic acid, azathioprine
	Women at ↑ risk	Halothane, minocycline, nitrofurantoin
Obesity	↑ hepatic fibrosis	Halothane, tamoxifen, methotrexate
Fasting	↑ hepatotoxicity	Acetaminophen
Pre-existing liver disease	↑ hepatotoxicity	Antituberculosis treatment (ATT), ibuprofen
Excessive alcohol intake[5]	↓ dose threshold, ↑ hepatotoxicity and fibrosis	Acetaminophen, INH, methotrexate
Drug-related factors		
Dose	Directly related to blood level	Acetaminophen
	↑ hepatotoxicity with ↑ dose and frequency	Vitamin A and methotrexate
History of drug reactions	Halothane, diclofenac, ibuprofen	↑ cross-sensitivity
Co-administration of other drugs [5]	Acetaminophen, valproic acid	INH, phenytoin: lower dose threshold and ↑ hepatotoxicity
		Other antiepileptics agents: ↑ risk of hepatotoxicity

Enzyme inducers

Some substances, such as phenobarbitone, phenytoin, ethanol, cigarette smoke and grape juice, induce hepatic enzymes and alter the plasma drug levels, which in turn can result in extrahepatic reactions, e.g. torsade de pointes and drug interaction.[5]

Role of enzyme inducers in drug toxicity

Enzyme inducers play a dynamic role in enhancing hepatotoxicity. Simultaneous ingestion of ethanol and acetaminophen exacerbates the toxic effects of acetaminophen in alcoholics. When both are taken simultaneously, there is substrate competition for the cytochrome P450 2E1 isomer (CYP2E1) between ethanol and acetaminophen. Ethanol blocks most of the CYP2E1 and acetaminophen remains unattached. Thus, initially the toxic metabolite N-acetyl p-benzoquinone-imine (NAPQI) of acetaminophen is decreased. Ethanol slows the degradation of CYP2E1, thus increasing the availability of CYP2E1 for a longer duration, from the usual 7 hours to 37 hours.

Once ethanol is withdrawn, more CYP2E1 sites are available to acetaminophen and therefore more NAPQI is formed, leading to further liver injury (Fig. 1).

MECHANISMS OF LIVER INJURY

Injury to the liver cells occurs in patterns specific to the intracellular organelles affected. There are multiple cellular pathways to cellular liver injury even in the case of a single drug.

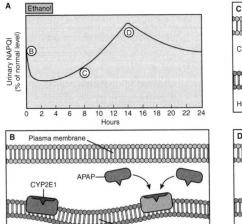
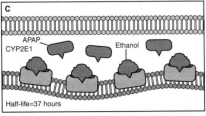
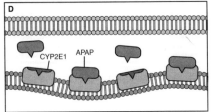

Fig. 1. The role of ethanol in the formation of N-acetyl-p-benzoquinone-imine (NAPQI), the toxic metabolite of acetaminophen, and the dynamics of enzyme induction. Panel A depicts the variation in the urinary levels of NAPQI over time, when ethanol competes with acetaminophen for CYP2E1. Panels B, C and D depict the 3 phases of this process. CYP2E1: cytochrome P450 2E1; APAP: acetaminophen

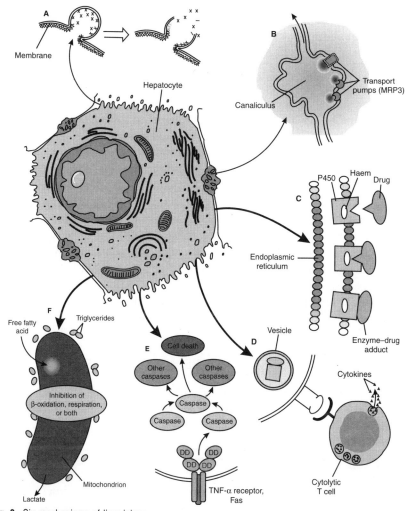

Fig. 2. Six mechanisms of liver injury
DD: death domain; TNF: tumour necrosis factor; MRP3: multidrug resistance-associated protein 3

The six mechanisms of liver injury are as follows (Fig. 2):

1. Disruption of intracellular calcium homeostasis leads to the disassembly of actin fibrils at the surface of the hepatocyte, resulting in blebbing of the cell membrane, rupture and cell lysis.
2. In cholestatic diseases, disruption of actin filaments may occur next to the canaliculus, the specialized portion of the cell responsible for bile excretion.[6] Loss of villus processes and the interruption of transport pumps such as multidrug resistance-associated protein 3 (MRP3) prevent the excretion of bilirubin and other organic compounds.
3. Drugs are relatively small molecules and, therefore, unlikely to evoke an immune response. Many hepatocellular reactions involve the haem-containing cytochrome P450 system, and generate high-energy reactions that

can lead to the covalent binding of drugs to enzymes, thus creating new, non-functioning adducts, which are large enough to serve as immune targets.

4. These enzyme–drug adducts migrate to the cell surface in vesicles to serve as target immunogens for cytolytic attack by the T cells, stimulating a multifaceted immune response involving both cytolytic T cells and cytokines.[7]

5. Activation of apoptotic pathways by the tumour necrosis factor-α (TNF-α) receptor or *Fas* may trigger a cascade of intercellular caspases, which results in programmed cell death with loss of nuclear chromatin.[8]

6. Certain drugs inhibit mitochondrial function by a dual effect on both β-oxidation (affecting energy production by inhibition of the synthesis of nicotinamide adenine dinucleotide [NAD] and flavin adenine dinucleotide [FAD], resulting in decreased ATP production) and the respiratory chain enzymes. Free fatty acids cannot be metabolized, and the lack of aerobic respiration results in the accumulation of lactate and reactive oxygen species. The presence of reactive oxygen species may further disrupt mitochondrial DNA. This pattern of injury is characteristic of a variety of agents, including nucleoside reverse-transcriptase inhibitors, which bind directly to mitochondrial DNA as well as valproic acid, tetracycline and aspirin.[9] Toxic metabolites excreted in the bile may damage the bile duct epithelium.

CLASSIFICATION OF DRUG-INDUCED HEPATIC DISORDERS

This is very difficult because many drugs exhibit similar manifestations, whereas a few drugs can cause various hepatic disorders. A simpler classification based on clinicopathological features is given in Table II.

ROLE OF LIVER BIOPSY IN DIAGNOSIS

Sometimes liver biopsy is required to exclude other diseases and provide further clues to a drug-induced aetiology. The following patterns of injury suggest a drug-induced aetiology but their absence does not exclude drug injury.[10]

- Zonal necrosis or fatty change;
- A disproportionately severe degree of necrosis in relation to the patient's clinical condition and biochemical changes;
- Fatty changes in a fully developed stage of hepatitis;
- Granuloma formation in the absence of an obvious cause in a patient who is not a drug addict;
- Mixed histological picture of hepatocellular necrosis and cholestasis;
- Destructive bile duct lesions; and
- Infiltration by numerous eosinophils and prominent neutrophils in the absence of an obvious cause.

Table II. Clinicopathological classification of drug-induced hepatic disorders

Category	Description	Examples
Hepatic adaptation	No symptoms, raised GGT and ALP Hyperbilirubinaemia	Phenytoin, warfarin rifampicin, flavaspidic acid
Dose-dependent hepatotoxicity	Symptoms of hepatitis, focal, bridging and massive necrosis ALT ↑ >5-fold normal	Acetaminophen, nicotinic acid
Other cytopathic, acute steatosis	Microvescicular steatosis, diffuse or zonal; partially dose-dependent, severe liver injury, features of mitochondrial toxicity (lactic acidosis)	Valproic acid, didanosine, highly active antiretroviral therapy (HAART)
Acute hepatitis	Symptoms of hepatitis, focal, bridging and massive necrosis ALT ↑ >5-fold normal; extrahepatic features of drug allergy in some cases	Isoniazid, nitrofurantoin, halothane, phenytoin, ketoconazole
Chronic hepatitis	Duration >3 months, features of CLD, mildly raised AST/ALT	Nitrofurantoin, diclofenac, minocycline
Granulomatous hepatitis	Hepatic granulomas with ↑ ALP, GGT and ALT	Allopurinol, carbamazepine, quinidine
Cholestasis without hepatitis	Cholestasis, no inflammation, ALP ↑ >2-fold normal	Oral contraceptives, androgens
Cholestatic hepatitis	Cholestasis with inflammation, raised ALT and ALP	Chlorpromazine, erythromycins, amoxi/clavulanic acid
Cholestasis with bile duct injury	Bile duct lesions and cholestatic hepatitis	Chlorpromazine, flucloxacillin
Chronic cholestasis	Cholestasis present >3 months	Chlorpromazine, flucloxacillin

CLD: chronic liver disease

CLINICAL DIAGNOSTIC APPROACH

It is difficult to be certain that a particular drug is responsible for the drug reaction. However, one should consider the possibility of a drug reaction as a cause of liver dysfunction in any patient presenting with abnormal LFT.

Assessment should include a careful history, which forms the cornerstone of the diagnosis. It includes a stringent check of the use of all prescribed drugs, and over-the-counter herbal or alternative medications that have been taken, because the latter two have been shown to be an important cause of liver injury.[11] In the case of multiple drug intake, the agent most likely to be implicated is the one used most recently before the injury.

The diagnosis is usually made by exclusion but it is of utmost importance that DILD should not be a 'dumping' diagnosis prior to the exclusion of other possible aetiological factors such as viral hepatitis. Hypotension and biliary tract disease or alcohol-related liver disease should be excluded by a detailed medical history, USG or appropriate serological tests.

The assessment of causality can often be difficult; many agents are used simultaneously and questions about other potential causes may be inadvertently omitted.

INTERNATIONAL CONSENSUS CRITERIA FOR DRUG-INDUCED HEPATOTOXICITY[12]

In a suspected case of drug-induced hepatitis, the international criteria provide a uniform approach to determine the likelihood of drug involvement.

The international consensus criteria for drug-induced hepatotoxicity are as follows:

1. Time of drug intake to the apparent onset of reaction is 'suggestive' (5–90 days), or 'compatible' (<5 days or >90 days from initial drug intake);
2. Course of reaction after cessation of the drug is 'very suggestive' (fall in liver enzymes by 50% of excess above upper limit of normal within 8 days), or 'suggestive' (fall in liver enzymes by 50% within 30 days for hepatocellular and 180 days for cholestatic injury);
3. Alternative causes of reaction excluded by detailed investigations, including liver biopsy; and
4. Positive response to rechallenge (at least doubling of liver enzymes), if possible. This is not ethical as it may be associated with a severe reaction.

A reaction is 'drug-related' if the first 3 criteria are met or if 2 of the first 3 criteria are met with a positive rechallenge test.

CLINICAL DIAGNOSTIC SCALE FOR THE DIAGNOSIS OF DRUG-INDUCED LIVER DISEASE

A clinical diagnostic scale (CDS) has been developed for the diagnosis of DILD and is considered suitable for clinical practice.[12] This scale considers seven different components and each of them is given a quantitative score (Table III).

The CDS scoring system correlates well with the international consensus criteria and may be a useful tool in the routine evaluation of suspected hepatotoxic drug reaction. Figure 3 shows the approach adopted for the diagnosis of DILD.

HEPATOTOXICITY IN PATIENTS WITH CHRONIC LIVER DISEASE

The use of toxic drugs in patients with established cirrhosis increases the risk of hepatic decompensation. Thus, extra caution should be taken in treating patients with underlying liver disease because of the potential for serious consequences.

Many enzyme systems are preserved even in advanced liver disease, particularly those involved in conjugation reactions. In severe liver disease, the activity of the cytochrome P450 2C19 isoenzyme is greatly decreased, whereas that of the 2D6 isoenzyme is intact.[13,14]

The rates of drug metabolism in patients with cirrhosis may be reduced by as much as 50%. Changes resulting from the increased fibrosis along the hepatic sinusoids in patients with cirrhosis further separate the blood stream and hepatocytes.[15]

In general, patients with liver disease are uniformly at increased risk for hepatic injury, but there are some exceptions. Patients with hepatitis C do appear

Table III. Clinical diagnostic scale for the diagnosis of drug-induced liver disease

Component	Score
Temporal relationship between drug intake and reaction	
Time from drug intake until the onset of the first clinical or laboratory manifestation	
4 days–8 weeks (or <4 days in the case of re-exposure)	3
<4 days or >8 weeks	1
Time from drug withdrawal to the onset of manifestations	
0–7 days	3
8–15 days	0
>15 days (except in the case of persistence of the drug in the body after	
withdrawal, e.g. amiodarone)	−3
Time from drug withdrawal to normalization of liver function parameters	
(decrease to values twice the upper limit of normal)	
<6 months (cholestatic or mixed pattern) or 2 months (hepatocellular)	3
>6 months (cholestatic or mixed pattern) or 2 months (hepatocellular)	0
Exclusion of alternative causes (viral hepatitis, alcoholic liver disease, billiary obstruction,	
pre-existing liver disease, ischaemic hepatitis)	
Complete exclusion	3
Partial exclusion	0
Possible alternative causes detected	−1
Probable alternative causes detected	−1
Extrahepatic manifestation (rash, fever, arthralgia, eosinophilia, cytopenia)	
4 or more	3
2 or 3	2
1	1
None	0
Intentional or accidental re-exposure to the drug	
Positive rechallenge test	3
Negative or absent rechallenge test	0
Previous reports in the literature of hepatotoxicity with the drug	
Yes	2
No (drug marketed for up to 5 years)	0
No (drug marketed for >5 years)	−3

Reactions are graded according to the final score as:
    Definite drug-induced hepatotoxicity: >17
    Probably drug-induced hepatotoxicity: 14–17
    Possibly drug-induced hepatotoxicity: 10–13
    Unlikely drug-induced hepatotoxicity: 6–9
    Drug-induced hepatotoxicity excluded: <6

to be at increased risk for veno-occlusive disease after myeloablative therapy, in preparation for bone marrow transplantation.[16] HIV-infected patients undergoing treatment with highly active antiretroviral therapy (HAART) may be at increased risk for hepatotoxic effects when they are coinfected with diseases such as hepatitis B and C.[17] Patients with cirrhosis are also prone to renal injury; aminoglycosides, radiocontrast agents and prostaglandin inhibitors must be used with extreme caution in this group.

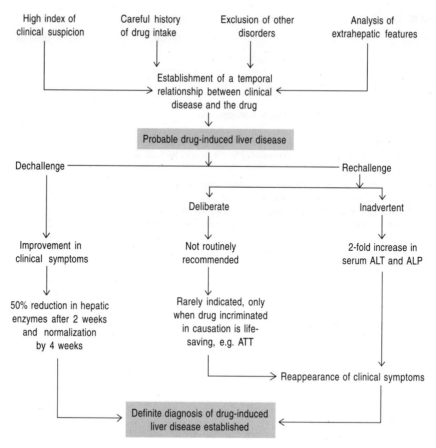

Fig. 3. Approach to the diagnosis of drug-induced liver disease

INDIVIDUAL DRUGS

Antituberculosis medications

Isoniazid

Isoniazid is a very common cause of drug-induced hepatitis, with an average frequency of about 21 per 1000 exposed. Isoniazid-induced hepatitis can be fatal in 5%–10% of patients. The risk and severity of hepatitis increases with the following parameters:[18]

- Age (≥60 years)
- Female sex
- High alcohol intake
- Hepatitis B, C and HIV infection
- Malnutrition
- Slow acetylators[18]
- BMI (<17.2±2.7)
- Other antituberculosis drugs used concomitantly.[19]

The usual latent period is 1 week to >6 months. Re-exposure causes an accelerated onset of hepatic drug injury. In Indians, for unknown reasons, reintroduction is possible without any major untoward adverse outcome. About 70% of patients present with prodromal features such as those seen in acute viral hepatitis (AVH).[20] Jaundice is usually a late feature. Biochemistry shows AST>ALT in more than 30% of exposed persons within 10 weeks. Isoniazid should be stopped if the ALT level is >250 U/L (>5 times the upper limit of normal). A rise in ALT level >10 times the upper limit of normal is a poor prognostic indicator. In the initial stage, recovery is rapid but in the later stages with advanced liver damage, the prognosis is poor. In one study, serious complications such as subacute hepatic failure (SHF) and hepatic encephalopathy (HE) developed in 16% of patients,[20] and the mean duration of treatment before the onset of hepatitis was significantly longer in the group of patients that died compared to those who survived (36 days *v.* 30 days).[20] Liver histology is not specific and is variable. Management depends on the stage of liver injury; in the initial stage, management is supportive and protocol screening is advised, whereas advanced-stage liver damage should be managed with liver transplantation.

Rifampicin and pyrazinamide

Liver toxicity is usually dose-dependent. There is cross-sensitivity and reactivity between isoniazid, pyrazinamide and ethionamide. The clinical features sometimes resemble those seen in AVH, and about 20%–30% of the patients show an alteration in the LFT. Patients are at greater risk of liver toxicity at high doses and concomitant multiple antituberculosis drug administration.

PREVENTION AND MANAGEMENT

The majority of DILD are idiosyncratic. Therefore, the prevention and early detection of liver injury are the most effective ways to minimize the incidence of adverse drug reactions.

For dose-dependent hepatotoxins, prevention is dependent on strict adherence to the dosage guidelines or the estimation of blood levels of the drugs. In cases with specific risk factors, a strategy to avoid toxicity is essential, e.g. avoidance of acetaminophen in moderate alcohol consumers.

Early detection is also critical. The appearance of any untoward symptoms such as nausea, malaise, right upper quadrant abdominal pain, lethargy or fever and prodromal features of hepatitis, are an indication to perform LFT and stop the medication.

Protocol screening is usually not recommended since its efficacy and cost-effectiveness are unknown. However, monthly or two-weekly screening is of some use for a few drugs, e.g. valproic acid, isoniazid, pyrazinamide, dantolene, tacrine, thioridazone, antidiabetics, synthetic retinoids and ketoconazole.

Active management includes discontinuation of the offending agent along with administration of antidotes, and anti-inflammatory and cytoprotective agents. For ingested dose-dependent hepatotoxic agents such as acetaminophen, removal of unabsorbed drugs and the use of antidotes (N-acetylcysteine) is recommended.

The management of drug-induced hepatitis and cholestasis is symptomatic and supportive. In severe cases, hepatic transplantation should be considered. Ursodeoxycholic acid holds some promise in the management of chronic cholestasis and pruritus. Glucocorticoids are usually reserved for atypical, refractory cases and those with vasculitis.

REFRENCES

1. Friis H, Andreasen PB. Drug-induced hepatic injury: An analysis of 1100 case reports to The Danish Committee on Adverse Drug Reactions between 1978 and 1987. *J Intern Med* 1992;**232:**133.
2. Stricker BHCH. *Drug-induced hepatic injury.* 2nd ed. Amsterdam: Elsevier; 1992.
3. Farrell OC. In: Farr GC (ed). *Drug-induced liver disease.* London: Churchill Livingstone; 1994.
4. Larrey D. Drug-induced liver diseases. *J Hepatol* 2000;**32** (Suppl):77–88.
5. Guengerich FP. Common and uncommon cytochrome P450 reactions related to metabolism and chemical toxicity. *Chem Res Toxicol* 2001;**14:**611–50.
6. Trauner M, Meier PJ, Boyer J. Molecular pathogenesis of cholestasis. *N Engl J Med* 1998;**339:**1217–27.
7. Robin M-A, Le Roy M, Descatoire V, Pessayre D. Plasma membrane cytochromes P450 as neoantigens and autoimmune targets in drug-induced hepatitis. *J Hepatol* 1997;**26** (Suppl):23–30.
8. Reed JC. Apoptosis-regulating proteins as targets for drug discovery. *Trends Mol Med* 2001;**7:**314–19.
9. Pessayre D, Berson A, Fromenty B, Man Souri A. Mitochondria in steatohepatitis. *Semin Liver Dis* 2001;**21:**57–69.
10. Hall PD. Histological diagnosis of drug induced liver disease. In: Farr GC (ed). *Drug-induced liver disease.* Edinburgh: Churchill Livingstone; 1994:15–51.
11. Chitturi S, Farrell GC. Herbal hepatoxicity: An expanding but poorly defined problem. *J Gastroenterol Hepatol* 2000;**10:**1093–9.
12. Benichou C. Criteria for drug induced liver disorder. Report of an International Consensus Meeting. *J Hepatol* 1990;**11:**272.
13. George J, Murray K, Byth K, Farrell GC. Differential alterations of cytochrome P450 proteins in livers from patients with severe chronic liver disease. *Hepatology* 1995;**21:**120–8.
14. Adedoyin A, Arns PA, Richards WO, Wilkinson GR, Branch RA. Selective effect of liver disease on the activities of specific metabolizing enzymes: Investigation of cytochromes P450 2C19 and 2D6. *Clin Pharmacol Ther* 1998;**64:**8–17.
15. Froomes PRA, Morgan DJ, Smallwood RA, Angus PW. Comparative effects of oxygen supplementation on theophylline and acetaminophen clearance in human cirrhosis. *Gastroenterology* 1999;**116:**915–20.
16. Strasser SI, Myerson D, Spurgeon CL, *et al.* Hepatitis C virus infection and bone marrow transplantation: A cohort study with 10-year follow-up. *Hepatology* 1999;**29:**1893–9.
17. Clark CJ, Creighton S, Portmann B, Taylor C, Wendon JA, Cramp ME. Acute liver failure associated with antiretroviral treatment for HIV: A report of six cases. *J Hepatol* 2002;**36:**295–301.
18. Singh J, Arora A, Garg PK, Thakur VS, Pande JN, Tandon RK. Antituberculosis treatment induced hepatotoxicity: Role of predictive factors. *Postgrad Med J* 1995;**71:**359–62.
19. Pande JN, Singh SP, Khilnani GC, Khilnani S, Tandon RK. Risk factors for hepatotoxicity from antituberculosis drugs: A case–control study. *Thorax* 1996;**51:**132–6.
20. Singh J, Garg PK, Tandon RK. Hepatotoxicity due to antituberculosis therapy: Clinical profile and reintroduction of therapy. *J Clin Gastroenterol* 1996;**22:**211–14.

CHAPTER 15

Jaundice in patients with haematological malignancy

USHA DUTTA

The liver *per se* does not have any organized lymphoid tissue although lymphocytes traverse the liver continually. Thus, secondary infiltration of the liver by haematological malignancies is far more common than primary haematological malignancies of the liver.[1] Hepatic involvement often poses problems in the diagnosis and management of these patients. Infiltration of the liver indicates the presence of advanced disease and thus has a grave prognosis. Among patients with hepatic infiltration, jaundice is present in only those with considerable liver involvement, and thus occurs in a small minority. However, jaundice due to reasons other than hepatic infiltration is often not related to the tumour load. The time at which jaundice develops during the course of the malignancy is an important indicator of the possible aetiology.[2] In this chapter, emphasis will be laid on the various mechanisms implicated in the pathogenesis of jaundice, various haematological conditions associated with liver involvement and the approach to ascertaining the aetiopathogenesis of jaundice in patients with haematological malignancies.

PATHOGENETIC MECHANISMS

Jaundice in patients with lymphoma may be due to a single or multiple aetiologies. Though it is often not possible to identify all the mechanisms operating in a patient, it is necessary to identify the dominant mechanism so that therapy can be directed against it. The prototype haematological malignancy in which jaundice is a striking manifestation is lymphoma. Thus, most of the discussion will be focused on this disease with reference to other malignancies whenever appropriate. Various possible mechanisms of jaundice among patients with lymphoma are listed in Table I.

Table I. Causes of jaundice in patients with lymphoma

Direct effect of the tumour	*Effect of antitumour therapy*
Diffuse hepatic infiltration	Chemotherapeutic agents
Focal mass	Hepatic irradiation
Extrahepatic biliary obstruction by the tumour	Graft-versus-host disease
Lymph nodes: porta hepatis/	Veno-occlusive disease
peripancreatic group	*Immunosuppression and parenteral exposure-related*
Gallbladder	Hepatitis: HBV, HCV, CMV, Epstein–Barr virus,
Common bile duct	Cryptosporidium
Ampulla of Vater	*Miscellaneous causes*
Indirect effects of the tumour	Sepsis
Intrahepatic cholestasis	Antibiotics
Haemolysis (autoimmune haemolytic	Total parenteral nutrition
anaemia)	Allopurinol
Haemophagocytosis	

Direct effect of the malignancy

Hepatic infiltration

Jaundice is usually a late manifestation of tumour infiltration.[3] Diffuse infiltration results in jaundice due to a marked reduction in the functioning hepatocyte mass secondary to hepatocyte dysfunction/destruction. However, even small focal infiltrations in critical areas can result in jaundice due to compression of the biliary radicles. Jaundice is usually mild to moderate in severity. It is accompanied by hepatomegaly and elevated levels of serum ALP. USG examination may show evidence of hepatomegaly and altered echotexture of the liver with or without focal deposits. Liver biopsy reveals infiltration of the portal tracts by atypical lymphoid cells with evidence of cholestasis. Jaundice usually resolves on instituting appropriate chemotherapy. A small proportion of patients may present with features of acute hepatic failure, which has a high mortality. In contrast to viral hepatitis-induced acute liver failure (ALF), these patients have an enlarged liver at presentation and lactic acidosis with high levels of ALP.[4]

Hepatic infiltration leading to ALF needs to be differentiated from toxin and viral-induced ALF, as chemotherapy is the treatment of choice for patients with lymphoma rather than transplantation, which is the appropriate therapy for toxin- and viral-induced liver failure. Transjugular biopsy is useful in patients with ALF for establishing the aetiology. Biopsy usually shows infiltration of the portal tracts and, in advanced cases, involvement of the sinusoids. Portal tract infiltration may mimic the histology seen in patients with chronic hepatitis. However, the differentiating features are the absence of hepatic parenchymal destruction, cytologically uniform infiltrate and more circumscribed lesions compared to those seen in patients with chronic hepatitis.

Biliary tract obstruction

Among patients with jaundice due to extrahepatic obstruction, compression by the lymph nodes at the porta hepatis is the most common.[5] Other causes are primary involvement of the CBD, gallbladder and ampulla of Vater, or extrinsic compression by a pancreatic mass or the peripancreatic lymph nodes.[2,6] USG examination in these patients confirms the presence of biliary radicle dilatation and identifies the site of obstruction. These patients may present with fever, which may be due to the primary disease or cholangitis. The presence of polymorphonuclear leucocytosis, fever with rigors of recent onset, change in the pattern of fever, presence of cholangitic abscesses and transient but markedly elevated transaminase levels suggest the presence of cholangitis. Biliary stenting is indicated in the presence of cholangitis and for the palliation of intractable pruritus. Routine stenting to reduce bilirubin levels before instituting chemotherapy is controversial.

Indirect effects of tumour

In some patients, jaundice may be due to certain mediators released by the tumour or immunological processes initiated by the tumour. These effects are usually disproportionate to the tumour load. Moreover, these effects may antedate the other characteristic features of an underlying malignancy.[2] Thus, a careful search and close follow-up would be necessary in these patients to ascertain the underlying aetiology.

Idiopathic intrahepatic cholestasis

Patients with lymphoma may present with cholestatic jaundice without any evidence of hepatic tumour infiltration or extrahepatic obstruction. It is a paraneoplastic phenomenon and is not related to the tumour bulk. In some patients, the cholestasis may be severe and fatal. The mechanism of development of the cholestasis is not yet completely understood. However, an increasing number of such patients have recently been documented to have vanishing bile ducts in the portal tracts.[7-9] What initiates this phenomenon is not clear. Idiopathic cholestasis needs to be differentiated from rapid tumour infiltration, which may also result in deep jaundice, fever and liver failure. The ALP level does not help in differentiating between these conditions as it is elevated in both. The presence of massive hepatomegaly, evidence of diffuse infiltration at other sites, elevated transaminase levels and lactic acidosis are suggestive of infiltration as the possible underlying mechanism rather than idiopathic cholestasis.[10] Chemotherapy may not have any predictable effect on idiopathic cholestasis; however, it plays a definite role in the management of hepatic infiltration-induced jaundice.[2] Thus, liver biopsy is required to differentiate between these two entities.

Haemolysis

Haemolysis is usually due to a warm antibody of the IgG type.[2] The dominant mechanism of RBC destruction is through phagocytosis of the IgG-coated RBCs by macrophages. If phagocytosis is not possible, part of the cell membrane is chipped off, resulting in the formation of spherocytes, which are destroyed in the spleen. The other rare mechanism of destruction is through complement-mediated lysis. Splenomegaly in these patients may be secondary to haemolysis or splenic infiltration. Haemolytic anaemia could be the presenting manifestation of lymphoma and thus a careful search for an underlying occult disease should be made in such patients. Investigations reveal the presence of unconjugated hyperbilirubinaemia, anaemia with increased reticulocytes and the presence of spherocytes in the peripheral blood film. The direct Coombs test is positive in 98% of cases and usually IgG antibodies are detected on the surface of the RBCs with or without C3. There may be an associated presence of immune-mediated thrombocytopenia, when the condition is labelled as the Evan syndrome. The clinical severity of the haemolysis may be variable, ranging from isolated Coombs positivity to frank, severe, life-threatening haemolysis. In these patients, jaundice may get exaggerated after blood transfusion for anaemia. An algorithm for the management of haemolysis-induced jaundice is given in Table II.

Haemophagocytosis-induced jaundice

Among patients with haematological malignancies, haemophagocytosis may be triggered, resulting in cytopenia along with jaundice. Histiocytes/macrophages are activated in genetically susceptible hosts to phagocytose RBCs, WBCs and platelets, resulting in pancytopenia. These histiocytes with phagocytosed material are found to infiltrate the lymph nodes, liver, spleen and bone marrow. Evaluation of any of these organs would help to establish the diagnosis. Jaundice in these patients is usually marked, predominantly conjugated and accompanied by marked elevation of the transaminase levels. The cause of jaundice in these patients is excessive RBC turnover and hepatocyte destruction. The surrogate

Table II. Management of haemolysis-induced jaundice

Evaluation
    Haemogram
    Reticulocyte count
    Renal and liver function tests
    Direct Coombs test
    Assess for aetiology: malignancy, drugs, systemic lupus erythematosus

Management of acute phase
  General
    Hydration
    Blood transfusion: Slow transfusion of washed ABO-compatible RBCs; closely watch for transfusion reaction
    Watch for renal failure

  Specific measures
    Mild: Watch
    Moderate: Start oral steroids 1 mg/kg/day
    Severe haemolysis: Oral steroids + intravenous immunoglobulin ± splenectomy

Maintenance therapy
  Assess response at 3 weeks
  Good response: taper steroids to 20 mg/day rapidly and slowly to 5 mg/day, and then stop
  Poor response/relapse: Oral steroids on alternate days/immunosuppressive drugs/splenectomy

---

markers for the presence of haemophagocytosis are elevated levels of serum ferritin and triglyceride, and reduced levels of fibrinogen. The malignancy *per se* or an intercurrent infection may initiate haemophagocytosis, which should be suspected in any patient who has jaundice, cytopenia and fever. This combination of symptoms could also occur in patients with sepsis secondary to neutropenia. However, in patients with sepsis-induced jaundice, this is usually of the cholestatic type with elevated serum ALP levels and minimal/no elevation of transaminase levels, in contrast to haemophagocytosis in which transaminase levels are markedly elevated.

Treatment-related jaundice

After the institution of therapy, patients may develop jaundice due to toxicity of the chemotherapeutic agents, hepatic irradiation, reactivation of dormant hepatitis, development of post-transfusion hepatitis or graft-versus-host disease (GVHD) in patients undergoing bone marrow transplantation.[2,10] It is important to differentiate between these possibilities as the treatment options are drastically different.

Chemotherapy-induced jaundice

As the liver is the major site of drug metabolism, it is not surprising that hepatotoxicity is so common. The majority of these agents cause centrilobular necrosis. Liver injury manifests as hepatocellular inflammation, necrosis, fibrosis, cholestasis, fatty infiltration, veno-occulsive disease (VOD), granulomatous infiltration or a combination of these. The type of hepatic injury produced by some commonly used drugs is given in Table III.

Liver injury is usually asymptomatic. However, severe hepatotoxicity occurs when high-dose intensive regimens are used during bone marrow transplantation. Commonly used drugs that result in hepatotoxicity include 6-mercaptopurine, methotrexate, cytosine arabinoside, procarbazine and vincristine.[11] Combination chemotherapy is notorious for causing hepatotoxicity even when the individual component drugs are not hepatotoxic.[11] Patients undergoing chemotherapy should be monitored by regular LFT. Any abnormality detected should be carefully analysed to exclude other causes for derangement of the LFT. An important differential diagnosis is hepatitis due to reactivation of the hepatitis B virus, which occurs during withdrawal of chemotherapy, in contrast to chemotherapy-induced hepatotoxicity, which would occur during therapy. Serological markers for the presence of active viral infection and estimation of viral DNA/RNA levels would be useful in such situations.[2] Although histological examination may occasionally be useful, often it is not possible due to the risk associated with an invasive procedure. Most of these derangements are transient and recover on stopping the offending agent. The decision to stop or modify therapy should be individualized. Reintroduction of the drugs may result in the recurrence of jaundice, which establishes the aetiology; however, this may be risky in some patients and is thus not advocated.

Table III. Hepatic injury produced by chemotherapeutic agents and other treatment-related causes

Type of liver injury	Chemotherapeutic agent	Other treatment-related causes
Cholestasis	6-mercaptopurine Carboplatin Androgens	Acute graft-versus-host disease (GVHD) Chronic GVHD Prochlorperazine
Steatosis	Methotrexate Asparaginases Steroids	Total parenteral nutrition
Granuloma	Allopurinol	
Hepatocellular necrosis	Chlorambucil 6-mercaptopurine Etoposide Retinoids	Mithramycin Allopurinol Acetaminophen Antifungal agents
Veno-occlusive disease	Dacarbazine 6-thioguanine Carmustine Busulfan Mitomycin-C Dactinomycin	Chronic GVHD Radiotherapy
Peliosis	6-thioguanine Tamoxifen Androgens	
Fibrosis	Methotrexate	Total parenteral nutrition
Cirrhosis	Methotrexate	Chronic GVHD
Sclerosing cholangitis	Floxuridine (intra-arterial)	
Neoplastic	Androgens	

Radiotherapy

Hepatic irradiation causes dose-related injury to the liver, which histologically manifests as VOD. Factors associated with an increased risk of hepatic injury are total dose >3500 cGy, higher individual dose fractions, concurrent/ sequential administration of dactinomycin, vincristine or doxorubicin.[11,12] Intra-arterial mitomycin-C and 5-fluorouracil in combination with lower doses of radiotherapy are also associated with abnormalities of LFT. Clinical and laboratory evidence of liver injury is usually seen at 1–3 months after completion of treatment. Most patients recover within 3 months.[11]

Biological response modifiers

Various biological response modifiers are now being tried in the management of various malignancies. Alpha-, beta- as well as gamma-interferons cause dose-related, reversible elevation in transaminase levels, which occurs within the first week of therapy. Resolution takes place within 2 weeks. Rarely, fatality has been reported. The other agents that result in hepatic injury are tumour necrosis factor (TNF), interleukin (IL)-6, IL-4, granulocyte–macrophage colony stimulating factor (GM-CSF) and vitamin A derivatives. BCG, *Corynebacterium parvum* and other bacterial adjuvants also result in the formation of granulomas.[11–14]

Graft-versus-host disease

This occurs in patients who have undergone bone marrow transplantation. GVHD may be acute or chronic in presentation.[11] Manifestations include hepatomegaly, hyperbilirubinaemia, and elevated ALP and aminotransferase levels. Liver biopsy shows evidence of bile duct injury, cholestatic changes and periportal lymphocytic infiltrate.[15] Patients with chronic GVHD have progressive loss of the interlobular bile ducts, resulting in the vanishing bile syndrome.

Veno-occlusive disease

VOD is characterized by the development of hepatomegaly, ascites, abdominal pain and unexplained weight gain.[11,16] LFT initially show a rise in bilirubin followed by an elevation in transaminase levels. Liver biopsy initially shows centrizonal haemorrhagic necrosis followed by central venular sclerosis. VOD occurs due to direct injury to the vascular endothelium. The overall mortality is about 33%–45%. Histological examination may show a mixed picture of VOD and GVHD. The other causes of VOD are related to the use of drugs and radiotherapy (Table III).

Reactivation of hepatitis B

The immunosuppression that occurs during the administration of chemo-therapy results in unchecked proliferation of HBV inside the hepatocytes. However, as immune-mediated destruction is not possible, these hepatocytes cannot be destroyed. When chemotherapy is withdrawn or tapered, there is a resurgence of immunity.[2] This triggers the immune-mediated destruction of hepatocytes which are loaded with HBV, resulting in a marked increase in the transaminase levels. If the withdrawal is rapid, severe hepatic necrosis manifesting as ALF may occur in some patients.[17] Thus, HBsAg-positive patients are assessed before and during therapy for any evidence of reactivation. If the markers of reactivation (HBeAg positivity, increase in HBV DNA and trans-aminase levels) suggest active replication, the use of lamivudine is currently recommended to suppress HBV replication.[2] It is also recommended that myelosuppressive therapy or steroids be slowly tapered in these patients. According to the recent recommendations of European Association for the Study of Liver Diseases (EASLD), lamivudine therapy should be instituted prophy-lactically in patients who are HBsAg-positive prior to starting chemotherapy.

Post-transfusion hepatitis

Due to multiple parenteral exposures and blood transfusion, these patients are at high risk of developing hepatitis B or C infection. Moreover, due to an immune-suppressed state, they are less likely to clear an acquired virus, resulting in the development of chronic infection. Most of these patients are asymptomatic and the infection is detected only incidentally during screening. However, some may manifest features of hepatitis when the immune system bounces back during the phase of chemotherapy withdrawal. Careful monitoring of these patients during the withdrawal phase of chemotherapy is thus necessary. The treatment of hepatitis C infection is difficult as the standard therapy with IFN is either contraindicated or ineffective in most of these patients. Treatment with ribavarin alone is not effective. However, hepatitis B infection can be managed with lamivudine therapy. CMV infection can occur due to either reactivation or parenteral transmission.[2,18] Intravenous gingiclovir is useful in these patients. Positive IgM serology specific for these viral infections would help in establishing the diagnosis. Although markers for viral replication are also of immense use, their utility is restricted as they are expensive.

Sepsis

Patients suffering from haematological malignancies are more predisposed to infection due to an immunocompromised state. Septicaemia can manifest as jaundice in these patients. Among patients with extrahepatic biliary obstruction who present with jaundice, the possibility of cholangitis should be considered. Though fever may also be a manifestation of the primary disease itself, a careful search for a focus of infection should be made before attributing the fever to the malignancy *per se*.

Antibiotics

Various antibiotics have been implicated in the causation of jaundice. The important ones relevant to this situation are amoxycillin–clavulanic acid, cephalosporins, itraconazole, fluconazole and nitrofurantoin. Antitubercular therapy for reactivation tuberculosis among these patients can result in hepatotoxicity, which may present as jaundice. Usually, discontinuation of these drugs leads to the resolution of jaundice. The presence of a temporal relationship between jaundice and drug intake often provides a clue to the diagnosis. Recurrence of jaundice on an inadvertent rechallenge establishes the diagnosis. However, deliberate rechallenge should preferably be avoided.

AETIOLOGY

Lymphomas and leukaemias are the most common haematological malignancies affecting the liver. All the haematological malignancies that affect the liver are listed in Table IV. Certain haematological conditions that occur secondary to or mimic malignancy are also given.

Hodgkin disease

Hepatic infiltration in Hodgkin disease (HD) is regarded as evidence of stage IV disease and the prevalence of infiltration increases with the duration of the disease.[10] Hepatic infiltration is seen in 5%–14% of liver biopsies at the time of diagnosis, 30% of biopsies obtained during the course of the disease and 60% at the time of autopsy.[10] Hepatic infiltration is more common in the lymphocyte-

Table IV. Haematological malignancies associated with involvement of the liver

Secondary involvement of the liver	*Primary hepatic lymphomas*
Lymphoma	Hepatosplenic T-cell lymphomas
Leukaemia	T-cell or histiocyte-rich B-cell lymphoma
Paraproteinaemia	Follicular dentritic cell tumours
Polycythaemia vera	MALTomas
Essential thrombocythaemia	Plasmacytomas
Myelofibrosis	Angiocentric lymphoma
Sēzary syndrome	Post-transplant lymphoproliferative disease
Aetiologies that mimic haematological malignancies	*Haematological conditions secondary to malignancy*
Angioimmunoblastic lymphadenopathy	Amyloidosis
Myelodysplasias	Extramedullary haematopoiesis
Systemic mastocytosis	Haemophagocytosis
Langerhans cell histiocytosis (histiocytosis X)	

depleted and mixed-cellularity variety, and least common in the lymphocyte-predominant type.[18] Patients with hepatic involvement invariably have splenic involvement. There is only one instance reported of a patient who had hepatic involvement without evidence of splenic involvement.[19] Hepatic involvement may be diffuse, or occur as focal masses (yellow in colour) or just as infiltrates at the portal tracts. Histological involvement characteristically comprises multifocal infiltration of the portal tract with Reed–Sternberg cells admixed with lymphocytes, plasma cells, eosinophils, atypical histiocytes and proliferating fibroblasts. Non-specific findings include non-caseating epithelioid granulomas, non-specific infiltrates in the portal tracts, sinusoidal dilatation, steatosis, haemosiderosis, cholestasis and peliosis hepatis. Granulomas occur in 10% of cases and are often seen in patients in whom there is no evidence of hepatic infiltration by the tumour.[2,3,11,20] Occasionally, caseating granulomas without any evidence of tuberculosis have been reported. Among patients with non-specific infiltrates in the portal tracts, a careful search for Reed–Sternberg and atypical cells should be made and, if required, immunostaining used to aid in making an appropriate diagnosis. Cholestasis may again be an isolated finding without evidence of hepatic infiltration.

Most patients with hepatic infiltration are asymptomatic and have non-tender hepatomegaly. Jaundice is a frequent late manifestation of the disease. Rarely, it may be a manifestation of idiopathic cholestasis and can occur early in the course of the disease. LFT usually show an elevation in serum ALP and GGT levels with or without elevation in transaminase levels. USG and CT scan may show hepatomegaly with or without focal masses. Liver biopsy is usually essential to establish the diagnosis of hepatic infiltration. Guided liver biopsies using USG or CT when a focal lesion is identifiable, and laparoscopy when the focal lesion is not identifiable, yield better results than a blind biopsy. However, a negative needle biopsy does not exclude hepatic involvement. Liver biospy may show evidence of amyloidosis, haemophagocytosis or extramedullary erythropoiesis. Bile ductular proliferation, cholangitis, portal oedema and portal infiltrates >1 mm may be seen in patients with extrahepatic biliary obstruction.[11]

Aggressive treatment of the lymphoma would result in regression of these features. The presence of jaundice does not alter the choice of therapy for the primary disease. However, if extrahepatic obstruction results in considerable jaundice or cholangitis, the placement of a biliary stent would be of use. In patients with persistent jaundice, local irradiation may achieve some palliation. If drug toxicity is the offending cause, withdrawal/modification of the drug dose may be useful. Surgical resection is of use only in patients with a focal lesion due to primary lymphoma, though chemotherapy remains the mainstay even in these patients.

Non-Hodgkin lymphoma

Involvement of the liver in non-Hodgkin lymphoma (NHL) is similar to that in HD except for certain differences. The prevalence of liver infiltration at presentation is slightly more common in NHL than in HD (15%–20% v. 8%–14%).[2,3,11] However, at autopsy, the prevalence of involvement is similar. Jaundice is less common in patients with NHL than in those with HD. Jaundice due to extrahepatic obstruction is more common in NHL than HD. Hepatic granulomas are less common among patients with NHL than HD. Hepatic infiltration is more common in low-grade, lymphocytic lymphomas rather than high-grade, large-cell, histiocytic lymphomas. The well-differentiated low-grade, lymphocytic and follicular lymphomas, mantle cell and marginal zone lymphomas, and lymphoid leukaemias tend to produce multiple, small, nodular deposits predominantly at the portal tracts in contrast to the poorly differentiated lymphomas, which produce larger, irregular deposits involving the portal tracts and sinusoids. Immunophenotyping is useful in establishing the diagnosis. Occasionally, Burkitt lymphoma can present with subcapsular deposits due to direct spread from the peritoneum. Rarely, hepatic infiltration can present as ALF. Lymphoma should be considered in patients presenting with ALF if it is accompanied by hepatic enlargement and lactic acidosis, which are not the features of toxin- or viral-induced liver failure. Differentiation is important as chemotherapy rather than transplantation should be the appropriate therapy in these patients. Transjugular biopsy is useful in establishing the diagnosis. Biopsy usually shows infiltration of the portal tracts and, in advanced cases, involvement of the sinusoids. Portal tract infiltration may mimic the histological picture found in patients with chronic hepatitis. However, differentiating features are the absence of hepatic parenchymal destruction, cytologically uniform infiltrates and more circumscribed lesions compared to those seen in patients with chronic hepatitis.

Acute leukaemias

Leukaemias frequently involve the liver but seldom to the extent of causing hepatic dysfunction. In contrast to lymphomas, the leukaemic cells in myeloid leukaemias predominantly infiltrate the sinusoids and, rarely, in advanced cases, involve the portal tracts.[3,11] The immature cells lie outside the sinusoids and in direct contact with the hepatocytes. The leukaemic deposits compress the hepatic cords. In lymphoid leukaemias, the infiltrates are only in the portal tract and not the sinusoids. The liver cells are uninvolved in lymphoid leukaemias. In hairy cell leukaemias, infiltration of the portal tracts and sinusoids is present. The characteristic finding in these cases is the presence of dilated angiomatous lesions with destruction of the endothelial lining and the presence of hairy cells (mononuclear clear cells) in the space of Disse. These leukaemic cells may be overlooked on an H&E stain, but can be identified by their content of tartrate-resistant acid phosphatase or immunochemical methods. The enlarged liver is usually smooth and firm. The LFT are usually only mildly deranged.

Chronic leukaemias

In chronic leukaemias, involvement of the liver is a late phenomenon and hepatic infiltrates are predominantly seen only in the portal tracts. Sinusoidal involvement occurs during blast crisis, especially in chronic myeloid leukaemias. Rarely, hepatic venous outflow tract obstruction has been recorded in chronic lymphocytic leukaemia due to tumour cell infiltration.

Primary hepatic lymphomas

Primary lymphoma of the liver usually affects the middle-aged, and presents with abdominal pain and B symptoms (fever, weight loss, night sweats and pruritus) without any ascites or jaundice. The criteria for the diagnosis of primary hepatic lymphoma are: the absence of lymphadenopathy, splenomegaly, normal thoracic and abdominal CT scan, and normal bone marrow and peripheral counts.[2-23] Primary lymphomas usually have focal lesions in the liver that are hyper- or hypoechoic on USG examination and hypodense on CT scan. A targeted liver biopsy establishes the diagnosis. Elevation of the serum ALP is characteristic; however, transaminase levels may not be elevated.

Rarely, primary lymphomas of the CBD, gallbladder and sphincter of Oddi are reported. Their association with hepatitis C has been increasingly reported recently. In these patients, the lymphoma is usually of the B-cell type and of intermediate grade. Hepatosplenic T-cell lymphoma is associated with the consistent presence of iso-chromosome 7q. It is usually confined to the liver and spleen where sinusoidal permeation by small lymphoid cells is detectable. The cells usually show a clonal T-gamma/delta receptor gene arrangement and, rarely, alpha/beta-clonal expansion. This may develop in a setting of immunosuppression. T-cell or histiocyte-rich B-cell lymphomas may mimic HD, and frequently present with B symptoms and marked derangement in LFT. Histologically, this tumour is characterized by a florid reactive stromal response, which may mask the presence of malignant cells. Follicular dentritic cell tumour is very rare and is characterized by a pseudotumour-like histology with fascicles of bland spindle cells. This tumour seems to be related to Epstein–Barr virus (EBV) infection.

Angioimmunoblastic lymphoproliferative disease

This disorder is characterized by generalized lymphadenopathy, elevated serum transaminase levels, lymphocytosis, splenomegaly and autoimmune phenomena.[2] The underlying defect appears to be an impaired lymphocyte apoptosis due to an inherited mutation on the CD95 (*Fas*) gene. These patients have lymphocytic infiltrates in the portal tract with fibrosis and extramedullary erythropoiesis.

Paraproteinaemias

About 40% of patients with advanced multiple myeloma (MM) and Waldenström macroglobulinaemia (WM) have hepatic involvement.[2,3] These patients show evidence of portal and sinusoidal infiltrates. Involvement of the liver can occur in the absence of plasma cell leukaemia and may manifest as focal lesions in the liver. These patients may also develop amyloid deposits in the space of Disse. Rarely, peliosis hepatitis, nodular hyperplasia of the liver and portal hypertension due to infiltration of the portal vein can occur.

APPROACH TO A PATIENT WITH JAUNDICE

The aetiology of jaundice may be multifactorial in some patients. However, there is usually a single dominant mechanism that needs to be identified so that appropriate therapy can be instituted. A methodical approach is required for the assessment of these patients. Evaluation includes clinical, radiological and laboratory parameters. The time at which jaundice develops during the course of therapy is an important pointer towards the aetiology. It is important to ascertain whether there is some temporal relationship between the development of jaundice and the introduction/withdrawal of any agent. A history of blood or blood product transfusion may indicate the presence of hepatotropic viral illnesses as the possible aetiology. It is important to assess whether the jaundice is intrahepatic or extrahepatic as the differential diagnoses to be considered are significantly different. In patients with extrahepatic obstruction, the site, nature and presence/absence of associated cholangitis should be specifically ascertained. Cholangitis in these patients is associated with a high mortality unless appropriate antibiotics are started early and drainage of the biliary tract performed. Associated clinical features such as the presence or absence of hepatomegaly, ascites, anaemia, thrombocytopenia and lymphadenopathy provide clues towards the possible aetiology (Tables V and VI). LFT and USG examination are the two key investigations in the evaluation of these patients. However, liver biopsy and markers for viral hepatitis may be required in selected patients. A careful analysis of these parameters can help in arriving at a diagnosis and directing the management of these patients. Jaundice in most patients is

Table V. Differential diagnosis of various clinical presentations of jaundice

Cholestasis
    Infiltration
    Idiopathic intrahepatic cholestasis
    Extrahepatic biliary obstruction
    Sepsis
    Drug-induced
Elevated transaminase levels
    Hepatitis
    Cholangitis
    Hepatic infiltration
    Graft-versus-host disease (GVHD)
Acute liver failure
    Reactivation hepatitis
    Post-transfusion hepatitis
    Massive hepatic infiltration
Ascites
    Veno-occlusive disease (VOD)
    Budd–Chiari syndrome
    Acute portal vein thrombosis

Unconjugated hyperbilirubinaemia
    Haemolysis
Cytopenias
    Drug-induced
    Haemophagocytosis
    Bone marrow infiltration
    Immune-mediated destruction
Fever
    Malignancy
    Systemic sepsis
    Cholangitis
    Haemophagocytosis
Abdominal pain
    VOD
    Budd–Chiari syndrome
    Hepatic infiltration

Table VI. Evaluation of a patient with jaundice

Mechanism	Characteristic features	Liver biopsy
Diffuse hepatic infiltration	Massive hepatosplenomegaly, ↑ serum ALP	Portal/sinusoidal infiltration
Focal infiltration	SOL of liver compressing bile ducts	Cholestasis
Extrahepatic obstruction	IHBR dilatation, mass at the site of obstruction	Cholestasis
Drug-induced	Temporal relationship	Varied patterns
Hepatitis	Viral markers, ↑↑ ALT/AST	Specific markers
Veno-occlusive disease	Hepatomegaly, ascites	Centrilobular haemorrhagic necrosis
Budd–Chiari syndrome	Hepatomegaly, ascites HV block on Doppler study	Centrilobular haemorrhagic necrosis
Haemolysis	Anaemia, Coombs test positive, ↑ reticulocytes	Hyperplasia of the reticuloendothelial system
Idiopathic cholestasis	↑ ALP and normal ALT/AST	Paucity of the bile ducts
Hepatic irradiation	Temporal relationship	Centrilobular haemorrhagic necrosis

SOL: space-occupying lesion; IHBR: intrahepatic biliary radicle; HV: hepatic vein

mild and self-limiting. However, in a small proportion, it may be fatal, especially when associated with liver failure, cholangitis, progressive cholestasis and massive hepatic infiltration or reactivation of hepatitis B. The presence of such conditions should be recognized early so that appropriate management can be immediately instituted. Whenever the aetiology of jaundice cannot be established definitely, therapy should be directed against the most probable and treatable cause of jaundice.

REFERENCES

1. Walz-Mattmuller R, Homy HP, Ruck P, Kaiseling E. Incidence and pattern of liver involvement in haematological malignancies. *Pathol Res Pract* 1998;**194**:781–9.
2. Sherlock S, Dooley J. Liver in myelo- and lymphoproliferative diseases. In: Sherlock S, Dooley J (eds). *Diseases of the liver and biliary system.* 11th ed. London: Blackwell Science; 2002:56–65.
3. Birrer MJ, Young RC. Differential diagnosis of jaundice in lymphoma patients. *Semin Liver Dis* 1987;**7**:269–77.
4. Woolf GM, Petrovic LM, Rojter SE, *et al.* Acute liver failure due to lymphoma: A diagnostic concern when considering liver transplantation. *Dig Dis Sci* 1994;**39**:1351–8.
5. Feller E, Schiffman FJ. Extrahepatic biliary obstruction by lymphoma. *Arch Surg* 1990;**125**:1507–9.
6. Maymind M, Mergelas JE, Seibert DG, Hotsetter RB, Chang WW. Primary non-Hodgkin's lymphoma of the common bile duct. *Am J Gastroenterol* 1997;**92**:1543–6.
7. Hubscher SG, Lumley MA, Elias E. Vanishing bile duct syndrome: A possible mechanism for intrahepatic cholestasis in Hodgkin's lymphoma. *Hepatology* 1993;**17**:70–7.
8. de Medirios BC, Lacerda MA, Telles JE, da Silva JA, de Medirios CR. Cholestasis secondary to Hodgkin's disease: Report of two cases of vanishing bile duct syndrome. *Haematologica* 1998;**83**:1038–40.
9. Lefkowitch JH, Falkow S, Whitlock RT. Hepatic Hodgkin's disease simulating cholestatic hepatitis with liver failure. *Arch Pathol Lab Med* 1985;**109**:424–6.
10. Bruguera M. The effect of haematological and lymphatic diseases on the liver. In: Bircher J, Benhamou P, McIntyre N, Rizzetto M, Rodes J (eds). *Oxford textbook of clinical hepatology.* Oxford, UK: Oxford University Press; 1999:1709–14.
11. Mario Sznol, Ohnuma T. Hepatotoxic effects of cancer and its treatment. *Cancer medicine.* 4th ed. Holland: Williams and Wilkins; 1997:2358–70.
12. Ingold JS, Reed GB, Kaplan HS, Bagshaw MA. Radiation hepatitis. *Am J Roentgenol Radium Ther Nucl Med* 1965;**93**:200–8.
13. Heinrich PC, Castell JV, Andus T. Interleukin-6 and acute phase response. *Biochem J* 1990;**265**:621–36.
14. Sparks FC, Silverstein MJ, Hunt JS, Haskell CM, Pilch YH, Morton DL. Complications of BCG immunotherapy in patients with cancer. *N Engl J Med* 1973;**289**:827–30.
15. Deeg HJ, Storb R. Graft-versus-host disease. Pathophysiological and clinical aspects. *Ann Rev Med* 1984;**35**:11–24.
16. McDonald GB, Sharma P, Matthews DE, Shulman HM, Thomas ED. Veno occlusive disease of the liver after bone marrow transplantion: Diagnosis, incidence, and predisposing factors. *Hepatology* 1984;**4**:116–22.
17. Bird GL, Smith H, Portmann B, Alexander GJ, Williams R. Acute liver decompensation on withdrawal of cytotoxic chemotherapy and immunosuppressive therapy in hepatitis B carriers. *Q J Med* 1989;**73**:895–902.
18. Jaffe ES. Malignant lymphomas: Pathology of hepatic involvement. *Semin Liver Dis* 1987;**7**:257–68.
19. Colby TV, Hopper RT, Warnke RA. Hodgkin's disease: A clinicopathological study of 659 cases. *Cancer* 1982;**49**:1848–58.
20. Abt AB, Kirschner RH, Belliveau RE, *et al.* Hepatic pathology associated with Hodgkin's disease. *Cancer* 1974;**33**:1564–71.
21. Anthony PP, Sarsfield P, Clarke T. Primary lymphoma of the liver: Clinical and pathological features of 10 patients. *J Clin Pathol* 1990;**43**:1007–13.
22. Zafrani ES, Gaulard P. Primary lymphoma of the liver. *Liver* 1993;**13**:57–61.
23. Ohsawa M, Aozasa K, Horiuchi K, *et al.* Malignant lymphoma of the liver: Report of five cases and review of the literature. *Dig Dis Sci* 1992;**37**:1105–9.

CHAPTER 16

Jaundice and pancreatic diseases

PRAMOD KUMAR GARG

Jaundice is not a typical symptom of pancreatic disorders and does not *per se* suggest the presence of any pancreatic disease. However, jaundice may give useful clues to the aetiology, diagnosis and prognosis in a variety of pancreatic diseases. For example, the presence of jaundice may suggest a biliary cause of acute pancreatitis; its presence denotes biliary stricture as a complication in chronic pancreatitis; and it is often a presenting symptom in patients with pancreatic cancer, indicating a grave prognosis. Thus, jaundice is often associated with pancreatic diseases. This chapter reviews the aetiopathogenesis of jaundice and its implications with regard to the diagnosis, treatment and prognosis of various pancreatic diseases.

JAUNDICE IN ACUTE PANCREATITIS

Acute pancreatitis is a potentially serious condition that may be associated with significant morbidity and mortality. The commonest cause of acute pancreatitis in western countries as well as in India is gall stones.[1,2] The pathogenesis of gall stone-induced pancreatitis is not well understood. However, the most likely mechanism is related to the passage of a gall stone from the gallbladder through the bile duct into the duodenum. The landmark studies by Opie[3] and Acosta *et al.*[4] have made important contributions in this regard. Opie[3] hypothesized that gall stones cause acute pancreatitis by obstruction at the level of the ampulla of Vater. Acosta *et al.*[4] showed that gall stones could be recovered in the stool in up to 70% of patients with acute pancreatitis within 48 hours, suggesting that it is the migration of gall stones from the gallbladder via the CBD to the duodenum that causes acute pancreatitis. Subsequent studies have shown that transient obstruction of the pancreatic duct by a stone during its passage results in the initiation of a chain of events culminating in acute pancreatitis.[5,6]

Liver function tests (LFT) are typically abnormal in acute biliary pancreatitis, with a rise in serum bilirubin, ALT and/or AST during the initial phase. Such an abnormality in LFT basically reflects acute transient biliary obstruction, thus lending support to the obstructive theory regarding the pathogenesis of gall stone pancreatitis. The presence of an abnormal LFT is a sensitive marker of gall stone-induced acute pancreatitis.[7] If the stone does not pass out into the duodenum, then it may cause an overt obstructive type of jaundice. This may be further complicated by the development of acute cholangitis which worsens the prognosis of acute pancreatitis. If the obstruction of the bile duct is important in the pathogenesis of acute pancreatitis and may result in acute cholangitis, it is conceivable that relieving the biliary obstruction may help to decrease the severity of acute pancreatitis and thus mortality. Indeed, studies have shown that ERCP and endoscopic sphincterotomy may decrease the morbidity and even mortality in patients with severe acute pancreatitis if performed within 48 hours of the onset of acute pancreatitis.[8,9] It has also been shown that endoscopic therapy decreases the incidence of acute cholangitis in these patients.[10] Thus, the presence of jaundice may be a marker of the biliary (gall stones) aetiology of acute pancreatitis, has implications with regard to the prognosis and is an indication for endoscopic therapy in patients with acute pancreatitis.

Many case reports have shown that acute viral hepatitis may be associated with acute pancreatitis. Thus, in addition to biliary pancreatitis, jaundice may also suggest the viral aetiology of acute pancreatitis. The hepatitis B, hepatitis A and, lately, hepatitis E viruses have been shown to cause both acute hepatitis and acute pancreatitis in the same patient.[11–13] This may in fact create a diagnostic dilemma. The distinction between gall stone-induced pancreatitis and viral hepatitis-associated pancreatitis may be difficult initially. The history of a viral prodrome, nausea, aversion to food and anorexia may clinically suggest the presence of acute hepatitis in such a situation. On laboratory investigations, much higher levels of serum AST and ALT, and no or minimal rise in ALP would suggest hepatitis-associated pancreatitis. Moreover, the LFT abnormality is more persistent and takes much longer to resolve in viral hepatitis-associated pancreatitis, unlike that seen in gall stone-induced pancreatitis. Thus, careful analysis of the clinical picture and judicious interpretation of the various tests may lead to the correct diagnosis. Furthermore, positive results of acute serological markers of viral infection and an ultrasound of the abdomen will help to confirm the diagnosis. The management of patients with viral hepatitis-associated acute pancreatitis remains essentially conservative but calls for close monitoring and intensive/supportive treatment. Whether or not the development of acute pancreatitis in addition to acute viral hepatitis affects the outcome is not known, although all the cases of hepatitis-associated acute pancreatitis reported in the literature recovered.

JAUNDICE IN CHRONIC PANCREATITIS

Jaundice is usually not associated with chronic pancreatitis. Although alcohol may cause both chronic pancreatitis and alcoholic hepatitis, it is uncommon, if not rare, for the two to occur together. The commonest cause of jaundice in patients with chronic pancreatitis is biliary stricture occurring as a complication.

This may occur in 3.2%–45.6% of patients with chronic pancreatitis.[14] Such a wide variation is mainly on account of differences in the criteria for the diagnosis of biliary stricture, e.g. only biochemical evidence, imaging evidence and/or clinical evidence (presence of jaundice). Clinically, a patient with biliary stricture presents typically with features suggestive of obstructive jaundice. The cause of biliary obstruction is fibrosis of the intrapancreatic part of the bile duct in the region of the pancreatic head. Patients with chronic pancreatitis and biliary stricture have predominant disease in the head of the pancreas. The differential diagnosis in such a patient is pancreatic cancer either *de novo* or superimposed on chronic pancreatitis. Differentiating between focal pancreatitis affecting mainly the head of the pancreas and pancreatic cancer is difficult, and the only way to do so is by histological examination. The tissue for histology can be obtained by an ultrasound/CT/endoscopic ultrasound (EUS)-guided FNAC. The diagnosis of biliary stricture is made on the basis of biochemical investigations and imaging tests. Serum ALP is raised with or without a rise in serum bilirubin. USG of the abdomen shows a dilated bile duct in addition to the features of chronic pancreatitis, i.e. a dilated pancreatic duct and pancreatic calcification. The diagnosis may be confirmed by either ERCP or MRCP. Cholangiography shows a benign smooth stricture of the intrapancreatic CBD. The management of biliary stricture is either endoscopic or surgical. Endoscopic therapy involves dilatation of the stricture and stenting of the bile duct with the insertion of multiple stents for around 12 months. Several studies have shown that endoscopic therapy may be effective in up to 80% of patients with biliary stricture due to chronic pancreatitis.[15,16] However, a few studies have shown that endoscopic therapy is not effective and the treatment of choice is surgery.[17] Surgery is in the form of a bilioenteric bypass such as choledochojejunostomy with or without pancreaticoduodenectomy.[18] The long-term results of surgery are promising.[19]

Tropical pancreatitis, a special type of chronic pancreatitis seen in India, has been shown to be associated with cirrhosis in some patients in an earlier series on tropical pancreatitis.[20] However, most such patients do not present with jaundice.

Another special type of chronic pancreatitis, a rather recently described entity, is known as autoimmune pancreatitis. Most of the reports on autoimmune pancreatitis are from Japan.[21] Autoimmune pancreatitis is characterized by recurrent episodes of biliary obstruction and a mass lesion in the head of the pancreas. The histological features are marked by lymphoplasmacytic infiltration of the pancreatic parenchyma, pancreatic acinar atrophy and fibrosis. The CBD is stenosed in the intrapancreatic part of the pancreatic head, thus causing an obstruction. The aetiology is autoimmune-mediated inflammation of the pancreas. The IgG 4 class of antibodies is usually elevated. Autoimmune pancreatitis is commonly associated with other types of autoimmune diseases. The diagnosis is supported by the presence of autoantibodies to carbonic anhydrase, and antinuclear and antithyroid antibodies. ERCP shows a narrow and irregular main pancreatic duct, and a benign stricture of the lower end of the bile duct. The biliary histology also shows lymphoplasmacytic infiltration. Treatment with steroids is effective and may result in complete resolution.[22]

JAUNDICE AND CARCINOMA OF THE PANCREAS

Carcinoma of the pancreas is one condition wherein jaundice is often the presenting symptom. However, it denotes an advanced stage of the cancer and is associated with a poor prognosis. Carcinoma of the pancreas involves the head of the pancreas in about 90% of cases, and thus involves the intrapancreatic part of the CBD and causes obstructive jaundice.[23] Carcinoma of the pancreas is the commonest cause of obstructive jaundice in the West and the second commonest in India (cancer of the gallbladder being the commonest).[24,25]

The clinical features of carcinoma of the pancreas are pain in the upper abdomen and back, jaundice associated with pruritus and light-coloured stools, and hepatomegaly with a palpable gallbladder lump. The presence of a palpable gallbladder in a patient with jaundice militates against the diagnosis of a parenchymal cause (hepatitis) of jaundice and almost always suggests malignant obstruction of the bile duct as the cause of jaundice. In patients with obstructive jaundice, the level of obstruction is at the lower end of the bile duct if the gallbladder is palpable; the two important causes are carcinoma of the pancreas and periampullary carcinoma. A periampullary carcinoma is generally painless, and the jaundice has a waxing and waning course due to tumour necrosis. Thus, if a patient presents with features of obstructive jaundice that has a progressive course, pain in the abdomen and a palpable gallbladder, the diagnosis is carcinoma of the pancreas unless proved otherwise. The diagnosis can be confirmed by LFT, which typically show an obstructive pattern, and imaging tests such as USG and CT scan, which may show the presence of a pancreatic mass. CT is also helpful in staging the tumour; it identifies nodal involvement, vascular invasion and distant metastasis, all of which suggest an advanced, unresectable tumour. Although the histological confirmation can be done by FNAC, it is usually not performed for fear of seeding of the needle tract in a patient with a potentially resectable tumour. However, if the tumour is deemed unresectable on imaging studies, then the diagnosis should be confirmed by FNAC before the patient is either subjected to palliative treatment or is advised no treatment.

Overall, only about 10%–20% of patients with carcinoma of the pancreas who present with jaundice have a resectable tumour, indicating that jaundice is a sign of an advanced tumour.[26] The definitive treatment of resectable carcinoma of the pancreas is Whipple operation in which pancreaticoduodenectomy is performed along with 3 anastomoses—pancreaticojejunostomy, choledocho-jejunostomy and gastrojejunostomy. The postoperative mortality is around 5%–15%.[27] If the tumour is unresectable, then palliative treatment should be offered. Palliative treatment is basically required for relieving pain, pruritus associated with jaundice and gastric outlet obstruction due to duodenal involvement by the tumour. Pain relief is generally obtained by narcotic analgesics, but the patient may require a coeliac nerve plexus block for intractable pain. Pruritus may be very intense and disabling in patients with obstructive jaundice due to carcinoma of the pancreas. Relief of pruritus is the main indication for palliating obstructive jaundice in such patients.

Palliation of biliary obstruction is achieved by biliary drainage. Biliary drainage can be performed either surgically by a bilioenteric bypass such as choledochojejunostomy or by endoscopic biliary stenting. Randomized controlled trials have shown that endoscopic stenting is better than surgical bypass in terms of complications and 30-day mortality.[28] The success of endoscopic stenting approaches 90% in providing symptomatic relief with a complication rate of 10%–15% and a 30-day mortality of around 5%.[29] For gastric outlet obstruction, surgical gastrojejunostomy is the standard procedure. Of late, some studies have shown good results of palliative endoscopic stenting of the gastroduodenal area (usually the first and second parts of the duodenum) obstructed by the tumour.[30] The role of chemoradiotherapy in the management of carcinoma of the pancreas remains limited.

Another uncommon cause of jaundice in patients with carcinoma of the pancreas could be multiple metastases in the liver, especially in patients with carcinoma of the body or tail of the pancreas, which does not involve the bile ducts.

PSEUDOCYST OF THE PANCREAS AND JAUNDICE

Pseudocyst of the pancreas can develop following an attack of acute pancreatitis or in patients with chronic pancreatitis.[31] A pseudocyst may be located anywhere in relation to the pancreas. Those located in the head region may compress the bile duct by virtue of its proximity. This may result in obstructive jaundice; however, the occurrence of clinically overt jaundice is rather uncommon, although one may frequently find abnormal LFT with a predominant rise in ALP and a minimal rise in serum bilirubin, AST and ALT levels. USG is ideal for diagnosing both the presence and location of the pseudocyst and biliary obstruction. Treatment is directed towards the drainage of the pseudocyst, with abatement of jaundice following soon afterwards due to relief of the obstruction. Pseudocyst drainage can be done surgically, endoscopically or percutaneously. Endoscopic drainage is preferred if the cyst is in close contact with the stomach or duodenum and produces an internal bulge inside the stomach or duodenum. The success rate of endoscopic drainage is similar, i.e. around 90%, and the complication rate is less than that of surgical drainage.[32]

MISCELLANEOUS PANCREATIC DISEASES AND JAUNDICE

The pancreas may be involved in other systemic diseases, such as tuberculosis and lymphoma.[33,34] If the head of the pancreas is involved in the disease process, then it may lead to biliary obstruction similar to that seen in cancer of the pancreas. The diagnosis is suspected by the involvement of other sites by the disease process, such as the lungs, lymph nodes, spleen, etc. and is confirmed by obtaining tissue for histology. If there is isolated involvement of the pancreas, it may mimic carcinoma of the pancreas and the diagnosis may be very difficult. The dilemma can only be resolved by histological examination. Thus, there is a definite need for tissue diagnosis if there is a suspicion of carcinoma of the pancreas and the lesion seems unresectable, thereby precluding surgery. In such cases, one may detect potentially treatable conditions, such as tuberculosis or lymphoma.

Thus, jaundice, though an uncommon symptom in patients with pancreatic diseases (except carcinoma of the pancreas), often gives an important clue to the aetiology of acute pancreatitis, suggests the presence of biliary obstruction as a complication in a variety of pancreatic diseases, indicates a bad prognosis in patients with pancreatic cancer and may direct the choice of treatment in different pancreatic disorders.

REFERENCES

1. Steinberg W, Tenner S. Acute pancreatitis. *N Engl J Med* 1994;**330**:1198–210.
2. Bohidar NP, Garg PK, Khanna S, Tandon RK. Incidence, etiology and impact of fever in patients with acute pancreatitis. *Pancreatology* 2003;**3**:9–13.
3. Opie EL. The etiology of acute hemorrhagic pancreatitis. *Bull Johns Hopkins Hosp* 1901; **12**:182–8.
4. Acosta JM, Ledesma CL. Gallstone migration as a cause of acute pancreatitis. *N Engl J Med* 1974;**290**:484–7.
5. Weber CK, Adler G. From acinar cell damage to systemic inflammatory response: Current concepts in pancreatitis. *Pancreatology* 2001;**1**:356–62.
6. Raraty MG, Pope IM, Finch M, Neoptolemos JP. Choledocholithiasis and gallstone pancreatitis. *Baillieres Clin Gastroenterol* 1997;**11**:663–80.
7. Davidson BR, Neoptolemos JP, Leese T, Carr-Locke DL. Biochemical prediction of gallstones in acute pancreatitis: A prospective study of three systems. *Br J Surg* 1988;**75**:213–15.
8. Neoptolemos JP, London N, Slater ND, Carr-Locke DL, Fossard DP, Moosa AR. A prospective study of ERCP and endoscopic sphincterotomy in the diagnosis and treatment of gallstone in acute pancreatitis. A rational and safe approach to management. *Arch Surg* 1986;**121**:697–702.
9. Folsch UR, Nitsche R, Ludtke R, Hilgers RA, Creutzfeldt W. Early ERCP and papillotomy compared with conservative treatment for acute biliary pancreatitis. The German Study Group on Acute Biliary Pancreatitis. *N Engl J Med* 1997;**336**:237–42.
10. Fan ST, Lai EC, Mok FP, Lo CM, Zheng SS, Wong J. Early treatment of acute biliary pancreatitis by endoscopic papillotomy. *N Engl J Med* 1993;**328**:228–32.
11. Sood A, Midha V. Hepatitis A and acute pancreatitis. *J Assoc Physicians India* 1999;**47**:736–7.
12. Mishra A, Saigal S, Gupta R, Sarin SK. Acute pancreatitis associated with viral hepatitis: A report of six cases with review of literature. *Am J Gastroenterol* 1999;**94**:2292–5.
13. Maity SG, Ray G. Severe acute pancreatitis in acute hepatitis E. *Indian J Gastroenterol* 2002;**21**:37–8.
14. Tandon RK, Sato N, Garg PK. Chronic pancreatitis: Asia-Pacific consensus report. *J Gastroenterol Hepatol* 2002;**17**:508–18.

15. Vitale GC, Reed DN Jr, Nguyen CT, Lawhon JC, Larson GM. Endoscopic treatment of distal bile duct stricture from chronic pancreatitis. *Surg Endosc* 2000;**14:**227–31.

16. Draganov P, Hoffman B, Marsh W, Cotton P, Cunningham J. Long-term outcome in patients with benign biliary strictures treated endoscopically with multiple stents. *Gastrointest Endosc* 2002;**55:**680–6.

17. Eickhoff A, Jakobs R, Leonhardt A, Eickhoff JC, Riemann JF. Endoscopic stenting for common bile duct stenoses in chronic pancreatitis: Results and impact on long-term outcome. *Eur J Gastroenterol Hepatol* 2001;**13:**1161–7.

18. Vijungco JD, Prinz RA. Management of biliary and duodenal complications of chronic pancreatitis. *World J Surg* 2003;**27:**1258–70.

19. Smits ME, Rauws EA, van Gulik TM, Gouma DJ, Tytgat GN, Huibregtse K. Long-term results of endoscopic stenting and surgical drainage for biliary stricture due to chronic pancreatitis. *Br J Surg* 1996;**83:**764–8.

20. Narendranathan M. Chronic calcific pancreatitis of the tropics. *Trop Gastroenterol* 1981;**2:**40–5.

21. Ito T, Nakano I, Koyanagi S, *et al.* Autoimmune pancreatitis as a new clinical entity. Three cases of autoimmune pancreatitis with effective steroid therapy. *Dig Dis Sci* 1997; **42:**1458–68.

22. Kojima E, Kimura K, Noda Y, Kobayashi G, Itoh K, Fujita N. Autoimmune pancreatitis and multiple bile duct strictures treated effectively with steroid. *J Gastroenterol* 2003;**38:**603–7.

23. Carter DC. Cancer of the pancreas. *Gut* 1990;**31:**494–6.

24. Rossi RL, Traverso LW, Pimentel F. Malignant obstructive jaundice. Evaluation and management. *Surg Clin North Am* 1996;**76:**63–70.

25. Kar P, Kumar R, Kapur BM, Tandon BN, Tandon RK. Surgical obstructive jaundice in India: A clinical profile. *J Assoc Physicians India* 1986;**34:**115–18.

26. Cooperman AM, Kini S, Snady H, Bruckner H, Chamberlain RS. Current surgical therapy for carcinoma of the pancreas. *J Clin Gastroenterol* 2000;**31:**107–13.

27. Sorensen MB, Lundemose JB, Rokkjaer M, Jacobsen NO. Whipple's operation for carcinoma of the pancreatic head and the ampullary region. Short- and long-term results. *Scand J Gastroenterol* 1998;**33:**759–64.

28. Smith AC, Dowsett JF, Russell RC, Hatfield AR, Cotton PB. Randomised trial of endoscopic stenting versus surgical bypass in malignant low bile duct obstruction. *Lancet* 1994;**344:**1655–60.

29. Garg PK, Tandon RK. Non-surgical drainage for biliary obstruction. *Indian J Gastroenterol* 1994;**13:**118–27.

30. Nassif T, Prat F, Meduri B, *et al.* Endoscopic palliation of malignant gastric outlet obstruction using self-expandable metallic stents: Results of a multicenter study. *Endoscopy* 2003;**35:**483–9.

31. Kozarek RA. Endoscopic treatment of pancreatic pseudocysts. *Gastrointest Endosc Clin North Am* 1997;**7:**271–83.

32. Howell DA, Elton E, Parsons WG. Endoscopic management of pseudocysts of the pancreas. *Gastrointest Endosc Clin North Am* 1998;**8:**143–62.

33. Franco-Paredes C, Leonard M, Jurado R, Blumberg HM, Smith RM. Tuberculosis of the pancreas: Report of two cases and review of the literature. *Am J Med Sci* 2002;**323:**54–8.

34. Boni L, Benevento A, Dionigi G, Cabrini L, Dionigi R. Primary pancreatic lymphoma. *Surg Endosc* 2002;**16:**1107–8.

CHAPTER 17

Parasitic infections causing jaundice

MANISHA DWIVEDI, SRI PRAKASH MISRA

Liver parasites may involve the hepatocytes, reticuloendothelial cells, portal venous system or bile ducts. The pathological changes that occur depend on how well the parasite is adapted to the host organ. Severe injury results if the parasite is poorly adapted to the host organ, e.g. *Echinococcus* tapeworms cause severe hepatic injury in human beings, and *Entamoeba histolytica* and *Ascaris lumbricoides* cause acute injury to the liver parenchyma and bile ducts, respectively.

On the other hand, well-adapted parasites, such as malarial parasites, schistosome worms and bile duct flukes, cause minimal acute injury to the liver, but produce progeny in large numbers. These have the potential to infect other hosts.

Hosts with compromised immune responses may have severe disease manifestations. In HIV-infected persons, there may be reactivation of subclinical *Leishmania* infection or the development of advanced visceral leishmaniasis or disseminated strongyloidiasis. Parasitic diseases of the liver which cause jaundice are listed in Table I.

AMOEBIASIS

Amoebiasis affects 10% of the world's polulation, and is commonest in the tropical and subtropical regions.[1]

Entamoeba histolytica causes dysentery, colitis and amoebic liver abscess (ALA) in man, whereas its morphologically indistinguishable counterpart *E. dispar* is not associated with symptomatic disease.[2] ALA is the commonest manifestation of extraintestinal amoebiasis. In developed countries, if ALA occurs in a person who has not travelled to, or is not residing in, an endemic area, underlying immune supression, especially AIDS, should be considered.[3]

Table I. Parasitic diseases of the liver causing jaundice

Disease (cause)
Protozoa
Amoebiasis (*Entamoeba histolytica*)
Malaria (*Plasmodium falciparum, P. malariae, P. vivax, P. ovale*)
Visceral leishmaniasis (*Leishmania donovani*)
Nematodes
Ascariasis (*Ascaris lumbricoides*)
Hepatic capillariasis (*Capillaria hepatica*)
Strongyloidiasis (*Strongyloides stercoralis*)
Trichinosis (*Trichinella spiralis*)
Trematodes
Fascioliasis (*Fasciola hepatica*)
Clonorchiasis/opisthorchiasis (*Clonorchis sinensis, Opisthorchis viverrini, O. felineus*)
Cestodes
Echinococcosis (*Echinococcus granulosus, E. multilocularis*)

Life cycle

E. histolytica exists in the trophozoite or cystic forms. After infection, the cysts pass through the GI tract to change into trophozoites in the colon, where they invade the mucosa to produce typical 'flask-shaped' ulcers. From here, the organism may be carried to the liver via the portal circulation, and further to the lungs and brain.

Clinical features

Amoebic liver abscess is commonly found in men between 20 and 40 years of age. Gender differences may be because of alcohol consumption, as alcohol impairs Kupffer cell function and both cellular and humoral immune responses, rendering the liver more prone to the development of ALA.[4] Less than 10% of patients with ALA give a past history of bloody diarrhoea. The patient presents with abdominal pain, usually localized to the right upper quadrant, fever, malaise, myalgias and arthralgias. The pain frequently radiates to the scapular region and right shoulder, but if the abscess is in the left lobe, the pain may radiate to the left shoulder. Nearly 30% of patients also develop a non-productive cough.

On physical examination, patients are found to have tender hepatomegaly. Digital pressure in the right lower intercostal spaces causes pain. Jaundice is present in about 10% of patients. Ventilation is usually diminished on the right side.[5] Most commonly, the abscesses are single rather than multiple, ranging in size from 5 to 15 cm, and are found in the right lobe of the liver. However, 35% of patients may present with an abscess in the left lobe and 16% develop multiple abscesses.[6] Rupture of the abscess into the thoracic cavity may produce pain in the right shoulder and an irritating, hacking cough. Anchovy sauce pus may be expectorated and dyspnoea may occur.

Diagnosis

Leucocytosis is found in >90% of patients, whereas 5% may show a leukaemoid reaction. Nearly half the patients have elevated ALP values, with a mild increase in serum bilirubin. Increase in aminotransferase values and hypoalbuminaemia are occasionally seen.[7]

Indirect haemagglutination (IHA) and ELISA are most commonly used for serology. The most sensitive and specific method is IHA, which is positive in 85%–95% of patients. A cut-off of 1:512 is diagnostic. Techlab *E. histolytica* II, a commercially available test, detects *E. histolytica* Gal/Gal/Nac lectin antigen with nearly 100% sensitivity in invasive amoebiasis before starting treatment with metronidazole.[8] Salivary adherence lectin antigen is an effective tool to detect invasive amoebiasis.[9] More controlled trials are under way to establish the sensitivity and specificity of the lectin antigens. PCR may be done on material aspirated from an ALA.[10]

The first choice in imaging tests for ALA is USG. A hypoechoic space-occupying lesion is seen in nearly 75%–95% of patients. On CT scan, the abscess may show a contrast-enhancing peripheral rim. MRI does not add to the USG findings.[10] Chest X-ray usually shows elevation of the right side of the diaphragm, minimal right-sided pleural effusion and an infiltrate in the right lower lobe.

Treatment

Metronidazole in a dose of 1 g twice daily for 10–15 days is the treatment of choice. The intravenous dose for adults is 500 mg 6 hourly for 10 days. This treatment results in a cure rate of 95%. When on oral metronidazole, alcohol should not be consumed to avoid an antabuse-like effect. Tinidazole or ornidazole in a dosage of 2 g orally for 10 days is also effective.

Other drugs which may be used are dehydroemetine 1 mg/kg/day intra-muscularly for 10 days to a maximum of 60 mg/day and chloroquine 1 g/day for 2 days, followed by 500 mg/day for 2–3 weeks orally.

Ultrasonography-guided aspiration of an ALA should be done if the risk of rupture is high, response to medication is slow or secondary infection is suspected. Peritoneal irrigation and drainage of the abscess should be done in case of a ruptured ALA.

Vaccines are being developed against the *E. histolytica* Gal/Gal/Nac lectin antigen, which is an antigenically conserved surface molecule in distinct isolates of *E. histolytica*.[11]

MALARIA

Life cycle

Human infection by the malarial parasite begins when a female anopheline mosquito inoculates plasmodial sporozoites from its salivary gland during a blood meal. These microscopic motile forms of the malarial parasite are carried rapidly by the blood stream to the liver, where they invade the hepatic parenchymal cells and begin a period of asexual reproduction. Direct binding of sporozoites to hepatocyte membranes is mediated by a surface protein expressed during the sporozoite stage.[12] Sporozoites mature into schizonts that rupture to release merozoites into the circulation which enter the erythrocytes. Sporozoite uptake and maturation is influenced by the metabolic state of the hepatocyte, being favoured by iron overloading.[13] By intrahepatic or pre-erythrocytic schizogony or merogony, a single sporozoite may release 10 000 or more than 30 000 daughter merozoites into the blood stream. At this stage, the symptomatic stage of infection begins. The various species of *Plasmodium* differ with respect to the release of merozoites and maturation times. In *P. vivax* and *P. ovale* infection, a proportion of intrahepatic forms do not divide immediately but remain dormant for months to years before reproduction begins. These dormant forms or hypnozoites are the cause of relapses that characterize infection with these two species.

Clinical features

The cyclic fever, haemolysis, vascular stasis, shock and multiple organ failure seen in severe malaria are the clinical result of synchronized multiplication and release of parasites in the erythrocytic stage. Kupffer cells take up the released degradation product of haemoglobin, known as the malarial pigment, which appears as dark cytoplasmic granules in the liver. The highest risk of severe illness and death is with *P. falciparum* infection. Malaria due to *P. falciparum* often produces clinical and laboratory evidence of multiple organ dysfunction. Hepatic involvement is commonly due to haemolysis but hepatocyte dysfunction can also result, leading to conjugated hyperbilirubinaemia. Hyperglycaemia and lactic acidosis may be serious complications of *P. falciparum* infection. Reversible reduction in the portal venous blood flow may result in acute *falciparum* malaria due to occlusion of the portal venous branches by parasitized red blood cells.[14]

Severe liver injury in malaria has been reported only infrequently in patients with a heavy *P. falciparum* load, and is commonly associated with acute renal failure, altered sensorium and coma. In a report from India of 7 such patients who presented with acute onset of jaundice, asterixis or impaired sensorium, bleeding with prolonged PT and partial thromboplastin time (PTT), and aminotransferase levels elevated to 4 times the normal values, *P. falciparum* infection was evident in the blood.[15,16]

Laboratory findings

Diagnosis

Demonstration of the parasite: The diagnosis of malaria rests on the demonstration of asexual forms of the parasite in peripheral blood smears.

Giemsa stain at pH 7.2 is preferred. Wright, Field or Leishman stains can be used. Both thin and thick smears should be examined.

Simple, sensitive and specific antibody-based diagnostic stick or card tests which detect *P. falciparum*-specific histidine-rich protein (HRP) 2 or lactic dehydrogenase antigens in finger-prick blood samples have been introduced.

The relationship between parasitaemia and prognosis is complex; in general, patients with >100 000 parasites/µL are at an increased risk of dying, but non-immune patients may die with much lower counts and semi-immune persons may tolerate much higher parasitaemia levels with only minor symptoms. In severe malaria, a poor prognosis is indicated by the predominance of more mature *P. falciparum* parasites (i.e. >20% of parasites with visible pigments), presence of circulating schizonts in peripheral blood smears or presence of phagocytosed malarial pigment in >5% of neutrophils. Gametocytes may remain detectable for several days after treatment has begun; unless trophozoites are also visible in blood films, their presence does not constitute evidence of drug resistance.

Staining of the parasite with the fluorescent dye acridine orange allows rapid diagnosis of cases in which the level of parasitaemia is low.

Normocytic normochromic anaemia is usually present. The leucocyte count is generally low to normal, although it may be raised in very severe infection. The ESR, degree of plasma viscosity and level of C-reactive protein are high. The platelet count is usually reduced to 100 000/µL. Severe infection may be accompanied by prolonged PT and PTT.[17] Findings of severe malaria may include metabolic acidosis with a low plasma concentration of plasma glucose, sodium, bicarbonate, calcium, phosphate and albumin, together with elevation of lactate, blood urea nitrogen, creatinine, urate, muscle and liver enzymes, and unconjugated bilirubin. Hypergammaglobulinaemia is usual in immune and semi-immune-sufficient subjects, and urinalysis is generally normal.

Histopathology

In acute *falciparum* malaria, the hepatic macrophages (Kupffer cells) hypertrophy and are seen to contain large quantities of malarial pigment produced by the degradation of haemoglobin from parasitized and non-parasitized red blood cells.[18] Hepatocyte oedema, mononuclear cell infiltration and focal necrosis may be seen. Post-mortem liver specimens from patients with severe *falciparum* malaria were shown to have submassive necrosis.[18]

Treatment

Treatment of malaria depends on the species of the parasite. Chloroquine is usually effective for all species in areas where the parasite is sensitive. Resistant *falciparum* infection can be treated with mefloquine alone, quinine, doxycycline or clindamycin, pyrimethamine–sulphadoxine or a combination of atovaquone and proguanil. In *P. vivax* or *P. ovale* infection, the residual exoerythrocytic hypnozoites are treated with primaquine in addition to chloroquine or

Table II. Geographical distribution of the various species of *Leishmania*

Species causing visceral leishmaniasis	Geographical region
L. donavani	India, China, Pakistan, sub-Saharan Africa
L. infantum	Middle-East Asia, southern Europe (Spain, France, Italy), north and sub-Saharan Africa
L. archibaldi	East Africa
L. chagasi	Latin America

mefloquine to prevent relapses. Primaquine should not be administered to patients with glucose-6-phosphate dehydrogenase (G6PD) deficiency as severe haemolysis may be precipitated.

VISCERAL LEISHMANIASIS (KALA-AZAR)

This is an infection of the reticuloendothelial cells of the liver, spleen, bone marrow and other organs by the intracellular protozoan parasite *Leishmania*.[19] The geographical distribution of the various species is given in Table II.

Mode of transmission

Visceral leishmaniasis involving the liver normally results from infection of children and young adults with *L. donovani*. In the Indian subcontinent, the parasite is transmitted by sandflies that have bitten infected humans. Besides infection from the bite of sandflies in endemic areas, clinical studies show that *Leishmania* can be transmitted by transfused blood or needles shared for drug abuse, sexual contact or the transplantation of infected organs.

Life cycle

Leishmania are obligate intracellular parasites of macrophages in mammalian hosts. They exist in nature in 2 distinct morphological stages. The extracellular promastigote is a flagellated parasite, 10–15 µm in length, which develops to maturity in the gut of the sandfly.[20] During a blood meal, the sandflies generate a small pool of blood in the mammalian skin into which the promastigotes are regurgitated. In the mammalian skin, the promastigotes quickly attach to and are taken up by local tissue macrophages (Langerhans cells). They transform intracellularly into obligate intracellular amastigotes. Subsequently, amastigote-infected macrophages either remain in the skin to cause cutaneous leishmaniasis or disseminate throughout the reticuloendothelial system to cause clinical symptoms of visceral leishmaniasis. Amastigote-infected macrophages are taken up during the blood meal of an uninfected sandfly, whereupon they convert back to promastigotes within the gut of the sandfly.

Host response and immunology

After infection of the blood stream and uptake of the parasite by the reticulo-endothelial cells, the amastigotes multiply within the Kupffer cells and macrophages, infect new cells, and trigger cellular and humoral host responses. Uptake of promastigotes occurs due to their attachment to several macrophage receptors, including the CR1 and CR3 receptors, for complement components C3b and C3bi.[21,22] The macrophage mannose receptor and the fibronectin receptor also mediate promastigote binding.[23,24] The majority of immuno-competent persons respond to infection with a successful defence mediated by T-helper subtype-I (Th1) cells, which prevent clinical disease and suppress, but may not eliminate, the infection.[25] Such a cellular response, akin to that seen in tuberculoid leprosy or successfully contained initial *Mycobacterium tuberculosis* infection, involves the same CD4 cells and cytokines, such as IFN-γ, IL-2 and IL-12, which are critical for dealing with other intracellular organisms.

Humoral antibody responses, which are also regularly present, do not appear to modify the course of leishmanial infection, nor the Th2 type cellular responses seen in persons in whom clinically severe disease develops.

Pathology

Pathological examination of liver specimens shows findings that parallel the predominant host response. In persons with minimal disease, few parasites are visible in liver specimens. Epithelioid granulomas, including fibrin ring granulomas similar to those seen in Q fever, may be seen in the liver.[26]

The multiplication of numerous parasites within the activated Kupffer cells and macrophages, appearance of myofibroblasts, deposition of interlobular collagen and effacement of the space of Disse with connective tissue all accompany an ineffective response in persons with overt disease.[27,28] A pattern of severe intralobular liver fibrosis as the predominant finding was described by Rogers[29] as a peculiar cirrhosis in Indian patients with visceral leishmaniasis. However, patients with so-called Rogers cirrhosis have a normal liver architecture and no regenerative nodules.

Clinical manifestations

Most immunocompetent patients are asymptomatic. The incubation period is 3–8 months.[30] Predisposing factors include malnourishment, immunocom-promised states and genetic factors.[31,32]

At the site of inoculation of the *Leishmania*, a small papule may form.[33] The major clinical manifestations of visceral leishmaniasis include fever, weight loss, hepatomegaly, splenomegaly, pancytopenia and hypergammaglobulinaemia. All organs with reticuloendothelial cells may be involved, including the entire GI tract. The spleen becomes massively enlarged but may be soft on examination. The development of a firm, enlarged spleen should suggest an alternative diagnosis. Lymphadenopathy may sometimes occur.[34] The liver also becomes enlarged and jaundice with hepatic inflammation is occasionally present. The skin can become dark, explaining the Indian name for the disease—kala-azar or black fever. With progressive disease, fever, weight loss, peripheral oedema, epistaxis, gingival bleeding, petechiae and ecchymosis may result. Bacterial superinfection usually occurs in nearly 60% of infected patients, leading to the development of pyoderma, pneumonia, bronchitis or otitis caused by *Pseudomonas aeruginosa* or *Staphyloccocus*.[35] Treatment may lead to symptomatic relief; however, amastigotes may persist in the splenic aspirate.[36,37] Malnutrition, immunosuppressive therapy or HIV infection may precipitate overt visceral leishmaniasis in previously healthy people with latent infection.[38,39] Intracellular parasites may be obtained from a liver or intestinal biopsy specimen of patients with HIV being investigated for persistent fever or diarrhoea.[40] Visceral leishmaniasis may develop in immunosuppressed patients who have undergone renal, cardiac or hepatic transplantation.[41,42.]

Laboratory diagnosis

Laboratory abnormalities due to leishmaniasis include anaemia, neutropenia and thrombocytopenia. Low platelet and neutrophil counts are particularly associated with massive splenomegaly. Hypergammaglobulinaemia, immune complexes and a positive rheumatoid factor are common in visceral leishmaniasis. Modest elevations of aminotransferase and ALP levels may occur together with depressed albumin values. Liver biopsy may show intralobular fibrosis. There may be evidence of mild glomerulonephritis because of the deposition of immune complexes, although renal insufficiency is rare. Patients with visceral leishmaniasis typically develop high levels of non-specific and parasite-specific antibodies. Serology for the organisms (*L. chagas, L. donovani, L. infantum*) is usually positive during the period of the disease. Cellular immune responses are impaired; however, a delayed-type hypersensitivity testing leishmanin antigen (Montenegro test) is typically negative when the disease is active. A delayed type of hypersensitivity and positivity to the leishmanin skin test usually develops after the disease resolves. The procedure for diagnosing visceral leishmaniasis with the highest accuracy, close to 100%, is examination and culture of a splenic needle aspirate. In areas where the disease is not endemic and the level of experience required to perform splenic aspiration safely is lacking, examination and culture of the bone marrow and liver biopsy are performed more often. Either methods provide a yield of 50%–80%.

Treatment

Successful treatment requires both appropriate antibiotics and an adequate host response. Pentavalent antimonial compounds are the mainstay of therapy. In the US, the drug service of the Centers for Disease Control and Prevention provides sodium stibogluconate as an investigation drug. Daily intramuscular or intravenous injections for 3 weeks or longer are safe and generally effective. Second-line antileishmanial agents include pentamidine, amphotericin B, allopurinol, ketoconazole and related azole compounds.

A new strategy for drug delivery by incorporating amphotericin B into liposomes or lipid complexes appears to greatly enhance efficacy; a 5-day course of lipid-complexed amphotericin B at a total dose of 5–15 mg/kg is remarkably effective in patients who do not respond or relapse after antimonial therapy.

Other alternatives to antimonial therapy reported from India, where resistance to antimonials is a cause for concern, include an intramuscular injection of paromomycin for 21 days[43] and oral therapy with miltefosine, a phosphocholine derivative, for 28 days.[44] Although the clinical manifestations of visceral leishmaniasis resolve with antiparasite therapy, it remains unclear, especially in immunocompetent persons, whether the infection is truly eliminated or only suppressed below detectable levels.[45] Consistent with the importance of the Th1 cellular responses for the resolution of visceral leishmaniasis, the administration of Th1-related cytokines IFN-γ and IL-12 in animals with experimental leishmaniasis promotes recovery.[46] In a controlled evaluation of the addition of IFN-γ to antimonial therapy in Indian patients with visceral leishmaniasis, combined therapy accelerated cure and eliminated detectable parasites, suggesting the importance of appropriate adjunctive cytokine therapy. [46]

ASCARIASIS

This is a helminthic infection of man caused by the nematode *Ascaris lumbricoides*. The adult parasite enters and resides in the jejunum after the ingestion of embryonated eggs. The larvae penetrate the intestinal mucosa to enter the portal circulation, and thus reach the liver, pulmonary artery and lungs. They are regurgitated and swallowed to finally reach the intestine, where the adult worm is found.

Clinical presentation

Depending on the worm burden, the patient may be asymptomatic or have fever, cough, substernal pain, wheezing and hepatomegaly in the first 2 weeks. Chronic infection is characterized by episodic periumbilical pain. With a heavy worm burden, intestinal obstruction, volvulus, perforation or appendicitis may result.[47]

Hepatobiliary and pancreatic ascariasis (HPA) is the result of migration of the worm to the ductal system via the papillary opening. The clinical manifestation of HPA is in the form of biliary colic, acalculus cholecystitis, acute cholangitis or pancreatitis, and hepatic abscess. In the biliary tree, the fragmented worm may act as a nidus for stone formation.[48,49] HPA is more common in females, with a female-to-male ratio of 3:1 and a mean age of 35 years (range 4–70 years).[50]

Pregnant women[51] and those who have undergone previous surgery on the biliary tree, such as cholecystectomy, choledocholithotomy or sphincteroplasty, are particularly prone to HPA.[52] Recurrent pyogenic cholangitis (RPC) may be the aftermath of recurrent biliary invasion by *Ascaris*,[53] as ascariasis and RPC have a similar geographic distribution. Nearly 5% of patients with HPA develop RPC over a follow-up period of 2 years. Papillitis and motor abnormalities of the sphincter of Oddi may be related to mechanical injury to the papilla by worms invading the ampullary orifice.[54]

Diagnosis

The diagnosis of HPA is made by USG or ERCP. The characteristic USG findings are single or multiple echogenic structures, which may contain a central anechoic tube, representing the digestive tract of the worm, without acoustic shadowing seen in the bile duct.[55] USG examination may also show liver abscesses or oedematous pancreatitis. A history of regurgitating the adult worm may be obtained and characteristic *Ascaris* eggs may be found in stool specimens, sputum or gastric washings.

Treatment

Cholangitis is treated conservatively, and the worms are paralysed by the oral administration of antihelminthic agents, after which they are expelled by effective peristalsis. Endoscopic intervention from the ampullary orifice is successful in all patients and from the bile or pancreatic duct in nearly 90% of patients, resulting in a rapid amelioration of symptoms; 6% of patients may develop cholangitis and hypotension after the endoscopic procedure.[56]

STRONGYLOIDIASIS

Strongyloides infestation is common in the tropical regions, the US, and southern and Eastern Europe.

The life cycle of the parasite is characterized by the filariform larva penetrating the skin in humans, reaching the lungs, migrating through the alveoli and being swallowed to reach the intestine, where maturation occurs. The adult worms release rhabditiform larvae in the intestine, resulting in autoinfection.

The infestation is usually asymptomatic, unless a heavy infectious burden occurs or the host is immunocompromised, when a hyperinfection syndrome results. In this situation, filariform larvae are disseminated into tissues not normally infected.[57] Corticosteroid administration, which may convert low-grade strongyloidiasis into a fulminant disease with a high mortality, is a major risk factor. This may be because of the ability of corticosteroids to deplete eosinophils, which are considered to be important for the containment of *Strongyloides* infection. Corticosteroids may also promote the transformation of rhabditiform to filariform larvae, resulting in autoinfection.

Common clinical manifestations are fever, cough, wheezing, abdominal pain, diarrhoea and eosinophilia. The liver may be involved in the hyperinfection syndrome, resulting in jaundice with or without cholestasis. Liver biopsy shows periportal inflammation or eosinophilic granulomatous hepatitis. *Strongyloides* larvae may be seen in the intrahepatic bile canaliculi or small branches of the portal vein.

Diagnosis is made by the identification of larvae in the stool or an intestinal biopsy specimen. Dissemination of the infection must be considered if cholestatic jaundice develops in a patient diagnosed with strongyloidiasis. Serological tests are also available to diagnose the infection.

The treatment of choice in the acute phase is ivermectin 200 μg/kg/day for 2 days. Albendazole 400 mg/day for 3 days may be given to adults. However, this drug is less effective for disseminated disease and re-treatment may be needed.

TRICHINOSIS

Trichinella spiralis may infect human beings through the consumption of raw or undercooked pork containing larvae that penetrate the small intestinal mucosa and disseminate in the systemic circulation. Larvae are commonly found in the myocardium and cerebrospinal fluid, and less commonly in the liver and gallbladder. Encapsulation of the larvae occurs in the striated muscle when the larvae re-enter the circulation.[58]

Clinical manifestations include fever, diarrhoea, muscle pain, periorbital oedema and marked eosinophilia. Hepatic involvement may be characterized by biliary obstruction or sinusoidal involvement.

The infection can be diagnosed by a muscle biopsy. Serological studies showing antibodies against *Trichinella* may be positive after 2 weeks.

Corticosteroids are given to relieve allergic symptoms and albendazole is given in a dose of 400 mg/day for 3 days.

HEPATIC CAPILLARIASIS

Humans are infected with *Capillaria hepatica* by eating raw fish which has acquired the infection from migratory birds through faecal passage. Human faeces containing infective stages of the organism further contaminate the habitats of fish, thus increasing fish–human transmission. Epizootics including other fish-eating mammals could also be involved. Larvae develop into adults in the small intestine. Females shed eggs or live larvae in the stools which embryonate in water. Larvae in the intestine of man maintain the parasite burden by autoinfection, and reach the liver through the portal venous circulation after penetrating the intestinal mucosa. In the liver, the adult worm degenerates after 4 weeks, releasing eggs which produce a severe inflammatory reaction in the liver parenchyma consisting of macrophages, eosinophils and giant cells. Resolution is indicated by marked peri-egg fibrosis.

The clinical manifestations include acute or subacute hepatitis characterized by fever, nausea, vomiting, arthralgias, myalgias, and tender hepatomegaly and splenomegaly, with a mild derangement of liver functions.

Liver biopsy may show necrosis, fibrosis or granuloma formation and the presence of the adult worm or eggs of *Capillaria hepatica* in the liver.

The treatment of hepatic capillariasis has generally been unsuccessful. Anecdotal benefit has been reported with dithiazanine iodide, thiabendazole and sodium stibogluconate.[59]

FASCIOLIASIS

Fasciola hepatica (sheep liver fluke) infects humans accidentally in Asia, Africa, Europe and the Americas, where sheep are intensively raised.[60] The mode of infection is by consuming watercress on which the larval stages of *F. hepatica* are present.

Most cases of acute fascioliasis present with fever for up to 3 months, right upper quadrant discomfort and hepatomegaly.[60-62] In the liver, the track along which the worm moves is characterized by coagulation necrosis in association with an intense eosinophilic response.[63] At laparoscopy, characteristic yellowish-white, subcapsular serpiginous cords are seen,[64] whereas on CT scan the tracks look like linear arrays of small 1–3 cm abscess-like lesions.[65-68] Eosinophilia is a predominant feature in the majority of patients. Due to penetration of the ductal system, haemobilia or abscess formation may occur.[69] Subcutaneous nodules may be present due to eosinophilic infiltrate surrounding a dead worm; eosinophilic pericarditis or pleuritis may also occur.

Chronic fascioliasis results from irritation of the bile duct epithelium by proline produced by the adult worm in the bile ducts. Proline is a major nitrogen excretion product and a key precursor of collagen. Chronic irritation results in ductal hyperplasia, fibrosis and episodes of acute cholangitis.[60] USG, CT scan or cholangiography may show dilated ducts in addition to adult flukes.

Diagnosis is made on the basis of the dietary history, clinical presentation, eosinophilia and suggestive findings on imaging. Serology testing by ELISA using cathepsin L1 (purified *Fasciola*-specific protease) as antigen could detect 20 out of 26 patients with fascioliasis with no false-positive results. A 97% sensitivity and high specificity was seen for the detection of fascioliasis when a crude *Fasciola* worm antigen was used.[69] Stool examination for eggs may be negative in acute fascioliasis and also at times in chronic disease.

Drug treatment for this condition is with bithionol and triclabendazole. The latter is better tolerated and more effective than the former.[62,70] Bithionol may result in GI irritation, rash, leucopenia and photosensitivity. The dose is 25 mg/kg for 10 days.

OPISTHORCHIASIS, CLONORCHIASIS

Bile duct flukes may be acquired by humans who eat raw fish containing the parasite in the infective metacercaria stage. The life cycle is completed when human hosts excrete eggs that hatch in water, and pass through the snail and fish stages to infect other humans and animals. The major liver flukes that infect human beings are *Clonorchis sinensis, Opisthorchis viverrini* and *O. felineus*. The adult flukes are about 1 cm in size and have a ventral sucker with which they attach themselves to the bile duct epithelium. These flukes have a life span of nearly 10 years. Nearly 25% of Chinese immigrants to the US have been shown to have active infection with *C. sinensis*,[71] while 33% of the population in north-eastern Thailand is infected with *O. viverrini*.[72] *O. felineus* infects cats and humans in some parts of Russia and Eastern Europe.

Pathogenesis

Adult *Opisthorchis* and *Clonorchis* flukes inhabit the bile ducts of humans and cause mechanical irritation of the bile ducts. Metabolic products secreted by them cause desquamation of the biliary epithelium, later leading to hyperplasia, dysplasia, and eventual fibrosis and cancer. [73] Increased activity of P450 2A6, an enzyme that promotes the activation of carcinogenic nitrosamines, was seen with *O. viverrini* infection.[74] As the adult flukes are long-lived, symptoms can occur even after the host has emigrated from an endemic area. Strong evidence exists to show that bile duct fluke infection is associated with chronic biliary tract abnormalities and cholangiocarcinoma in areas of endemicity. [73]

Clinical manifestations

Mild liver fluke infections are usually asymptomatic. The worm burden increases with age and symptoms usually manifest in adults more than 30 years of age. Mild symptoms include epigastric pain, anorexia and nausea. With heavy infection, relapsing cholangitis is a common presentation, especially with opisthorchiasis. Cholangitis occurs due to secondary bacterial infection and stone formation in chronically infected, strictured bile ducts. Oriental cholangiohepatitis is a chronic illness characterized by attacks of cholangitis and multiple pigment stones in the bile ducts, which are strictured and irregularly dilated. Cholangitis due to clonorchiasis is a common indication for emergency abdominal surgery in bile ducts that harbour adult liver flukes in Hong Kong.[75] Chronic opisthorchiasis can account for a sizeable chunk of hepatobiliary disease in endemic areas, resulting in jaundice, pancreatitis and cholangiocarcinoma.[76] In many patients with severe distortion of the ductal system, recurrent episodes of cholangitis appear to be self-perpetuating in the absence of active parasitic infection.

The diagnosis is made by demonstrating typical eggs in the stool, duodenal fluid or bile. On USG, fluke aggregates can be seen as non-shadowing echogenic foci in the bile ducts.

Treatment

Residents from areas with a high prevalence of infection and cholangio-carcinoma should modify their dietary habits and eliminate existing infection with praziquantel at a dose of 25 mg/kg every 8 hours for a total of three doses.

ECHINOCOCCOSIS

The metacestodes of all four species of the genus *Echinococcus* cause various forms of echinococcosis in man. However, the two important clinical forms are cystic echinococcosis (CE) caused by *Echinococcous granulosus* and alveolar echinococcosis (AE) caused by *E. multilocularis*. Progress in the management of these conditions has been possible due to the availability of better imaging modalities and better immunodiagnostic tests.

Life cycle

The adult tapeworm inhabits the small intestine of a definitive host; dogs or other canines in the case of *E. granulosus*, and foxes and rarely cats in the case of *E. multilocularis*. Dogs get infected by eating the infected viscera of sheep, cattle or other livestock. Human beings get infected by eating vegetables contaminated by dog faeces containing embryonated eggs. On hatching in the small intestine, the eggs liberate oncospheres that penetrate the mucosa and migrate via the blood vessels or lymphatics to distant sites. The liver is the commonest visceral site involved (70%). The lungs are involved in 20% of cases and other sites of involvement, including the kidney, spleen, brain and bone,[77] constitute the remaining 10%.

In these visceral sites, the parasites develop into metacestodes. The life cycle is completed when the intermediate host containing fertile metacestodes with protoscolices is eaten by a definitive host. Direct human-to-human transmission of *Echinococcus* is impossible, as it requires two mammalian hosts to complete its life cycle.

Organ localization and cyst characteristics

Primary echinococcosis results due to the metacestode cysts inhabiting nearly all anatomical sites after oral ingestion of the eggs of *E. granulosus*. Secondary echinococcosis results due to rupture of the cysts into the peritoneum, pleural space, bile ducts or bronchial tree, or release of viable parasitic material during invasive procedures. Rupture of the cyst into the hepatic vein or inferior vena cava may result in pulmonary emboli. In most series of hydatid cysts due to *E. granulosus*, single organ involvement, usually with a solitary cyst, was found. Simultaneous involvement of more than one organ was seen in only 13% of cases.[78]

The liver cysts range in size from 1 to 15 cm, and commonly involve the right lobe of the liver. The usual rate of growth of hydatid cysts as documented by serial USG was shown to be 1–5 mm per year.[78] The triple-layered hydatid cyst consists of a pericyst, which is derived from the host tissue; an endocyst of metacestode origin, which forms daughter cysts; and an acellular middle layer. Protoscolices or daughter cysts usually take 0–12 months or longer to form after infection.[79]

Clinical features

The initial phase of infection is always asymptomatic. Cysts of E. granulosus grow in the liver resulting in low-grade fever and tender hepatomegaly. Rupture of the cyst into the lungs presents as acute asthma or haemoptysis, rupture into the peritoneal cavity may result in anaphylactic shock and rupture into the biliary tree results in biliary colic, cholangitis, liver abscess, pancreatitis or obstructive jaundice.[80–82] Uncommonly, anaphylactic reactions such as asthma or anaphylactic shock, which can be life-threatening, may be the first clinical manifestation.[83]

E. multilocularis forms solid granulomatous lesions in the liver, which may mimic cirrhosis or carcinoma with a fatality rate of nearly 90%. E. vogeli infection presents as multiple fluid-filled cysts with protoscolices, and may show some local invasion.

Diagnosis

Diagnosis is based on X-ray and serology. ELISA and IHA, which may be used for diagnosis, have a sensitivity of 90%.[84,85] The Casoni skin test is no longer recommended due to its lack of specificity. On plain X-ray of the abdomen, ring-like calcifications are visible in nearly 25% of hepatic cysts. Both CT scan and USG have high sensitivity and specificity in confirming the diagnosis.[86,87] Structures of mixed echogenicity are seen in the cysts, with folded membranes seen in 7%–8% of cysts. Internal septations in the cysts may produce a 'cartwheel' appearance. This is typical of multiple daughter cysts within a large mother cyst. Contrast-enhanced CT may show vascular cysts with ring enhancement.

Though not routinely recommended, the cyst may be aspirated under controlled conditions using a thin needle after giving the patient antihelminthic therapy. The presence of protoscolices and acid-fast hooklets in the cyst fluid will confirm the diagnosis.[88]

In E. multilocularis infection, scattered areas of calcified necrotic tissue are seen on CT, whereas in E. vogeli infection, polycystic lesions are seen in the liver. Plain X-ray of the abdomen may show a ring-like calcification in nearly 25% of cases.

Treatment

The treatment of Echinococcus cysts is by surgical means, medical therapy or the PAIR procedure, which involves percutaneous puncture of the cyst, aspiration of fluid, injection of the scolicidal agent and reaspiration.

Surgical treatment

Surgical therapy consists of resection of the cyst after aspiration of the cyst fluid and injection of a scolicidal agent, such as hypertonic saline or silver nitrate, if the cyst fluid is clear.[89,90] If there is a suspicion that the cyst is in communication with the biliary tree, as evidenced by a turbid fluid in the cyst, sclerosants are avoided. The surrounding pericyst is usually left untouched while the cyst and its membrane are removed.[91] Other surgical approaches are cystectomy, omentoplasty or marsupialization. Hemihepatectomy or hepatic lobectomy may be needed in complicated cases. However, long-term recurrences occur in 2%–25% of cases.

Medical treatment

Albendazole is rapidly metabolized in the liver after intestinal absorption to its main metabolite albendazole sulphoxide, which has potent antihelminthic activity. The dose is 10–15 mg/kg/day. According to WHO recommendations, chemotherapy should be recommended for patients with inoperable disease and to prevent secondary echinococcosis after spontaneous or traumatic rupture of the cysts. After chemotherapy with albendazole, 30% of cysts disappear, 30%–35% show considerable reduction in size and 20%–40% remain unchanged. In nearly 25% of patients, cysts may recur after regression or resolution. Due to the risk of teratogenicity, albendazole should not be given to pregnant females. Alopecia, insomnia and leucopenia may occur, but these are usually mild and transient. If aminotransferase levels increase more than 4 times the normal value or marked leucopenia develops, the drug should be discontinued.[92–94]

Albendazole therapy is also given to stabilize unresectable *E. multilocularis* disease of the liver. Liver transplantation achieved good results in 12 patients with alveolar and 4 with cystic disease.[95]

The PAIR technique

This procedure is safe and useful for the long-term control of echinococcal cysts.[96–99] One or more days of percutaneous catheter drainage may be needed for large cysts. The usual practice is to start oral albendazole several days before the PAIR procedure. Antihistamines and steroids are administered immediately pre-procedure to prevent anaphylaxis in the event of cyst leakage at puncture. Albendazole is continued for 2 months after the PAIR procedure. The advantages of the procedure are early return to activity and a low recurrence rate as compared to 25% for cysts treated only by medical means.[100] The PAIR procedure and laparoscopic cyst evacuation have shown good results in experienced centres. Anaphylaxis and the potential for haemorrhage should always be considered when treating hepatic hydatid disease.

REFERENCES

1. Martinez-Palomo A, Ruiz-Palacios G. Amebiasis. In: Warren SK, Mahmoud AAF (eds). *Tropical and geographic medicine.* New York: McGraw-Hill; 1990:327–44.
2. Ackers J, Clark CG, Diamond IS, *et al. Entamoeba* taxonomy. *Bull World Health Organ* 1997;**72:**97–100.
3. Hung CC, Chen PJ, Hsieh SM, *et al.* Invasive amoebiasis: An emerging parasitic disease in patients with HIV in an area endemic for amoebic infection. *AIDS* 1999;**13:**2421–8.
4. Seeto RK, Rockey DC. Amebic liver abscess: Epidemiology, clinical features, and outcome. *West J Med* 1999;**170:**104–9.
5. Hughes MA, Petri WA Jr. Amebic liver abscess. Infections of the liver. *Infect Dis Clin North Am* 2000;**14:**565–82.
6. Mufioz LE, Botello MA, Carrillo O, *et al.* Early detection of complications in amebic liver abscess. *Arch Med Res* 1992;**23:**251–3.
7. Sharma MP, Dasarathy S. Amoebic liver abscess. *Trop Gastroenterol* 1993;**14:**3–9.
8. Haque R, Mollah NU, Ali IK, *et al.* Diagnosis of amebic liver abscess and intestinal infection with the TechLab *Entamoeba histolytica* II antigen detection and antibody tests. *J Clin Microbiol* 2000;**9:**3235–9.
9. Abd-Alla MD, Jackson TF, Reddy S, *et al.* Diagnosis of invasive amebiasis by enzyme linked immunosorbent assay of saliva to detect amebic lectin antigen and anti-lectin immunoglobulin G antibodies. *J Clin Microbiol* 2000;**6:**2344–7.
10. Petri WA Jr, Singh U. Diagnosis and management of amebiasis. *Clin Infect Dis* 1999; **29:**1117–25.
11. Gaucher D, Chadee K. Immunogenicity of an optimized *Entamoeba histolytica* Gal-lectin DNA vaccine. *Arch Med Res* 2000;**31:**5307–8.
12. Cox FEG. Malaria. Getting into the liver. *Nature* 1992;**359:**361–2.
13. Goma J, Renia L, Miltgen F, *et al.* Iron overload increases hepatic development of *Plasmodium yoelii* in mice. *Parasitology* 1996;**112:**165–8.
14. Molyneux ME, Looareesuwan S, Menzies IS, *et al.* Reduced hepatic flow and intestinal malabsorption in severe *falciparum* malaria. *Am J Trop Med Hyg* 1989;**40:**470–6.
15. Davies MP, Brook GM, Weir WRC, *et al.* Liver function tests in adults with *Plasmodium falciparum* infection. *Eur J Gastroenterol Hepatol* 1996;**8:**873–5.
16. Lalitha Murthy G, Sahay RK, Sreenivas DV, *et al.* Hepatitis in *falciparum* malaria. *Trop Gastroenterol* 1998;**19:**152–4.
17. Srivastava A, Khanduri A, Lakhtakia S, *et al. Falciparum* malaria with acute liver failure. *Trop Gastroenterol* 1996;**17:**172–4.
18. Dunn MA. Parasitic diseases. In: Schiff ER, Sorrell MF, Maddrey WE (eds). *Diseases of the liver.* 8th ed. Philadelphia: Lippincott-Raven; 1999:1533–48.
19. Magill AJ. Visceral leishmaniasis (kala-azar). In: Strickland GT (ed). *Hunter's tropical medicine and emerging infectious diseases.* 8th ed. Philadelphia: WB Saunders; 2000:670–9.
20. Ward RD. Vector biology and control. In: Chang KP, Bray RS (eds). *Leishmaniasis.* New York: Elsevier; 1985:199–204.
21. da Silva R, Hall BF, Joiner KA, *et al.* CRI, the C3b receptor, mediates binding of infective *Leishmania major* metacyclic promastigotes to human macrophages. *J Immunol* 1989; **143:**617–22.
22. Cooper A, Rosen H, Blackwell JM. Monoclonal antibodies that recognize distinct epitopes of the macrophage type three complement receptor differ in their ability to inhibit binding of *Leishmania* promastigotes harvested at different phases of their growth cycle. *Immunology* 1988;**65:**511–14.
23. Blackwell JM, Ezekowitz RAB, Roberts MB, *et al.* Macrophage complement and lectin like receptors bind *Leishmania* in the absence of serum. *J Exp Med* 1985;**162:**324–31.

24. Wilson ME, Pearson RD. Roles of CR3 and mannose receptors in the attachment and ingestion of *Leishmania donovani* by human mononuclear phagocytes. *Infect Immunol* 1988;**56**:363–9.

25. Miralles GD, Stoeckle MY, McDermorr DF, *et al.* Induction of Th1 and Th2 cell-associated cytokines in experimental visceral leishmaniasis. *Infect Immun* 1994;**62**:1058–63.

26. Marazuela M, Moreno A, Yebra M, *et al.* Hepatic fibrin-ring granulomas: A clinicopathologic study of 23 patients. *Hum Pathol* 1991;**22**:607–13.

27. Corbett CEP, Duarte MIS, Bustamante SE. Regression of diffuse intralobular liver fibrosis associated with visceral leishmaniasis. *Am J Trop Med Hyg* 1993;**49**:616–24.

28. El Hag IA, Hashim FA, El Toum IA, *et al.* Liver morphology and function in visceral leishmaniasis (kala-azar). *J Clin Pathol* 1994;**47**:547–51.

29. Rogers L. A peculiar intralobular cirrhosis of the liver produced by the protozoal parasite of kala-azar. *Ann Trop Med Parasitol* 1908;**2**:147–52.

30. Oren R, Schnur LF, Ben Yehuda D, *et al.* Visceral leishmaniasis: A difficult diagnosis and unusual causative agent. *J Infect Dis* 1991;**164**:746–9.

31. Cerf BJ, Jones TC, Badaro R, *et al.* Malnutrition as a risk factor for severe visceral leishmaniasis. *J Infect Dis* 1987;**156**:1030–3.

32. Portoles J, Prarts D, Torralbo A, Harrero J, Torrente J, Barrientos A. Visceral leishmaniasis: A cause of opportunistic infection in renal transplant patients in endemic areas. *Transplantation* 1994;**57**:1677–9.

33. Manson-Bahr PEC, Southgate BA, Harvey AEC. Development of kala-azar with special reference to the pathology, prophylaxis and treatment. *Trans R Soc Trop Med Hyg* 1959;**53**:123–6.

34. Zijlstra EE, Ali MS, El-Hassan AM, *et al.* Clinical aspects of kala-azar in children from the Sudan: A comparison with the disease in adults. *J Trop Pediatr* 1992;**38**:17–21

35. Andrade TM, Carvalho EM, Rocha H. Bacterial infections in patients with visceral leishmaniasis. *J Infect Dis* 1990;**162**:1354–9.

36. Aebischer T. Recurrent cutaneous leishmaniasis: A role for persistent parasites. *Parasitol Today* 1994;**10**:25.

37. Aebischer T, Moody SF, Handman E. Persistence of virulent *Leishmania major* in murine cutaneous leishmaniasis: A possible hazard for the host. *Infect Immun* 1993;**61**:220–6.

38. Badaro R, Carvalho EM, Rocha H, *et al.* Visceral leishmaniasis: An opportunistic microbe associated with progressive disease in three immunocompromised patients. *Lancet* 1986;**1**:647–8.

39. Berenguer J, Moreno S, Cercenado E, *et al.* Visceral leishmaniasis in patients infected with human immunodeficiency virus (HIV). *Ann Intern Med* 1989;**111**:129–32.

40. Hofman V, Marty P, Perrin C, *et al.* The histological spectrum of visceral leishmaniasis caused by *Leishmania infantum* MON-1 in acquired immune deficiency syndrome. *Hum Pathol* 2000;**31**:75–84.

41. Horber FF, Lerut JP, Reichen J, *et al.* Visceral leishmaniasis after orthotopic liver transplantation: Impact of persistent splenomegaly. *Transplant Int* 1993;**6**:55–7.

42. Hernandez-Perez J, Yebra-Bango M, Jiminez-Martinez E, *et al.* Visceral leishmaniasis (kala-azar) in solid organ transplantation: Report of five cases and review. *Clin Infect Dis* 1999;**29**:918–21.

43. Jha TK, Olliaro P, Thakur CPN, *et al.* Randomised controlled trial of aminosidine (paramomycin) versus sodium stibogluconate for treating visceral leishmaniasis in North Bihar. *India BMJ* 1998;**316**:1200–5.

44. Sundar S, Gupta LB, Makharia MK, *et al.* Oral treatment of visceral leishmaniasis with miltefosine. *Ann Trop Med Parasitol* 1999;**93**:589–97.

45. De Rossill RA, de Duran RJ, Rossell O, *et al.* Is leishmaniasis ever cured? *Trans R Soc Trop Med Hyg* 1992;**86**:251–3.

46. Murray HW, Hariprashad J. Interleukin 12 is effective treatment for an established systemic intracellular infection: Experimental visceral leishmaniasis. *J Exp Med* 1995;**181**:387–91.

47. Hlaing T. A profile of ascariasis morbidity in Rangoon Children's Hospital, Burma. *J Trop Med Hyg* 1987;**90**:165–7.

48. Schulman A. Non-western patterns of biliary stones and the role of ascariasis. *Radiology* 1987;**162**:425–30.

49. Uflacker R, Duarte D, Silva P. Association of congenital cystic dilatation of the common bile duct and congenital diverticulum of the hepatic duct with concomitant ascariasis. *Gastrointest Radiol* 1978;**3**:407–9.

50. Khuroo MS, Zargar SA, Mahajan R. Hepatobiliary and pancreatic ascariasis in India. *Lancet* 1990;**335**:1503–6.

51. Khuroo MS, Zargar SA, Yattoo GN, *et al*. Sonographic findings in galbladder ascariasis. *J Clin Ultrasound* 1992;**20**:587–91.

52. Khuroo MS, Mahajan R, Zargar SA, *et al*. Biliary and pancreatic ascariasis: A long-term follow-up. *Natl Med J India* 1989;**2**:4–6.

53. Schulman A. Intrahepatic biliary stones: Imaging features and a possible relationship with *Ascaris lumbricoides*. *Clin Radiol* 1993;**47**:325–32.

54. Khuroo MS, Zargar SA, Yattoo GN, *et al*. Oddi's sphincter motor activity in patients with recurrent pyogenic cholangitis. *Hepatology* 1993;**17**:53–8.

55. Khuroo MS, Zargar SA, Mahajan R, *et al*. Sonographic appearances in biliary ascarasis. *Gastroenterology* 1987;**93**:267–72.

56. Khuroo MS, Zargar SA, Yattoo GN, *et al*. Worm extraction and biliary drainage in hepato-biliary and pancreatic ascariasis. *Gastrointest Endosc* 1993;**39**:680–5.

57. Mahmoud AA. Strongyloidiasis. *Clin Infect Dis* 1996;**23**:949–52.

58. Capo V, Despommier DD. Clinical aspects of infection with *Trichinella spiralis*. *Clin Microbiol Rev* 1996;**9**:47–54.

59. Berger T, Degremont A, Gebbers JO, *et al*. Hepatic capillariasis in a 1-year-old child. *Eur J Pediatr* 1990;**149**:333–6.

60. Arjona R, Riancho JA, Aguado JM, *et al*. Fascioliasis in developed countries: A review of classic and aberrant forms of the disease. *Medicine* 1995;**74**:13–23.

61. Price TA, Tuazon CU, Simon GL. Fascioliasis: Case reports and review. *Clin Infect Dis* 1993;**17**:426–30.

62. Stark ME, Herrington DA, Hillyer GV, *et al*. An international traveler with fever, abdominal pain, eosinophilia and a liver lesion. *Gastroenterology* 1993;**105**:1900–8.

63. Meeusen E, Rickard MD, Brandon MR. Cellular responses during liver fluke infection in sheep and its evasion by the parasite. *Parasite Immunol* 1995;**17**:37–45.

64. Moreto M, Barron J. The laparoscopic diagnosis of the liver fascioliasis. *Gastrointest Endosc* 1980;**26**:147–9.

65. Van Beers B, Pringot J, Guebel A, *et al*. Hepatobiliary fascioliasis: Noninvasive imaging findings. *Radiology* 1990;**174**:809–10.

66. Puspeiro JR, Armesto V, Varela J, *et al*. Fascioliasis: Findings in 15 patients. *Br J Radiol* 2001;**64**:798–801.

67. Han JK, Chol BI, Cho JM, *et al*. Radiological findings of human fascioliasis. *Abdom Imaging* 1993;**18**:261–4.

68. Kim JB, Kim DJ, Huh S, *et al*. A human case of invasive fascioliasis asociated with liver abscess. *Korean J Parasitol* 1995;**33**:395–8.

69. Maher K, El Redi R, Elhoda AN, *et al*. Parasite-specific antibody profile in human fascioliasis: Application for immunodiagnosis of infection. *Am J Trop Med Hyg* 1999;**61**:738–42.

70. Bacq Y, Besnier J-M, Duong T-H, *et al.* Successful treatment of acute fascioliasis with bithionol. *Hepatology* 1991;**14**:1066–9.
71. Schwartz DA. Cholangiocarcinoma associated with liver fluke infection: A preventable source of morbidity in Asian immigrants. *Am J Gastroenterol* 1986;**81**:76–9.
72. Sithithaworn P, Haswell-Elkins M, Mairiang P, *et al.* Parasite-associated morbidity: Liver fluke infection and bile duct cancer in northeast Thailand. *Int J Parasitol* 1994;**24**:833–43.
73. Leung JWC, Sung Y, Banez VP, *et al.* Endoscopic cholangiopancreatography in hepatic clonorchiasis—a follow-up study. *Gastrointest Endosc* 1990;**36**:360–3.
74. Satarug S, Lang MA, Yongvanit P, *et al.* Induction of cytochrome P450 2A6 expression in humans by the carcinogenic parasite infection *Opisthorchiasis viverrini. Cancer Epidemiol Biomarkers Prev* 1996;**5**:795–800.
75. Stock FE, Fung JHY. Oriental cholangiohepatitis. *Arch Surg* 1962;**84**:409–12.
76. Watanapa P. Cholangiocarcinoma in patients with opisthorchiasis. *Br J Surg* 1996; **83**:1062–4.
77. Grove DI, Warren KS, Mahmoud AAF. Algorithm in the diagnosis and management of exotic diseases: Echinococcosis. *J Infect Dis* 1976;**133**:354–8.
78. Schantz PM, Brandt FH, Dickinson CM, *et al.* Effects of albendazole on *Echinococcus multilocularis* infection in the Mongolian jird. *J Infect Dis* 1990;**162**:1403–7.
79. Ammann RW, Eckert J. Clinical diagnosis and treatment of echinococcosis in humans. In: Thompson RCA, Lymbery AJ (eds). *Echinococcus and hydatid disease.* Wallingford, Oxon/UK: CAB International; 1995:411–15.
80. Van Steenbergen W, Fevery J, Broechaert L, *et al.* Hepatic echinococcosis ruptured into the biliary tract: Clinical, radiological and therapeutic features during five episodes of spontaneous biliary rupture in three patients with hepatic hydatidosis. *J Hepatol* 1987; **4**:133–9.
81. Werczberger Gohlman J, Wertheim G, Gunders AE, *et al.* Disseminated echinococcosis with repeated anaphylactic shock treated with mebendazole. *Chest* 1979;**76**:482–4.
82. Schantz PM, Okelo GBA. Echinococcosis (hydatidosis). In: Warren KS, Mahmoud AAF (eds). *Tropical and geographical medicine.* New York: McGraw-Hill; 1990:505–18.
83. Akinoglu A, Demiyurek H, Guzel C. Alveolar hydatid disease of the liver: A report on thirty-nine surgical cases in eastern Anatolia, Turkey. *Am J Trop Med Hyg* 1991;**45**:182–9.
84. Gottstein B. Molecular and immunological diagnosis of echinococcosis. *Clin Microbiol Rev* 1992;**5**:248–61.
85. Baba H, Messedi H, Masmoudi S, *et al.* Diagnosis of human hydatidosis: Comparison between imagery and six serological techniques. *Am J Trop Med Hyg* 1994;**50**:64–8.
86. Schaefer JW, Khan MY. Echinococcosis (hydatid disease): Lessons from experience with 59 patients. *Rev Infect Dis* 1991;**13**:243–7.
87. Kalovidouris A, Pissiotis C, Pontifex C, *et al.* CT characterization of multivesicular hydatid cysts. *J Comput Assist Tomogr* 1986;**10**:428–31.
88. Hira PR, Lindberg LG, Francis I, *et al.* Diagnosis of cystic hydatid disease: Role of aspiration cytology. *Lancet* 1988;**1**:655–7.
89. Fenton-Lee D, Morris DL. The management of hydatid disease of the liver: Part 1. *Trop Doctor* 1996;**26**:173–6.
90. Alonso Casado O, Moreno Gonzalez E, Loinaz Segurola C, *et al.* Results of 22 years of experience in radical surgical treatment of hepatic hydatid cysts. *Hepatogastroenterology* 2001;**48**:235–43.
91. Bastani B, Dehdeshti F. Hepatic hydatid disease in Iran, with review of the literature. *Mt Sinai J Med* 1995;**62**:62–9.
92. Steiger U, Corting J, Reichen J. Albendazole treatment of echinococcosis in humans: Effects on microsomal metabolism and drug tolerance. *Clin Pharmacol Ther* 1990;**47**:347–53.

93. Gil-Grande LA, Rodriguez-Caabeiro F, Prieto JG, *et al.* Abdominal hydatid disease. *Lancet* 1993;**342**:1269–72.

94. Ammann RW, Ilitsch N, Marincek B, *et al.* Swiss Echinococcosis Study Group. Effect of chemotherapy on the larval mass and the long-term course of alveolar echinococcosis. *Hepatology* 1994;**19**:735–42.

95. Bresson-Hadni S, Franza A, Miguet JP, *et al.* Orthotopic liver transplantation for incurable alveolar echinococcosis of the liver. Report of 17 cases. *Hepatology* 1991;**13**:1961–70.

96. Khuroo MS, Dar MY, Yattoo GN, *et al.* Percutaneous drainage versus albendazole therapy in hepatic hydatidosis: A prospective, randomized study. *Gastroenterology* 1993; **104**:1452–9.

97. Salama HM, Ahmed NH, el Deeb N, *et al.* Hepatic hydatid cysts: Sonographic follow-up after percutaneous sonographically guided aspiration. *J Clin Ultrasound* 1998;**26**:455–60.

98. Ustunsoz B, Akhan O, Kamiloglu MA, *et al.* Percutaneous treatment of hydatid cysts of the liver: Long-term results. *AJR Am J Roentgenol* 1999;**172**:91–6.

99. Odev K, Paksoy Y, Arslan A, *et al.* Sonographically guided percutaneous treatment of hepatic hydatid cysts: Long-term results. *J Clin Ultrasound* 2000;**28**:469–78.

100. Franchi C, di Vico B, Teggi A. Long-term evaluation of patients with hydatidosis treated with benzimidazole carbamates. *Clin Infect Dis* 1999;**29**:304–9.

CHAPTER 18

Space-occupying lesions of the liver causing jaundice

S.S. SIDDHU

A variety of diseases may cause space-occupying lesions of the liver, which may lead to jaundice. These may be classified as follows:

Congenital
  Polycystic liver disease
Infective
  Amoebic liver abscess
  Echinococcosis
  Tuberculosis
Neoplasms
  Benign
    Haemangioma
    Cystadenoma
  Malignant
    Lymphomas—Hodgkin, non-Hodgkin, primary intrahepatic lymphoma
    Hepatocellular carcinoma (HCC)
    Intrahepatic cholangiocarcinoma
    Hepatic metastases

CONGENITAL CAUSES

Polycystic liver disease

This is a rare disease in which multiple cysts develop within the liver parenchyma. It occurs in association with autosomal dominant polycystic kidney disease as well as in isolation.

Complications

These include portal hypertension presenting as variceal bleeding,[1] hepatic venous outflow tract obstruction with development of ascites[2] and obstructive jaundice resulting from direct obstruction of the biliary tree by a cyst.

Investigations

ERCP is helpful in identifying the obstructing cyst and decompressing the dilated biliary duct.

Treatment

Percutaneous drainage and sclerosing therapy[3] or surgery are the available treatment options.[3]

INFECTIVE CAUSES

Amoebic liver abscess

Escherichia histolytica is the cause of dysentery, colitis and liver abscess. The amoebae bind host cells via a galactose-binding lectin. The amoebae then lyse the target cell by means of pore-forming molecules called amoebapores and phospholipases.[4]

Clinical features

The condition is more frequent in men between 20 and 40 years of age. Clinical symptoms include fever (between 38 °C and 40 °C), right hypochondrial pain and non-productive cough (in 30%). At autopsy, the average size of an abscess ranges from 5 to 15 cm. Abscesses are mostly single and localized in the right lobe. Left lobe abscesses occur in 35% of patients and multiple abscesses in 16%.

Laboratory findings

Most patients (>90%) have leucocytosis (>15×10^9 cells/L). The serum ALP level is elevated in half of these patients. A mild increase in serum bilirubin is seen in 30% of patients and, occasionally, there may be hypoalbuminaemia (<3 g/dl).

Indirect haemagglutination (IHA) is the most sensitive and specific method of diagnosis, with positive results obtained in 85%–95% of patients. A test that detects serum *E. histolytica* Gal/Gal Nac lectin antigen is now available as Techlab *E. histolytica* II.

Imaging

On USG, a well-defined hypoechoic lesion is seen. On CT, an amoebic abscess shows low density, smooth margins and a contrast-enhancing peripheral rim. An abscess near the confluence of the major hepatic ducts can cause biliary obstruction.

Therapy

Drugs

Metronidazole can be given in a dose of 1 g b.i.d. orally or 500 mg intravenously q 6 hourly for 10 days. Alternative drugs are dehydroemetine 1 mg/kg daily intramuscularly for 10 days and chloroquine in a dose of 1 g/day orally for 2 days followed by 500 mg/day for 2–3 weeks.

Percutaneous aspiration/drainage

This is done when the risk of rupture is high, response to the drugs is slow or an association with pyogenic infection is suspected.[5]

Surgery

Rupture of a liver abscess into the surrounding intra-abdominal or thoracic organs is the indication for surgery.

Echinococcosis

Hydatid liver cysts caused by *E. granulosus* are usually silent. They are fluid-filled structures delimited by a parasite-derived membrane containing germinal epithelium that buds into viable scolices.

Imaging

USG, CT scan and MRI demonstrate the formation of daughter cysts and calcification of the cyst wall. Compression of the intrahepatic bile ducts and communication of the cyst with the biliary system are seen in complicated hydatid disease. Uncommon presentations include segmental portal hypertension secondary to splenic vein compression by a cyst in the splenic hilum,[6] and rupture of a hepatic hydatid cyst causing inferior vena cava thrombosis.[7]

Therapy

Drugs

Albendazole has strong scolicidal activity against *E. granulosus*. It is administered 2–3 times daily at doses of 10–50 mg/kg/day for 12–24 weeks.[8–10]

Surgery

This involves simple resection of the cyst and its membrane preceded by injection of hypertonic saline solution into the cyst.

Percutaneous drainage

The PAIR method—USG-guided process of puncture, aspiration, injection with hypertonic saline and re-aspiration—is the first-line standard of treatment in many centres.[11,12] Advantages include minimal disability and early return to full activity.

Tuberculosis

The clinical manifestations of hepatobiliary tuberculosis are those of extra-hepatic disease; hepatic involvement usually produces no symptoms.[13] An elevated serum ALP level suggests diffusely infiltrative hepatic tuberculosis.[14] The presence of jaundice suggests biliary involvement causing extrahepatic biliary obstruction.[15]

Imaging

A plain X-ray of the abdomen shows hepatic calcifications. USG and CT scan show complex hepatic masses, either solitary or multiple. Compression of the biliary tree by involved lymph nodes or rupture of a caseating granuloma into the lumen of the bile duct may cause obstructive jaundice. Bile duct tubercu-losis[16] may manifest as bile duct dilatation and common hepatic duct strictures.

Therapy

Experience with therapeutic ERCP biliary stenting has been variable. If ERCP fails, percutaneous biliary drainage can decompress the biliary obstruction.[17,18]

Drugs

At least four drugs including isoniazid, rifampicin, pyrazinamide and ethambutol[19] are given traditionally for 1 year.

NEOPLASMS OF THE LIVER

Benign neoplasms

Haemangioma

This is the most common benign mesenchymal hepatic tumour. The size varies from <1 cm to >20 cm. Lesions >4 cm are called giant haemangiomas.[20] They present most commonly in women (60%–80%) between the third and fifth decades of life.[21]

Pathogenesis

These are benign congenital hamartomas[22] and growth is a consequence of progressive ectasia. Growth during pregnancy or in patients receiving oral contraceptives suggests that oestrogens play a role in their development.[23]

Pathology

On gross examination, haemangiomas are compressible, dark-coloured, cystic lesions. Histological examination reveals a thin-walled lesion with vascular spaces lined by a single layer of endothelial cells and separated by fibrous septa.

Clinical features

Most often, the lesion is silent and located in the right lobe of the liver. Giant lesions cause symptoms in 40%–90% of cases. Common symptoms include abdominal pain, early satiety, anorexia and nausea.[24] Rarely, haemangiomas cause obstructive jaundice or gastric outlet obstruction.[25–27]

Imaging

USG shows a well-defined, hyperechoic lesion with posterior acoustic enhancement. Dynamic CT shows a hypodense lesion on plain scan, with early peripheral enhancement and progressive centripetal filling. The lesion remains isodense or hyperdense for up to 60 minutes after injection. MRI has a sensitivity >90%. The lesion is well-defined, homogeneous, with a low-signal intensity on T1-weighted images and a high-signal intensity on T2-weighted images. Single-photon emission CT (SPECT) with ^{99m}Tc-RBC is best used for lesions >2 cm in size.[28] On angiography, a cottonwool appearance is seen, which persists during and beyond the venous phase (>40 s).

Treatment

No treatment is needed for silent lesions. Surgical resection is indicated in severely symptomatic lesions.[29] Surgical enucleation is associated with less blood loss as compared to resection.

Cystadenoma

This is a benign tumour in which an epithelial layer surrounds a large, fluid-filled cyst in the hepatic parenchyma or, rarely, in the extrahepatic biliary tree. It accounts for <5% of cystic lesions of the liver. Approximately 80% of cases occur in middle-aged women. The clinical features are the result of compression of the expanding liver mass on adjacent structures. One-third of patients have compression of the biliary tree which leads to cholangitis or jaundice.[30] Treatment is by complete surgical resection.

Malignant neoplasms

Malignant lymphomas

Hepatic infiltrates may be massive, or present as space-occupying lesions. Large, intrahepatic deposits are the commonest cause of deep jaundice. Liver biopsy confirms the diagnosis. Obstructive jaundice is more frequent in non-Hodgkin lymphoma than in Hodgkin disease[31] and is due to enlargement of the hilar nodes. USG, CT scan, MRI, ERCP or percutaneous transhepatic cholangiography (PTC) along with cytology and biopsy gives the diagnosis. Lymphomas should be considered in patients with fever, jaundice, hepatosplenomegaly, and increase in serum ALP and GGT levels.

Primary hepatic lymphoma

By definition, this rare lymphoma affects only the liver. It presents with pain, hepatomegaly, a palpable mass, and elevated levels of ALP and bilirubin. There is no lymphadenopathy.

Imaging and diagnosis

USG and CT scan show a solitary mass in 60% of patients, multiple masses in 35% and diffuse disease in 5%.[32] Diagnosis is by liver biopsy. Histologically, it is a non-Hodgkin, large B-cell or, less often, T-cell lymphoma.

Hepatocellular carcinoma

This is the seventh commonest cause of cancer in men. The highest incidence is in the African and Oriental races in whom there is nearly always an associated cirrhosis. Hepatitis B and C are the most important aetiological factors for the development of HCC.

Pathology

Morphologically, HCC is of three types: expanding with discrete margins; spreading (infiltrative); and multifocal.[33] The expanding type occurs in a non-cirrhotic liver. Large hepatic or portal veins within the liver are often thrombosed and contain tumour tissue.

Clinical features

Males are affected more often than females, in a ratio of 4–6:1. Pain in the epigastrium, right hypochondrium, weight loss, low-grade fever and deterioration in the general condition of the patient with cirrhosis are common features. Jaundice is rarely deep and has little relation to the extent of hepatic involvement. Rarely, the tumour presents as an intrabiliary, pedunculated polyp causing obstructive jaundice.[34] The tumour may rupture into the CBD,[35] leading to haemobilia, which may be the immediate cause of death. Portal vein thrombosis and obstruction of the hepatic vein may occur, and ascites is found in half of the patients. Haemorrhage from oesophageal varices is frequent and terminal.

Imaging

On USG, the tumour is hypoechoic with ill-defined margins, or heterogeneous. CT scan shows a hypodense lesion,[36] or a mosaic pattern with many nodules of differing attenuation with enhancing septa within the masses. There may be invasion of the portal vein and arterioportal shunting. Lipiodol introduced into the hepatic artery is cleared from non-cancerous tissue but remains almost permanently in the tumour, so that lesions as small as 0.2–0.3 cm can be detected on CT scan 2 weeks later. MRI[37] is better than CT scan for identifying focal lesions. T1-weighted images show a hypointense peripheral ring and are isodense. T2-weighted images show good tumour–liver contrast, and can detect vascular invasion and satellite nodules. Gadolinium and magnesium contrast agents (MndPDP) are enhanced in HCC.[38] Supermagnetic iron oxide is useful in T2-weighted images.[39]

Needle liver biopsy

Biopsy is done under imaging control to confirm the diagnosis. FNAC using a 22 G needle will diagnose moderately and poorly differentiated tumours, but the cytological diagnosis of well-differentiated tumours is difficult by this method.

Treatment

Resection or transplantation offers the possibility of cure. Factors in favour of resection are size <5 cm, single lobe involvement, sparing of the capsule, absence of vascular invasion, good liver reserve, age <40 years and good general condition. The 1-year survival rate after resection is 55%–80%, and a 5-year survival rate of 25%–39% is reported. Orthotopic liver transplantation (OLT) is the best treatment modality for patients with a solitary HCC <5 cm in diameter and for patients with <3 tumours, each <3 cm (Milan criteria).[40]

Intrahepatic cholangiocarcinoma

Aetiological factors for cholangiocarcinoma include clonorchiasis, primary sclerosing cholangitis, fibrocystic diseases and the use of anabolic steroids. It is a glandular tumour arising from the intrahepatic bile ducts. Keratin is a good marker of biliary epithelium and is found in 90% of cholangiocarcinomas.[41] The clinical features are those of hepatic malignancy with prominent obstructive jaundice. The serum alpha-fetoprotein level is not increased. CT scan shows a space-occupying, hypovascular lesion of low attenuation, sometimes with calcification.[42] MRI may show vascular encasement. ERCP or percutaneous biliary drainage palliates the jaundice. The tumour does not responsed to chemotherapy.

Hepatic metastasis

The liver is the most frequent site of blood-borne metastases, irrespective of whether the primary is drained by the systemic or portal veins. It is involved in a third of all cancers, including half of the cancers of the stomach, breast, lung and colon. Other frequent primary sites include the oesophagus, pancreas and malignant melanoma.

Clinical features

These may be due to the hepatic metastases, the distant primary growth or a combination of both. There is weight loss, abdominal distension, fever and night sweats. The liver may be normal or very large in size. Splenomegaly is frequent. Jaundice is mild. Deep jaundice implies invasion of the major bile ducts. Obstructive jaundice is seen due to metastases from breast, colon or small-cell lung cancers.[43] Oedema of the legs suggests obstruction/invasion of the intrahepatic inferior vena cava. Ascites reflects peritoneal involvement and occasionally a thrombosed portal vein.

Biochemical tests

Even with enormous liver metastases, sufficient functioning tissue remains. The smaller intrahepatic bile ducts may be compressed, yet no jaundice develops. The area with the uninvolved ducts may excrete bilirubin from the occluded areas. Serum bilirubin values >2 mg/100 ml suggest involvement of the major bile ducts at the hilum. The levels of serum ALP, lactic dehydrogenase and transaminases are raised. If all of the above are normal, there is a 98% probability that metastases are absent.[44]

Imaging

USG shows echogenic lesions. A CT scan shows metastases as low-attenuation lesions. Colonic cancer metastases have a large avascular centre with a dense, peripheral, ring-like accumulation of contrast. T1-weighted MRI is the best method of detecting colorectal liver metastases.[45] T2-weighted images show oedema adjacent to the liver metastases.[46] Iron oxide- or gadolinium-enhanced MRI imaging is better than unenhanced MRI.[47]

Treatment

This is unsatisfactory. The various modalities are systemic chemotherapy, surgical resection, intratumoral ablation, chemoembolization and regional chemotherapy. In systemic chemotherapy, useful agents include 5-fluorouracil, leucovorin and irinotecan (CPT-II) for colorectal cancer with liver metastases.[48,49] Newer agents include oxaliplatin[50] and epidermal growth factor receptor-blocking monoclonal antibodies.[51] Intraoperative ultrasonography (IOUS) is the most sensitive modality currently available for detecting occult liver metastases.[52] IOUS has contributed to an improved survival rate among patients undergoing surgical resection of liver metastases, e.g. colorectal cancer. Local ablative therapies include radiofrequency ablation (RFA) in neuroendocrine metastatic liver disease,[53] microwave,[54] high-intensity focused USG,[55] laser thermotherapy [56]and Yttrium-90 seed implants.[57] Hepatic arterial chemoembolization provides palliation for hypervascular metastatic lesions from neuroendocrine tumours, melanoma and adrenal cancer.[58]

REFERENCES

1. Srinivasan R. Polycystic liver disease: An unusual cause of bleeding varices. *Dig Dis Sci* 1999;**44**:389–92.
2. Leconte I, Van Beers BE, Lacrosse M, *et al*. Focal nodular hyperplasia: Natural course observed with CT and MRI. *J Comput Assist Tomogr* 2000;**24**:61–6.
3. Lerner ME, Roshkow JE, Smithkline A, *et al*. Polycystic liver disease with obstructive jaundice: Treatment with ultrasound guided cyst aspiration. *Gastrointest Radiol* 1992; **17**:46–8.

4. Leippe M. Amoebapores. *Parasitol Today* 1997;**13**:178–83.

5. Rajak CL, Gupta S, Jain S, *et al.* Percutaneous treatment of liver abscesses: Needle aspiration versus catheter drainage. *AJR Am J Roentgenol* 1998;**170**:1035–9.

6. El Fortia M, Bendaoud M, Taema S, *et al.* Segmental portal hypertension due to a splenic *Echinococcus* cyst. *Eur J Ultrasound* 2000;**11**:21–3.

7. Anuradha S, Agarwal SK, Khatri S, Bhasin S, Singh NP, Chowdhury V. Spontaneous rupture of hepatic hydatid cyst causing inferior vena cava thrombosis. *Indian J Gastroenterol* 1999;**18**:34.

8. Ammann RW, Swiss *Echinococcus* Study Group. Improvement of liver resectional therapy by adjuvant chemotherapy in alveolar hydatid disease. *Parasitol Res* 1991;**77**:290–3.

9. Steiger U, Cotting J, Reichen J. Albendazole treatment of echinococcosis in humans: Effects on microsomal metabolism and drug tolerance. *Clin Pharmacol Ther* 1990;**47**:347–53.

10. Nahmias J, Goldsmith R, Soibelman M, *et al.* Three to seven year follow up after albendazole treatment of 68 patients with cystic echinococcosis (hydatid disease). *Ann Trop Med Parasitol* 1994;**88**:295–304.

11. Akhan O, Ozmen MN, Dincer A, *et al.* Liver hydatid disease: Long term results of percutaneous treatment. *Radiology* 1996;**198**:259–64.

12. Khuroo MS, Dar MY, Yattoo GN, *et al.* Percutaneous drainage versus albendazole therapy in hepatic hydatidosis: A prospective randomized study. *Gastroenterology* 1993;**104**:1452–9.

13. Alvarez SZ, Carpio R. Hepatobiliary tuberculosis. *Dig Dis Sci* 1983;**28**:193–200.

14. Essop AR, Posen JA, Hodkinson JH, *et al.* Tuberculosis hepatitis: A clinical review of 96 cases. *Q J Med* 1984;**53**:465–77.

15. Abascal J, Martin F, Abreu L, *et al.* Atypical hepatic tuberculosis presenting as obstructive jaundice. *Am J Gastroenterol* 1988;**83**:1183–6.

16. Kok KYY, Yap SKS. Tuberculosis of the bile duct: A rare cause of obstructive jaundice. *J Clin Gastroenterol* 1999;**29**:161–4.

17. Inal M, Aksungur E, Akgul E, *et al.* Biliary tuberculosis mimicking cholangiocarcinoma: A treatment with metallic biliary endoprosthesis. *Am J Gastroenterol* 2000;**95**:1069–71.

18. Bearer EA, Savides TJ, McCutchan JA. Endoscopic diagnosis and management of hepatobiliary tuberculosis. *Am J Gastroenterol* 1996;**91**:2602–4.

19. Raviglione MC, O' Brien RJ. Tuberculosis. In: Braunwald E, Fauci AS, Kasper DL, *et al.* (eds). *Harrison's principles of internal medicine.* New York: McGraw-Hill; 2001:1024–35.

20. Adam Y, Huvos A, Fortner J. Giant hemangiomas of the liver. *Ann Surg* 1970;**172**:239–45.

21. Reddy K, Kligerman S, Levi J, *et al.* Benign and solid tumours of the liver: Relationship to sex, age, size of tumours and outcome. *Am Surg* 2001;**67**:173–8.

22. Nichols F, Van Heerden J, Weiland L. Benign liver tumours. *Surg Clin North Am* 1989;**69**:297–315.

23. Zafrani E. Update on the vascular tumours of the liver. *J Hepatol* 1989;**8**:125–30.

24. Kuo P, Lewis W, Jenkins R. Treatment of giant hemangiomas of the liver by enucleation. *J Am Coll Surg* 1994;**178**:49–53.

25. Patersson D, Babany G, Belghiti J, *et al.* Giant hemangiomas of the liver with pain, fever and abnormal liver tests: Report of 2 cases. *Dig Dis Sci* 1991;**36**:524–7.

26. Roslyn J, Kuckenbecker S, Longmire W, *et al.* Floating tumour debris: A cause of intermittent biliary obstruction. *Arch Surg* 1984;**119**:1312–15.

27. Wakeley C. A large cavernous hemangioma of the left lobe of the liver causing obstruction to the cardiac orifice of the stomach. *Br J Surg* 1925;**12**:590–3.

28. Kudo M, Ikkekubo K, Yamamoto K, *et al.* Distinction between hemangioma of the liver and hepatocellular carcinoma: Value of labeled RBC-SPECT scanning. *AJR Am J Roentgenol* 1989;**152**:977–83.

29. Schwartz S, Cowles W. Cavernous hemangioma of the liver. *Ann Surg* 1987;**205**:456–65.

30. Akwari OE, Tucker A, Seigler HF, *et al.* Hepatobiliary cystadenoma with mesenchymal stroma. *Ann Surg* 1990;**211**:18–27.

31. Feller E, Schiffman FJ. Extrahepatic biliary obstruction by lymphoma. *Arch Surg* 1990; **125**:1507–9.

32. Ohsawa M, Aozasa K, Horiuchi K, *et al.* Malignant lymphoma of the liver: Report of 5 cases and review of the literature. *Dig Dis Sci* 1992;**37**:1105–9.

33. Okuda K and Liver Cancer Study Group of Japan. Primary liver cancers in Japan. *Cancer* 1980;**45**:2663.

34. Terada T, Nakanuma Y, Kawai K. Small hepatocellular carcinoma presenting as intrabiliary pedunculated polyp and obstructive jaundice. *J Clin Gastroenterol* 1989;**11**:578–83.

35. Chen MF, Jan YY, Jeng LB, *et al.* Obstructive jaundice secondary to ruptured hepato-cellular carcinoma into the common bile duct. *Cancer* 1994;**73**:1335–40.

36. Stevens WR, Johnson CD, Stephen DH, *et al.* CT findings in hepatocellular carcinoma: Correlation of tumour characteristics with causative factors, tumour size, and histologic tumour grade. *Radiology* 1994;**191**:531–7.

37. Rummeny E, Weissleder R, Stak DD. Primary liver tumours: Diagnosis by MR imaging. *AJR Am J Roentgenol* 1989;**152**:63–72.

38. Mirowitz SA, Gutierrez ER, Lee JKT, *et al.* Normal abdominal enhancement patterns with dynamic gadolinium-enhanced MR imaging. *Radiology* 1991;**180**:637–40.

39. Ros PR, Freeny PC, Harms SE, *et al.* Hepatic MR imaging with ferumoxides: A multicenter clinical trial of the safety and efficacy in the detection of focal hepatic lesions. *Radiology* 1995;**196**:481–8.

40. Mazzaferro V, Regalia E, Doci R, *et al.* Liver transplantation for the treatment of small hepatocellular carcinomas in patients with cirrhosis. *N Engl J Med* 1996;**334**:693–9.

41. Goodman ZD, Ishak KG, Langloss JM. Combined hepatocellular–cholangiocarcinoma: A histologic and immunohistochemical study. *Cancer* 1985;**55**:124–35.

42. Ros PR, Buck JL, Goodman ZD, *et al.* Intrahepatic cholangiocarcinoma: Radiologic–pathologic correlation. *Radiology* 1988;**167**:689–93.

43. Johnson DH, Hainsworth JD, Greco FA. Extrahepatic biliary obstruction caused by small cell lung cancer. *Ann Intern Med* 1985;**102**:487–90.

44. Kamby C, Dirksen H, Vejborg I, *et al.* Incidence and methodologic aspects of the occurrence of liver metastases in recurrent breast cancer. *Cancer* 1987;**59**:1524–9.

45. Ward BA, Miller DL, Frank JA, *et al.* Prospective evaluation of hepatic imaging studies in the detection of colorectal metastases: Correlation with surgical findings. *Surgery* 1989;**105**:180–7.

46. Lee MJ, Saini S, Compton CC, Malt RA. MR demonstration of edema adjacent to a liver metastasis: Pathologic correlation. *AJR Am J Roentgenol* 1991;**157**:499–50.

47. Hamm B, Thoeni RF, Gould RJ, *et al.* Focal liver lesions: Characterization with non-enhanced and dynamic contrast material-enhanced MR imaging. *Radiology* 1994;**190**: 417–23.

48. Saltz LB, Douillard JY, Pirotta N. Irinotecan plus fluorouracil/leucovorin for metastatic colorectal cancer: A new survival standard. *Oncologist* 2001;**6**:81–91.

49. Saltz LB, Cox JV, Blanke C, *et al.* Irinotecan plus fluorouracil and leucovorin for metastatic colorectal cancer. Irinotecan Study Group. *N Engl J Med* 2000;**343**:905–14.

50. Zori Comba A, Blajman C, Richardet E, *et al.* A randomized phase II study of oxaliplatin alone versus oxaliplatin combined 5 fluorouracil and folinic acid (Mayo Clinic regimen) in previously untreated metastatic colorectal cancer patients. *Eur J Cancer* 2001;**37**:1006–13.

51. Mendelsohn J. The epidermal growth factor receptor as a target for cancer therapy. *Endocr Relat Cancer* 2001;**88**:3–9.

52. Cervone A, Sardi A, Conaway GL. Intraoperative ultrasound (IOUS) is essential in the management of metastatic colorectal liver lesions. *Am Surg* 2000;**66**:611–15.
53. Siperstein AE, Berber E. Cryoablation, percutaneous alcohol injection and radiofrequency ablation for treatment of neuroendocrine liver metastases. *World J Surg* 2001;**25**:693–6.
54. Matsukawa T, Yamashita Y, Arakawa A, *et al.* Percutaneous microwave coagulation therapy in liver tumours, *Acta Radiol* 1997;**38**:410–15.
55. Prat F, Centarti M, Sille A, *et al.* Extracorporeal high intensity focused ultrasound for VX2 liver tumours in the rabbit. *Hepatology* 1995;**21**:832–6.
56. Muralidharan V, Christophi C. Interstitial laser thermotherapy in the treatment of colorectal liver metastases. *J Surg Oncol* 2001;**76**:73–81.
57. Lau WY, Leung WT, Ho S, *et al.* Treatment of inoperable hepatocellular carcinoma with intrahepatic arterial Yttrium-90 microspheres: A phase I and II study. *Br J Cancer* 1994;**70**:994–9.
58. Kim YH, Ajani JA, Carrasco CH, *et al.* Selective hepatic arterial chemoembolization for liver metastases in patients with carcinoid tumour or islet cell carcinoma. *Cancer Invest* 1999;**17**:474–8.

CHAPTER 19

Surgical obstructive jaundice

GOURDAS CHOUDHURI

Obstruction of the large bile ducts, such as the common bile duct, common hepatic duct or the major intrahepatic bile ducts, is a common cause of obstructive jaundice. Although the term 'surgical obstructive jaundice' came to be applied to this condition as surgery was the only method of treatment available till a few decades back; with the recent advent of several non-surgical treatment methods, such as endoscopic or percutaneous techniques, it is a misnomer today. The term 'extrahepatic biliary obstruction', though preferred, is also inaccurate as some parts of the major bile ducts lie within the liver.

PATHOPHYSIOLOGY OF OBSTRUCTIVE JAUNDICE

Obstruction of bile flow or cholestasis (*chole*: bile, *stasis*: lack of flow) increases biliary pressure leading to dilatation of the biliary tree. Bile regurgitates into the circulation by passage across the hepatocytes, through increased paracellular flow and via the lymphatics.

The hepatocytes show features of injury and damage; the albumin levels in the serum fall even in the absence of sepsis, indicating reduced hepatocellular synthetic functions. The prothrombin time is prolonged due to deficient absorption of vitamin K and reduced synthesis of prothrombin; however, this can be rapidly corrected by parenteral administration of the vitamin.

The clinically apparent systemic effects are jaundice and itching, and complications include renal failure, sepsis, cardiovascular changes, delayed wound healing and GI bleeding. While the cause of these complications is probably multifactorial, the four key suspects are bilirubin, bile acids, lipids and endotoxins.[1]

Bilirubin can be toxic to the tissues, as seen in kernicterus, wherein the brain cells of infants undergo permanent damage due to hyperbilirubinaemia. Bile acids are detergents and, in excess, may damage lipid membranes. The elevated blood lipids seen in obstructive jaundice have been shown to alter the composition and function of the cell membrane. Also, systemic endotoxaemia, often detected in these patients, produces deleterious effects on the renal vasculature and systemic coagulation cascade.[2]

Patients with obstructive jaundice are predisposed to prerenal renal failure and hypotension, in which several mechanisms seem to play a role. The peripheral vascular resistance is decreased and the response of blood vessels to vasoconstrictors impaired. Further, bradycardia, prolonged PR and QT intervals, along with ultrastructural and functional myocardial involvement, make these patients vulnerable to cardiovascular instability.

Obstructive jaundice predisposes to renal impairment in several ways. Coupled with systemic vasodilatation and impaired cardiac function, vasoconstriction and underperfusion within the kidneys lead to marked renal ischaemia. High concentrations of conjugated bilirubin, bile acids and endotoxins activate pathways that cause these changes. Renal tubular dysfunction is frequent and often worsens with the use of aminoglycosides and sepsis.[3-5]

Due to mechanisms similar to those which reduce local blood flow, gastric mucosal ischaemia and bleeding from erosions is commonly encountered in these patients. Wound healing is impaired, perhaps due to a combination of poor nutrition and the systemic effects of jaundice. With weakness and debility, resistance to infection is poor. In patients with long-standing obstruction, deficiencies of fat-soluble vitamins (A, D, K) begin to manifest as night blindness, osteomalacia and bleeding diatheses.[6] Itching is one of the most vexing symptoms; its mechanism is not clear but increased bile acids or opiate antagonists are suspected to play an aetiological role.

CAUSES

The commonest causes of large bile duct obstruction can be grouped as occurring:[8,9]

1. within the lumen of the duct (usually benign). These can be
   - bile duct stones;
   - primary sclerosing cholangitis;
   - biliary ascariasis (roundworm in the bile duct); and
   - obstruction due to hydatid daughter cysts
2. in the duct or from adjacent structures. These can be
   - benign biliary strictures which are further grouped into
     —post cholecystectomy (upper bile duct)
     —due to chronic pancreatitis (mid or lower)
     —post liver transplant;
   - malignant bile duct obstruction, which may be at the upper or lower part of the bile duct
     (i) upper bile duct
         —gallbladder cancer
         —cholangiocarcinoma
         —compression due to the portal lymph nodes
     (ii) lower bile duct
         —cancer of the head of the pancreas
         —periampullary cancer.

HISTORY AND EXAMINATION

Features in the history and examination of patients may suggest a specific cause and line of management.

Fever, often with chills and rigors, suggests cholangitis, which is usually associated with biliary stones. It is uncommon in malignant obstruction except in patients with periampullary tumours or after biliary interventions. Severe episodic pain is common in patients with stone disease and rare in patients with benign or malignant strictures.

Pain occurs late in malignant obstruction, and is usually boring and continuous. Itching can occur with any cause of biliary obstruction, but is commonly observed in malignant obstruction and intrahepatic cholestasis, and infrequently in the fluctuating obstruction seen with stone disease. Loss of more than 10% of the body-weight over 6 months suggests a malignant cause of obstruction, as does a history of a previous malignancy such as colonic cancer. Painless jaundice coming on soon after a recent cholecystectomy arouses suspicion of bile duct injury, while its appearance with sudden, severe pain in a patient with a history of cholecystectomy suggests retained bile duct stones. A history of inflammatory bowel disease should raise the possibility of primary sclerosing cholangitis as the cause of jaundice or itching.

Jaundice, scratch marks and loss of body mass on examination are clearly non-specific. Signs of chronic liver disease (spider naevi, palmar erythema, oedema) and splenomegaly denote long-standing intrahepatic cholestasis and progression to liver cirrhosis rather than recent, large bile duct obstruction. Lymph node enlargement, especially in the left supraclavicular region, may indicate an intra-abdominal malignancy.

The liver is usually enlarged and palpable in patients with a bile duct obstruction. The presence of nodules indicates a tumour. The presence of a palpable cystic gallbladder under the lower margin of the right lobe of the liver is a very valuable sign, and suggests that the obstruction is unlikely to be due to stones (Courvoisier law), as the gallbladder is usually fibrosed and shrunken in such patients, but is due to the malignant obstruction of the lower end of the bile duct from a pancreatic or periampullary tumour.[1,7]

LABORATORY INVESTIGATIONS

A full blood count and estimation of serum electrolytes, serum creatinine, PT, and LFT should be done. There may be leucocytosis in cholangitis and marked anaemia due to chronic blood loss in periampullary tumours. The PT may be prolonged due to malabsorption of vitamin K; this is usually easily corrected by giving daily injections of 10 mg of the vitamin for 3 days. Liver tests characteristically show raised bilirubin (total and conjugated), ALP and GGT level, with little or no rise in the levels of aminotransferases. Overall, the LFT are not specific to any diagnosis, but are used in combination with the clinical history and examination to choose the next step in the diagnostic work-up. Imaging is usually the next and often definitive step in arriving at a diagnosis.[1,7]

IMAGING

Non-invasive imaging with a transabdominal ultrasound examination is usually the first test, and is used to see whether the bile ducts are dilated, and thus differentiate between 'surgical' and 'medical' jaundice. It is usually possible to also detect the site of block, such as the upper or lower end of the bile duct, and to detect the cause of obstruction, such as a stone or tumour. Further detailed evaluation with a contrast-enhanced CT scan (for suspected tumours, especially at the lower end) or MRCP (for upper biliary lesions) may be necessary in some patients.

At present, invasive imaging with ERCP or PTC is rarely required for making a diagnosis; it is usually undertaken at the time of planning for biliary drainage after ascertaining the cause and site of obstruction.

MANAGEMENT

General measures

Patients with obstructive jaundice must be kept well hydrated because of the increased susceptibility to acute renal failure (tubular necrosis). Other co-factors that could contribute to renal failure, such as aminoglycosides or other nephrotoxic drugs and sepsis (endotoxaemia), should be avoided or managed adequately. Itching can be a vexing problem. Although antihistamines are often prescribed, they are of little value. Ursodeoxycholic acid (10–15 mg/kg/day) in divided doses has been shown to help if given for long periods. The bile acid binding resin, cholestyramine (4 g, 6 or 8 hourly), rifampicin and opiate antagonists are sometimes useful. Vitamin K injections (10 mg/day for 3 days) should be given to correct hypoprothrombinaemia due to malabsorption of the vitamin.[1]

Specific measures

Bile duct stones

At present, most bile duct stones are removed endoscopically. In patients with cholelithiasis, if bile duct stones are detected or suspected, ERCP and stone removal prior to cholecystectomy is the preferred option. Cholecystectomy, usually laparoscopic, due to its minimally invasive nature, allows the patient a short hospital stay, minimal morbidity and early return to work. In post-cholecystectomy patients with common bile duct stones, ERCP and endoscopic stone extraction is the clear choice; most stones (80%) can be removed easily after an adequate endoscopic papillotomy, either with the use of a Dormia wire basket or with a balloon extractor. In a small proportion (10%–20%), large stones may need to be crushed with a mechanical lithotripter before extraction. With modern equipment and techniques, only a small number of patients need to undergo surgery for bile duct stones with the attendant morbidity of an abdominal incision and T-tube, as well as a long hospital stay.[10]

Biliary strictures

A quarter of biliary strictures are benign. Others are caused by an underlying malignancy. While the prevention of secondary biliary cirrhosis and consequent liver failure would be the goal of therapy in a young patient with a benign biliary stricture, relief of pruritus and cholangitis might be the aim of treatment in an elderly patient with advanced, unresectable malignancy of the pancreas. Therapy, therefore, needs to be individualized; endoscopic (through therapeutic ERCP) or percutaneous biliary drainage by the placement of a stent or catheter is an extremely effective method of decompressing the obstructed biliary tree and achieving adequate drainage of bile with relief of jaundice and pruritus. In unresectable obstructing cancers, this may be the only therapy required.[8,9]

CONCLUSION

Obstruction of the major bile ducts remains a common clinical problem. Recent advances in technology have revolutionized the diagnosis and management of this condition, with only a small proportion of patients requiring surgical management. The term 'surgical obstructive jaundice' is, however, still popular and likely to remain in use to denote a major bile duct obstruction. Timely treatment of this condition is effective and life-saving.

REFERENCES

1. Dooley JS. Extrahepatic biliary obstruction: Systemic effects, diagnosis and management. In: Bircher J, Benhamou JP, McIntyre N, Rizzetto M, Rodes J (eds). *Oxford textbook of clinical hepatology. Vol. 2.* 2nd ed. New York: Oxford Univesity Press; 1999:1581–90.
2. Harry DS, McIntyre N. Plasma lipoproteins and the liver. In: Millward-Sadler GH, Wright R, Arthur MJP (eds). *Liver and biliary disease.* 3rd ed. London: WB Saunders; 1992:61–78.
3. Green J, Better OS. Systemic hypotension and renal failure in obstructive jaundice— mechanistic and therapeutic aspects. *Am Soc Nephrol* 1995;**5**:1853–71.
4. Bomzon A, Jacob G, Better OS. Jaundice in the kidney. In: Epstein M (ed). *The kidney in liver disease.* Baltimore: Hanley & Belfus; 1996:423–46.
5. Fogarty BJ, Parks RW, Rowlands BJ, Diamond T. Renal dysfuncton in obstructive jaundice. *Br J Surg* 1995;**82**:877–84.
6. Hay JE. Bone disease in cholestatic liver disease. *Gastroenterology* 1995;**108**:276–83.
7. Kimmings AN, van Deventer SJH, Obertop H, Rauws EAJ, Gouma DJ. Inflammatory and immunologic effects of obstructive jaundice: Pathogenesis and treatment. *J Am Coll Surg* 1995;**181**:576–81.
8. Meenan J, Raus E, Huibregtse K. Endoscopic management of postoperative bile duct injury, benign strictures, and sclerosing cholangitis. In: Jacobson IM (ed). *ERCP and its applications.* Philadelphia: Lippincott-Raven; 1998:125–32.
9. Kochhar R. Benign biliary strictures. In: Goenka MK, Das K (eds). *Therapeutic endoscopy;* 1999:87–99.
10. Manoukian AV, Schmalz MJ, Geenan GE, *et al.* Endoscopic treatment of problems encountered after cholecystectomy. *Gastrointest Endosc* 1993;**39**:9–14.

CHAPTER 20

Liver failure

S.K. ACHARYA

Liver failure is usually a consequence of liver injury that causes a substantial loss in the mass of functional hepatocytes and indicates a life-threatening situation. The natural course of patients with liver failure is diverse, and depends on the severity of the underlying liver disease, type of liver injury (acute or chronic) and rapidity of onset of liver failure. This chapter discusses liver failure as a clinical problem.

DEFINITION AND CLASSIFICATION

Conceptually, the term 'liver failure' is used when 'liver dysfunction occurs subsequent to an acute or chronic liver injury resulting in metabolic and haemodynamic alteration, which threatens life'.[1] In a clinical setting of liver injury, which usually manifests as jaundice or persistent and prolonged fatigue, if encephalopathy, coagulopathy or ascites appear, then the patient is considered to have developed liver failure. Depending on the duration of liver injury and the rapidity with which liver failure ensues, it has been categorized into three distinct types:[2] (i) acute hepatic failure (AHF); (ii) subacute hepatic failure (SHF); and (iii) liver failure due to chronic liver disease (CLD).

In 1969, Trey and Davidson defined AHF as the occurrence of encephalopathy within 8 weeks of the onset of acute hepatitic illness in an individual without any pre-existing liver disease.[3] However, during subsequent years, this definition was not adequate to describe patients with AHF seen in both western and eastern populations. In the UK,[4] Japan[5,6] and France,[7] it was observed that patients with AHF presenting within 7–10 days of the onset of jaundice had significantly higher survival rates than similar patients presenting with encephalopathy after 7–10 days of the onset of jaundice. This observation influenced the selection of patients with AHF for liver transplantation.[8,9]

In contrast to these observations, all the patients in an Indian study presented with encephalopathy within 3 weeks of the onset of jaundice and 4 weeks of the onset of other symptoms.[10] In this series, the rapidity of onset of encephalopathy did not influence survival. At the All India Institute of Medical Sciences (AIIMS), we observed that liver failure occurring more than 4 weeks after the onset of an acute hepatic illness manifests with progressive ascites; encephalopathy is an extremely rare presenting feature at this stage. We identify such cases as having SHF because they are different from AHF, and the majority of patients do not survive beyond 6 months; thus, they cannot be described as having liver failure due to CLD. Similar patients have been described from the West as having late-onset hepatic failure (LOHF) with protracted viral hepatitis and impaired regeneration or subacute hepatic necrosis.[11–13]

To resolve the geographical differences among the issues of definition, nomenclature and subclassification, the International Association for the Study of the Liver (IASL) formed a subcommittee in 1996 which, after careful analysis, has recommended a new set of definitions and subclassifications of AHF and SHF (Table I).[14]

AHF and SHF usually occur subsequent to acute hepatitis or due to acute liver injury over a pre-existing silent chronic liver injury (acute-on-chronic). It is well known that often patients infected with chronic HCV/HBV present with AHF or SHF subsequent to superimposed viral hepatitis (HAV, HEV) or acute liver injury due to drugs such as antitubercular agents.[8,15] Wilson disease and autoimmune hepatitis may also present with AHF or SHF as their initial clinical manifestation.[8,15]

On the other hand, CLD usually denotes continuous or intermittent ongoing liver injury occurring beyond 6 months from the onset of initial hepatic insult.[15] Liver failure appearing in such patients due to the primary process of liver damage is usually recognized as 'liver failure due to CLD'.

Table I. Recommendations of the International Association for the Study of the Liver (IASL) Subcommittee for the definition and classification of acute and subacute hepatic failure

Nomenclature	Acute hepatic failure (AHF) (synonyms such as fulminant hepatitis, fulminant hepatic failure and acute yellow atrophy should not be used)
	Subacute hepatic failure (SHF) (synonyms such as subfulminant hepatitis, subacute hepatic failure and late-onset hepatic failure should not be used)
Diagnostic criteria of liver failure	AHF: encephalopathy SHF: encephalopathy and/or progressive ascites
Maximum interval between the onset of icterus and features of liver failure	AHF: ≤4 weeks SHF: >4 weeks to 24 weeks
Subclassification	(i) aetiological: indicates the specific cause of AHF (ii) temporal: indicates the rapidity of encephalopathy Hyperacute—encephalopathy within 10 days of icterus Fulminant—encephalopathy between 10 and 30 days of the onset of jaundice (iii) not otherwise specified
	Example (AHF, hyperacute — A)

Table II. Causes of liver failure

Causes	Acute hepatic failure	Subacute hepatic failure	Chronic liver failure
Viruses	HEV, HBV, HAV	HBV, HEV Mixed viral infection Viral superinfection	HBV, HCV, HDV
Toxins and drugs	Antitubercular drugs Mushroom poisoning Paracetamol NSAIDs Anticonvulsants	Antitubercular drugs	Chloropromazine Dilantin Tineleic acid Arsenic Alcohol
Others	Acute fatty liver of pregnancy Hepatic venous outflow obstruction Amoebic liver abscess Metastatic liver disease Wilson disease Autoimmune hepatitis Ischaemic hepatitis	Wilson disease Autoimmune hepatitis	Biliary cirrhosis α_1-antitrypsin deficiency Wilson disease Autoimmune hepatitis

MAGNITUDE AND AETIOLOGY

Globally, hepatitis viruses are the most common causes of AHF and SHF, whereas the causes of CLD differ from region to region. While alcohol-induced liver injury, autoimmune liver diseases such as primary biliary cirrhosis, primary sclerosing cholangitis, autoimmune hepatitis; and metabolic liver diseases such as Wilson disease are more prevalent causes in the West, HBV and HCV are more frequent aetiologies of CLD in the East.[16] Depending upon the prevalence and endemicity of these aetiologies, the magnitude and causes of liver failure may vary geographically. Unfortunately, prospective data on the exact magnitude of liver failure are scarce. Table II depicts the common causes of liver injury leading to liver failure. In India, approximately 250 000 people die annually due to liver failure.

About one-third of all inpatients at AIIMS over a period of 7 years were admitted because of liver failure, who constituted three-fourths of all patients with liver diseases hospitalized during this period. Among the 1600 patients with liver failure, 1020 (64%) were due to CLD, whereas 580 (36%) due to AHF and SHF (Fig. 1). During 1990–96, out of 5354 inpatients admitted, 1071 (20%) died; among those who died during hospitalization, 793/1071 (74%) were due to liver failure. Thus, in a tertiary care referral centre, three-fourths of the inpatient deaths in the Gastroenterology Unit were due to liver failure (Fig. 2).

DIAGNOSIS

Liver failure is a clinical entity. As mentioned earlier, patients with liver failure usually present with encephalopathy, coagulopathy and ascites. These three protean manifestations may be present either in isolation or in combination. The type of liver failure is categorized based on the rapidity of its onset after recognizable hepatic injury is seen. For example, if features of liver failure occur within a few weeks of the onset of acute hepatitis, it is categorized as AHF. In

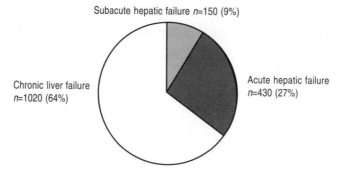

Fig. 1. Magnitude of each type of liver failure reported in patients admitted to the All India Institute of Medical Sciences during 1990–96

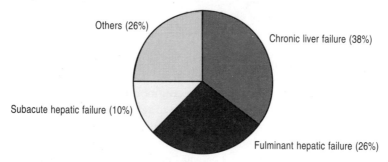

Fig. 2. Proportion of various types of liver failure (LF) present in patients who died due to LF at the All India Institute of Medical Sciences during 1990–96
Total patients n=5354; total deaths n=1071 (20%); deaths due to LF n=793 (74%)

contrast, when patients with known chronic hepatitis or compensated cirrhosis develop ascites or encephalopathy, they are categorized as having liver failure due to CLD.

The categorization of liver failure in a clinical situation is important because the natural course and cause of death due to each type of liver failure is different. For example, events are quick and stormy in patients with AHF. About 75% of deaths occur within 72 hours of the onset of AHF.[10] Therefore, in such patients, management is aggressive and early intervention is needed. In contrast, the median time between the onset and death among patients with SHF is about 4 months; thus, there is ample time for therapeutic manipulation.[1,2] Liver failure due to CLD may be protracted, repetitive and get precipitated by various factors such as variceal bleeding, sepsis, dyselectrolytaemia, constipation and superimposed hepatic injury due to viruses or drugs; among patients with chronic liver failure, removal or correction of the precipitating causes is important in managing them. Table III highlights the essential differences in the clinical, biochemical and natural course of the three types of liver failure.

Certain conditions may mimic liver failure, e.g. cerebral malaria and jaundice (due to intravascular haemolysis or hepatic involvement) may mimic AHF; septicaemia may cause hyperbilirubinaemia leading to an altered sensorium.

Table III. Essential differences between acute, subacute and chronic liver failure

Criteria	Acute hepatic failure	Subacute hepatic failure	Chronic liver failure
Onset after hepatitis*	4 weeks	>4 weeks to <24 weeks	>24 weeks
Dominant manifestation	Encephalopathy Jaundice Shrunken liver	Jaundice Ascites	Ascites/encephalopathy
Liver function tests	ALT ↑↑↑ Serum albumin normal	ALT ↑ Serum albumin ↓ normal	ALT ↑ /normal Serum albumin ↓
Prothombin time	Marked prolongation	Moderate prolongation	Mild prolongation
Complications	Cerebral oedema (70%) Sepsis	Sepsis Hepatorenal syndrome	Sepsis Bleed, renal failure
Cause of death	Cerebral oedema	Hepatorenal syndrome	Hepatorenal syndrome Sepsis Encephalopathy
Survivors	No chronicity	40% chronicity	Recurrence of encephalopathy

*Duration between the onset of liver disease and liver failure

Table IV. Differential diagnosis of acute and chronic liver failure

Acute hepatic failure	Chronic liver failure
• *Plasmodium falciparum* infection	• Cirrhosis with peritoneal tuberculosis
• Liver abscess with metastatic cerebral abscess	• Malignant surgical obstruction with metastatic peritoneal disease
• Septicaemia	• Uraemic encephalopathy with compensated chronic liver disease
• Enteric fever with encephalopathy and hepatitis	• Diabetic coma in a patient with cirrhosis
• Leptospirosis	

Ascites may occur in a patient with malignant surgical obstructive jaundice due to metastatic peritoneal disease. Cirrhosis with superadded tubercular peritonitis, or uraemic encephalopathy may mimic liver failure due to CLD. Table IV details the diffential diagnosis of liver failure.

COMPLICATIONS

Major complications include sepsis, cerebral oedema, renal failure and coagulopathy resulting in bleeding from various sites; these can lead to death.[1,2,5–8] Sepsis and cerebral oedema are the major complications reported as the predominant causes of death in more than two-thirds of patients with AHF,[1,2,10] whereas renal failure and sepsis are the major killers among patients with SHF.[2] Common complications among patients with CLD who develop liver failure include the hepatorenal syndrome (HRS), sepsis and variceal bleeding. Hypoglycaemia and dyselectrolytaemia may accompany any form of liver failure.[16]

Each of these complications may be fatal. Usually, patients with liver failure have encephalopathy. In such unconscious patients, none of the above complications has recognizable clinical parameters; therefore, close monitoring of these patients is necessary for the detection and management of such complications at the earliest. For example, patients with liver failure may develop sepsis without an overt manifestation of infection such as fever and leucocytosis.[2] On the other hand, infection in a patient with liver failure may manifest with the onset of HRS, haemodynamic instability, and deterioration of liver functions and coagulopathy status. At our institute, daily culture of the various body fluids forms an integral part of the protocol of management for liver failure. The causes of sepsis in patients with liver failure are multifactorial.[12] The liver produces opsonizing proteins such as fibronectin and vitronectin, which are necessary for the functioning of neutrophils and macrophages. Complement production is compromised in patients with advanced liver damage. The liver is the largest reticuloendothelial (scavenging function) organ in the body whose functions get compromised with the loss of liver volume. In a recent study, we reported that more than half of our patients with AHF had developed sepsis, and a quarter of them had systemic fungal infection.[2] About 20% of patients with cirrhosis admitted to AIIMS had spontaneous bacterial peritonitis.[17] Although GI bleeding and renal failure are rare among patients with AHF,[10] they are more frequent among patients with SHF and liver failure due to CLD.[17] In a recent study, we demonstrated that the pathophysiology of renal failure among patients with SHF was similar to that of HRS documented among patients with cirrhosis.[17]

MANAGEMENT

Patients with liver failure should be admitted to the ICU. The use of these specialized treatment centres is probably responsible for the modest improvement in survival of patients with liver failure receiving only medical therapy. Unfortunately, in India, the treatment of patients with liver failure in the ICU is not as good as of those with acute coronary insufficiency. Patients with liver failure, as mentioned earlier, may suffer from cerebral oedema, and hence need ventilatory support, which helps in preventing sudden respiratory arrest, provides an adequate oxygen supply, may assist in reducing cerebral oedema and prevents aspiration into the pulmonary cavity. Patients with liver failure may develop a hyperdynamic circulatory state and decreased systemic vascular resistance, and hence need haemodynamic monitoring—a crucial determinant of the cerebral perfusion pressure and cerebral blood supply.

The monitoring of blood glucose, electrolytes, acid–base imbalance and coagulopathy needs awareness, organization and facilities to correct these, which is best done in an ICU. Sepsis is a preventable cause of death and is probably better managed in an ICU set-up rather than a general ward. Essentially, the treatment of patients with liver failure by medical therapy means buying time for the liver inflammation to subside and liver cells to regenerate. Hence, it is extremely important to prevent metabolic disturbances that can cause death.

The treatment strategy for liver failure can be categorized into: (i) general supportive therapy; (ii) management of complications; and (iii) specific therapy.

Table V. Supportive therapy for patients with liver failure

Type of intervention	Purpose of intervention	Monitoring strategy
Artificial ventilation in grade III or IV encephalopathy	To prevent respiratory and CVS complications due to cerebral oedema	Estimate blood gases at least twice daily
Sterilization of the gut using an injectable such as ampicillin (4 g/day) or metronidazole (1.5–2 g/day) and neomycin (4–6 g/day)	To reduce the ammonia load	Estimate blood ammonia levels once in 1–3 days
Electrolyte replacement	To correct electrolyte deficiencies	Daily administration of electrolytes
Fluid/calorie intake	Hydration, nutrition	Maintenance of central venous pressure (between 8 and 10 cm of saline)
Detection of sepsis	Early institution of antibiotics	Barrier nursing Daily monitoring of blood and all other fluid cultures for bacteria and fungi, temperature and total leucocycte count
H_2-receptor blockers or sucralfate	To prevent stress-induced erosive mucosal disease	Intermittent nasogastric aspiration
Assessment of consciousness level, cerebral oedema, urinary output, chest condition, haemodynamics	To take early and appropriate action	Standard methods

General supportive therapy

Table V provides an outline of the essential constituents of supportive therapy.

Management of complications

Cerebral oedema

Cerebral oedema accompanies an advanced grade of encephalopathy. Overt cerebral oedema should be diagnosed if spontaneous decerebrate posturing or any two of the following four parameters are present:[10]

1. hypertension (supine blood pressure >150/90 mmHg);
2. bradycardia (pulse <10 beats/min from the expected pulse rate for the given body temperature);
3. pupillary changes; and
4. presence of central neurogenic hyperventilation in the absence of any metabolic or respiratory cause of hyperventilation.

In advanced centres, monitoring of the intracranial pressure (ICP) using extradural pressure devices is done if a raised ICP is suspected. It is recommended that the ICP be kept below 25 mmHg.[18] It is probably more important to keep the cerebral perfusion pressure (mean arterial pressure – ICP) above 50 mmHg. However, in the absence of ICP monitoring, when patients with liver failure develop grade IV encephalopathy or have overt features of cerebral oedema, mannitol at a dose of 0.5–1 g/kg body-weight is used, which can be repeated hourly as long as the renal functions are maintained.[10,18] If plasma osmolality is <310 mosm, mannitol cannot be repeated frequently. Other methods to reduce the ICP, such as hyperventilation, ultrafiltration using continuous venovenous haemodialysis (CVVH) or continuous arteriovenous haemodialysis (CAVH), steroids or diuretics, are not very effective. Intravenous thiopentone sodium at a dose of 5 mg/kg followed by an intravenous infusion rate of 1–3 mg/kg/hour has been used.[10,18,19] However, thiopentone causes hypotension, and monitoring of the intra-arterial pressure is mandatory if the drug is used.

Sepsis

As mentioned earlier, patients with liver failure may not manifest with fever or leucocytosis following bacterial or fungal infection. Therefore, daily monitoring of the blood and urine, and throat swab culture should be done to detect the presence of sepsis. Early detection of sepsis and specific antimicrobial therapy may help in improving the survival status of such patients. In patients with cirrhosis and SHF, examination of the ascitic fluid during initial hospitalization may detect the presence of spontaneous bacterial peritonitis. Urinary, pulmonary and other infections are not infrequent in such patients.

Coagulopathy

Prothrombin time, platelet count, APTT and fibrinogen degradation products should be monitored in such patients at regular intervals. However, correction of a prolonged PT by the routine use of fresh frozen plasma (FFP) is not recommended, as it has not been shown to decrease mortality; rather, it may lead to hypernatraemia, fluid overload and an increase in the ICP. Platelets and FFP should be used only when active haemorrhage occurs or if an invasive procedure is performed in a patient with liver failure.

Metabolic abnormalities

Close monitoring of the blood glucose (1–2 hourly using a bedside glucometer) to detect hypoglycaemia may be life-saving in these patients. Similarly, frequent monitoring of the acid–base balance and electrolytes is necessary for their correction. If necessary, haemodialysis may be used to correct severe metabolic acidosis and hyperkalaemia, particularly in the presence of renal failure.

Other complications

Pulmonary toilet is of utmost importance in patients with liver failure, particularly if the ICP is raised. Physiotherapy, bronchial suction, bronchoscopy and changing the patient's position may increase the ICP. Therefore, it is better to intubate all patients with higher than grade III encephalopathy.

A low urine output invariably responds to low-dose, continuous dopamine infusion (2–5 µg/kg/min), while maintaining the CVP at 10 cm of saline.

Specific therapy

Various therapies have been tried in patients with AHF to improve liver function or reduce hepatocyte necrosis. These include corticosteroids, prostaglandin E, insulin–glucagon infusion, N-acetylcysteine. None of these agents have been found to improve survival among patients infected with hepatotropic viruses causing AHF. N-acetylcysteine is the drug of choice in paracetamol-induced AHF,[18,20] the dose being 150 mg/kg IV over 15 min, followed by 50 mg/kg over 4 hours and then 100 mg/kg over 16 hours. British workers claim that N-acetylcysteine improves oxygen supply in patients with non-paracetamol-induced AHF.[18] The most specific therapy in AHF is liver transplantation and, in future, it will possibly include artificial liver support (ALS).

Liver transplantation

Patients who deteriorate despite intensive medical therapy or those with poor prognostic indicators should be considered for early referral to a transplant centre, if available. The survival rate following liver transplantation varies from 55% to 90%.[18,21] The procedure is relatively safe even in the presence of coagulopathy because coagulopathy gets corrected quickly when the new liver is grafted. Despite a lack of randomized controlled trials on orthotopic liver transplantation (OLT) in liver failure, liver transplantation is an established and probably the most effective form of therapy available to salvage these patients.

Artificial liver support[22]

As survivors of AHF are known to have few long-term sequlae, ALS has generated much interest and research in the hope that these patients might be maintained until spontaneous hepatic recovery can occur.[22] ALS may also be used to support rapidly deteriorating patients with other forms of liver failure awaiting liver transplantation. The initial approach to provide ALS using haemodialysis, extracorporeal liver perfusion, charcoal haemoperfusion and exchange transfusion did not succeed in improving survival. More recent attempts at developing ALS have focused on the use of a filter system containing isolated cultured hepatocytes in an extracorporeal liver-assisting device. Early experience with this technique is not very encouraging. In addition to possibly replacing the lost synthetic function of hepatocytes, these devices may result in clinical improvement through the removal of circulating toxins or inhibitors of hepatocyte regeneration. However, these artificial extracorporeal liver-assisting devices using hepatocytes have not been shown to improve survival or increase time to transplantation, and have therefore become unpopular.

Molecular adsorbents recirculating system

The extracorporeal liver support system—molecular adsorbents recirculating system (MARS) (Teraklin AG, Rostock, Germany)—is based on the principle of albumin dialysis (Fig. 3). Using a hollow-fibre dialysis module, the patient's blood is dialysed across an albumin-impregnated polysulphone membrane with a pore size of 50 kD, while at the same time maintaining a constant flow of albumin-rich (20%) dialysate in the extracapillary compartment.[23] The premise is that the albumin molecule has free binding sites, which compete with the toxins bound to proteins in the perfused blood. The toxins get detached from the plasma albumin and then attach to the binding sites of the albumin impregnated on the membrane. The dialysate is perfused through columns containing activated charcoal and anion exchange resin, where most of the albumin-absorbed toxins are given up, and albumin is thereby regenerated. Water-soluble substances are removed by perfusion through an additional haemofilter/haemodialysis column. Molecules larger than 50 kD (essential hormones bound to carrier proteins, growth factors, albumin) are not removed.[24] It is perfectly conceivable that the system would be equally efficacious utilizing single-pass albumin dialysis at a fast enough flow rate, without any of the other filters, but would probably require a considerable quantity of albumin. Closing the circuit using charcoal and ion-exchange filters is an innovation that makes the technique more practical and economical, without compromising the efficacy.[25]

The MARS system was first described 10 years ago, but has been evaluated only in the past 3–4 years and tried in several centres in Europe and, more recently, the US. Most of the preliminary data are encouraging, and these have been supported by the positive findings from the two controlled trials completed so far[26,27] as well as data from the International MARS Registry.[28] Although data from the Registry suggest that patients with a worse prognosis (as defined by a

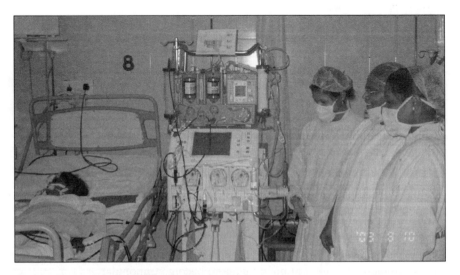

Fig. 3. Molecular adsorbents recirculating system (MARS)

higher Mayo end-stage liver disease score) are more likely to benefit from MARS treatment, this benefit is seen more among patients suffering from acute decompensation with cholestasis, with no (or minimal) end-organ failure, as evidenced from the studies by Stange *et al.*[29] and Heemann *et al.*[27] Patients with full-fledged acute-on-chronic liver failure may benefit as well, especially if there is an element of reversibility, as seen in a study of patients with alcoholic hepatitis.[30]

However, the most important lacuna that exists in the literature pertaining to MARS therapy is the lack of large, multicentre, randomized controlled trials. These are essential to provide the necessary evidence on the basis of which the widespread use of MARS in a clinical setting, as opposed to a research environment, can be recommended. At present, two such trials are in progress, one of which is investigating the role of MARS in hepatic encephalopathy (HE) in the US, while the other (MARS-Relief) is evaluating its impact on the survival of patients with acute-on-chronic liver failure with associated end-organ dysfunction (≥grade 2 HE and/or HRS). Hopefully, these studies will provide conclusive data on the use of MARS in liver failure.

CONCLUSION

Liver failure indicates severe liver dysfunction that threatens life. Identification of the type of liver failure and aggressive management in an ICU is the mainstay of therapy. MARS therapy may be the form of dialysis for liver failure that the clinician awaits for its wide availability, refined technique and affordability. Till date, liver transplantation seems to hold the best possible therapeutic outcome.

REFERENCES

1. Acharya SK. Liver failure—recent advances in pathophysiology and management. *J Anaesth Clin Pharmacol* 1993;**9**:179–82.
2. Acharya SK, Panda SK, Saxena A, Datta Gupta S. Acute liver failure in India: A perspective from the East. *J Gastroenterol Hepatol* 2000;**15**:473–9.
3. Trey C, Davidson C. The management of fulminant hepatic failure. In: Popper H, Schaffner F (eds). *Progress in liver disease. Vol. 3.* New York: Grune and Stratton; 1970:282–98.
4. O'Grady JG, Schalm SW, Williams R. Acute liver failure: Redefining the syndromes. *Lancet* 1993;**343**:273–5.
5. Takahashi Y, Shimuzu M. Aetiology and prognosis of fulminant viral hepatitis in Japan: A multicentric study. *J Gastroenterol Hepatol* 1991;**6**:159–64.
6. Muto Y. Present status of fulminant hepatitis in Japan (1989–1991). *Gastroenterol Jpn* 1993;**28** (Suppl):120–7.
7. Bernau J, Rueff B, Benhamaou JP. Fulminant and sub-fulminant liver failure: Definition and causes. *Semin Liver Dis* 1986;**6**:97–106.
8. Pelman RR, Gavaler JS, Vathiel DH, *et al.* Orthotopic liver transplantation for acute and subacute hepatic failure in adults. *Hepatology* 1997;**7**:484–9.
9. O'Grady JG, Alexander GJ, Thick M, Potter D, Calne RV, Williams R. Outcome of orthotopic liver transplantation in the aetiological and clinical variants of acute liver failure. *Q J Med* 1988;**69**:817–24.

10. Acharya SK, Dasarathy S, Longkumer T, et al. Fulminant hepatitis in a tropical population: Clinical course, cause, and early predictor of outcome. *Hepatology* 1996;**23**:1448–55.
11. Gimson AE, O'Grady J, Ede RJ, Portmann B, William R. Late onset hepatic failure: Clinical, serological and histological features. *Hepatology* 1986;**6**:288–94.
12. Boyer JL, Klatskin G. Patterns of necrosis in acute viral hepatitis: Prognostic value of bridging (subacute hepatic necrosis). *N Engl J Med* 1970;**283**:1063–71.
13. Peter RL, Omata M, Aschavai M, Liew CT. Protracted viral hepatitis with impaired regeneration. In: Vyas GN, Cohen SN, Schmid R (eds). *Viral hepatitis*. Philadelphia: Franklin Institute Press; 1978:79–84.
14. Tandon BN, Bernauau J, O'Grady J, et al. Recommendation of the International Association for the Study of the Liver Subcommittee on nomenclature of acute and subacute liver failure. *J Gastroenterol Hepatol* 1999;**14**:403–4.
15. Shawcross D, Deutz NEP, Olde Damink, Jalan R. Hepatic encephalopathy in liver failure. In: Arroyo V, Forns Z, Gracia-Pagan JC, Rhodes J (eds). *Progress in the treatment of liver disease*. Barcelona, Spain: Ars Medical; 2003:55–9.
16. Terracult NA. Hepatitis B virus and liver transplantation. *Clin Liver Dis* 1999;**3**:389–414.
17. Bal CS, Longkumer T, Dasarathy S, Panda SK, Datta Gupta S. Renal functions and structure in patients with subacute hepatic failure. *J Gastroenterol Hepatol* 2000;**15**:1318–24.
18. Riegler JL, Lake JR. Fulminant hepatic failure. *Med Clin North Am* 1993;**77**:1057–83.
19. Keys R, Grame J, Alexander M, Williams R. *Intracranial pressure monitoring and cerebral blood flow measurements in fulminant hepatic failure*. UK: SK & F Publication; 1991:46–7.
20. Trey C, Davidson C. The management of fulminant hepatic failure. In: Popper HH, Schaffner F (eds). *Progress in liver disease. Vol. 3.* New York: Grune and Stratton; 1970: 283–98.
21. Peleman RR, Gavaler JS, Van Thiel DH, et al. Orthotopic liver transplantation for acute and subacute hepatic failure in adults. *Hepatology* 1987;**7**:484–9.
22. Anand AC. Bioartifical liver support. *Trop Gastroenterol* 1996;**17**:202–12.
23. Stange J, Ramlow W, Mitzner S, Schmidt R, Klinkmann H. Dialysis against a recycled albumin solution enables the removal of albumin-bound toxins. *Artif Organs* 1993;**17**:809–13.
24. Stange J, Mitzner S. A carrier-mediated transport of toxins in a hybrid membrane. Safety barrier between a patient's blood and a bioartificial liver. *Int J Artif Organs* 1996;**19**:677–91.
25. Peszynski P, Klammt S, Peters E, Mitzner S, Stange J, Schmidt R. Albumin dialysis: Single pass vs recirculation (MARS). *Liver* 2002;**22** (Suppl):40–2.
26. Mitzner SR, Stange J, Klammt S, et al. Improvement of hepatorenal syndrome with extracorporeal albumin dialysis MARS: Results of a prospective, randomized, controlled clinical trial. *Liver Transpl* 2000;**6**:277–86.
27. Heemann U, Treichel U, Loock J, et al. Albumin dialysis in cirrhosis with superimposed acute liver injury: A prospective, controlled study. *Hepatology* 2002;**36**:949–58.
28. Steiner C. International MARS Registry: Analysis of 287 patients from 51 submitting centers. 4th International Symposium on Albumin Dialysis in Liver Disease, Ros-tock-Warnemunde, September 2002.
29. Stange J, Mitzner SR, Klammt S, et al. Liver support by extracorporeal blood purification: A clinical observation. *Liver Transpl* 2000;**6**:603–13.
30. Jalan R, Sen S, Steiner C, Kapoor D, Alisa A, Williams R. Extracorporeal liver support with molecular adsorbents recirculating system in patients with severe acute alcoholic hepatitis. *J Hepatol* 2003;**33**:24–31.

CHAPTER 21

Medical management of jaundice

M.P. SHARMA, K. MADAN

Jaundice can be the result of a variety of abnormalities of liver function and structure, involving different aspects of bilirubin metabolism. In this respect, the excess formation of bilirubin as well as excessive destruction of RBCs result in jaundice. Therefore, jaundice is a symptom that may point towards a number of diagnostic possibilities. The management of jaundice would thus include the management of individual conditions that result in jaundice, since jaundice is only a manifestation of that disease. The management of conditions such as sepsis and haemolytic anaemias is discussed in Chapters 10 and 11, respectively; in this chapter, the discussion will be restricted to the management of common liver conditions that produce jaundice.

CONGENITAL UNCONJUGATED HYPERBILIRUBINAEMIA

The most common condition producing unconjugated hyperbilirubinaemia is Gilbert syndrome, which is present in up to 7% of the general population.[1] In this condition, there is a defect in the conjugation of bilirubin to its glucuronide within the hepatocyte. The only symptom it produces is jaundice. Apart from the fear in the patient's mind of some chronic liver dysfunction, it rarely, if at all, is of any clinical consequence (see p. 12).

Treatment

The mainstay of therapy involves reassuring the patient about the benign nature of the disease and explaining the fact that the jaundice could be brought on by some intermittent illness, fasting and heavy physical exercise.

Various therapeutic options, such as phenobarbitone, glutethimide and tin-protoporphyrin, are available to reduce bilirubin levels but these are rarely, if ever, required[2] since the serum bilirubin level rarely rises above 3 mg/dl.

Crigler–Najjar syndrome

Crigler–Najjar syndrome types I and II are other causes of unconjugated hyperbilirubinaemia, and are more severe but rare defects of bilirubin conjugation (*see* p. 12).

Treatment of Crigler–Najjar syndrome type I

In Crigler–Najjar syndrome type I, there is an almost complete absence of the enzyme bilirubin uridyl glucuronyl transferase (UGT). If this condition is left untreated, death usually occurs within 18 months due to very high levels of unconjugated bilirubin.

The aim of therapy is to reduce the level of unconjugated bilirubin to a level at which it will not damage the basal ganglia (and cause kernicterus). The mainstay of therapy for this condition is exchange transfusion followed by daily sessions of phototherapy.[3] This therapy allows some neonates to grow till puberty.

However, the treatment of choice is liver transplantation, which abrogates the need for regular phototherapy.[4] Transplantation should be performed at an early age because the timing of onset of kernicterus cannot be predicted.

Enzyme inducers such as phenobarbitone have not been found to be useful because even if they are able to induce some amount of the enzyme, it is non-functional. Experimental therapy with tin-protoporphyrin has been found to be effective since it reduces the production of bilirubin by means of competitive inhibition of haem oxygenase.[5]

For the future, we hope that the routine application of gene therapy, which is only experimental at present, will become possible in humans.

Treatment of Crigler–Najjar syndrome type II

Crigler–Najjar syndrome type II is associated with a rise in bilirubin levels to less than 20 mg/dl; there is no risk of kernicterus. Therapy to reduce bilirubin levels is merely desirable but not at all essential for health; the benefit is mainly cosmetic.

Enzyme-inducing drugs such as phenobarbitone, phenytoin, glutethimide and phenazone are equally effective in reducing bilirubin levels. The drug of choice is phenobarbitone in doses of 60–180 mg/day. This results in a gradual reduction in the bilirubin level over 2–3 weeks.[6]

CONGENITAL CONJUGATED HYPERBILIRUBINAEMIA

This condition occurs as a result of two rare congenital defects of bilirubin excretion from the hepatocytes—the Dubin–Johnson and Rotor syndromes.[7,8] In the Dubin–Johnson syndrome, the molecular defect lies in the multidrug resistance-associated protein 2 (MRP2) gene, which is a membrane carrier that transports bilirubin across the hepatocyte canalicular membrane. This is a benign condition not associated with any liver dysfunction and the transaminase levels remain normal. Liver biopsy can be done in suspected cases to confirm the diagnosis; the characteristic finding is intracellular black pigmentation. There is also a diagnostic pattern of urinary coproporphyrin excretion, with more than 80% of the coproporphyrin being type I rather than the normal type III.

The molecular defect in Rotor syndrome has not yet been identified but is similar to that in the Dubin–Johnson syndrome. In Rotor syndrome, the liver does not contain the typical pigmentation and urinary coproporphyrin excretion is increased; however, the pattern is similar to that in other hepatobiliary disorders (*see* p. 13).

Treatment

Management of the Dubin–Johnson syndrome involves ruling out other causes of conjugated hyperbilirubinaemia and confirming the diagnosis of this entity. The bilirubin levels usually remain between 2 mg/dl and 5 mg/dl.

No active treatment is required; women should be reassured and cautioned regarding the exacerbation of jaundice following the use of oral contraceptives or other oestrogen-containing preparations.

The Rotor syndrome is a benign condition and requires no treatment except reassurance and ruling out other treatable causes.

ACUTE HEPATITIS

A variety of insults can lead to necrotic injury of the hepatocytes. These include viral illnesses, drugs and toxins, alcohol, ischaemia and sepsis. Of these, by far the most common cause of jaundice in the community is acute viral hepatitis caused by the hepatotropic viruses. The virus responsible for most of the cases in India is HEV followed by HBV and, rarely, HAV.[9] Hepatitis C virus rarely produces icteric hepatitis and the illness is usually subclinical in the acute phase (*see* the chapter on Acute viral hepatitis, pp. 105–21).

Treatment

The management of acute viral hepatitis is usually conservative and symptomatic with no specific therapy required for the disease since it runs a self-limiting course in more than 95% of cases.

First of all, the patient needs to be reassured that the jaundice is because of acute viral hepatitis and, whether or not therapy is taken, the illness will resolve spontaneously in 4–6 weeks' time. The patient should be advised to rest for the period of continuing liver inflammation. However, there is a controversy about the value of rest in this condition. Studies carried out on volunteers in the US army did not support any significant advantage of forced rest over mobilization.

Nausea may be treated with antiemetics on an 'as and when required' basis. If nausea and vomiting are troublesome, then round-the-clock use of antiemetics such as domperidone or metoclopramide may also help in improving food intake.

For patients who progress to the cholestatic phase of illness, therapy is required for troublesome itching (the management of itching is discussed on p. 171).

Hospitalization for acute viral hepatitis is required for specific indications such as a patient with incessant vomiting who is unable to eat and a patient with a disturbed sleep rhythm (such a patient may be in the early phase of encephalopathy). Patients who do not have a palpable liver or have a reduced liver span or those who have a prolonged PT are at increased risk of developing fulminant hepatitis and should, therefore, be kept under close follow-up or hospitalized.

No antiviral drug has been developed for hepatitis A or E since almost all these conditions have a self-limiting course with full recovery, except for a small percentage of patients who develop fulminant hepatitis. In acute hepatitis B, antiviral treatment with lamivudine has been tried[10] but is still not recommended. The role of antiviral treatment for acute hepatitis C is emerging but it will not be discussed here since hepatitis C rarely produces jaundice in the acute phase.

Myths that need to be dispelled[11]

A number of indigenous medicines and ill-founded treatment modalities are offered for this condition with variable results; sometimes, these agents may even be dangerous. The various hepatoprotective agents available in the market do not help in shortening or improving the course of the illness. Dietary advice should include dispelling the myth about unnecessary restrictions on food. All kinds of food are allowed with no specific restriction on fats. Fats may not be tolerated in the initial week or two due to increased nausea. There is also no logic behind prescribing a high-carbohydrate diet.

Corticosteroids have no place in the treatment of a classical attack of acute viral hepatitis; they do no good. On the other hand, they may aggravate or cause a flare-up of the disease, especially if the patient has hepatitis B or C.

The management of drug-induced hepatitis includes cessation of exposure to the offending agent; further management is symptomatic as is the case in acute viral hepatitis. A specific antidote (N-acetylcysteine) is required for acetaminophen poisoning. Often, drug-induced hepatitis progresses even after the drug is withdrawn as the injury is usually immunologically mediated (*see* the chapter on Drug-induced hepatitis, pp. 236–46).

Ischaemic hepatitis usually occurs in patients with underlying congestive heart failure who develop periods of hypotension. The treatment includes improvement of the haemodynamic status along with optimal management of the congestive heart failure.

SUBACUTE HEPATIC FAILURE

Subacute hepatic failure is used to describe the development of features of liver failure in the form of unequivocal ascites and/or encephalopathy 4 weeks after the onset of jaundice in a patient who does not have any underlying chronic liver disease. This condition is associated with a protracted course and higher short-term mortality, and most of the survivors go on to develop chronic liver disease (*see* p. 305).

Treatment

Treatment is generally supportive with building up of nutrition, diuretics and antibiotics to control infection. Specific therapy with a drug called SNMC (an interferon stimulator derived from *Glycyrrhiza*) has been used with significant improvement in short-term mortality as compared to retrospective controls (72.2% *v.* 31.1%).[12]

ACUTE ALCOHOLIC HEPATITIS

Alcoholic hepatitis is another important disease that presents with jaundice; however, it needs to be discussed separately because of the severity of the disease and the presence of underlying cirrhosis in the majority of patients with this condition (*see* the chapter on Jaundice in alcoholics, pp. 193–213).

Treatment

The management of acute alcoholic hepatitis starts with evaluation of the severity of the disease. The most commonly used parameter, Maddrey discriminant function, is calculated as $4.6 \times (PT\ patient - PT\ control) + serum\ bilirubin$. If this factor is ≥ 32, it signifies a high (>50%) 30-day mortality.[13]

Therapeutic agents used for the treatment of acute alcoholic hepatitis include glucocorticoids, pentoxiphylline, nutritional supplementation, propyl thiouracil and colchicine, apart from other experimental therapies.

About 13 randomized controlled trials have been carried out of glucocorticoids in severe acute alcoholic hepatitis, of which 6 have shown benefit and 7 have not shown any effect. Three meta-analyses of these studies and the only two prospective randomized controlled trials have shown the benefit of using steroids for reducing short-term mortality in these patients, especially those with severe disease with encephalopathy.[14,15]

A single, randomized, placebo-controlled trial of pentoxiphylline in 101 patients with severe alcoholic hepatitis showed that the mortality rate was significantly lower in patients who received pentoxiphylline (24% *v.* 46%).[16]

Patients with alcoholic liver disease are malnourished and have a high metabolic requirement, which led to trials of nutritional therapy in these patients. Both parenteral amino acid infusions and enteral feeding supplements have been used with variable results in terms of improvement in mortality, bilirubin levels and encephalopathy.[17]

Recently, however, a study has shown that the role of nutrition and glucocorticoids in alcoholic hepatitis may be synergistic, with steroids being helpful in reducing short-term mortality and nutrition in the long term.[18]

Apart from these, other therapies that are either experimental or have not proven to be of much use in this condition are colchicine, insulin–glucagon infusion and anabolic steroids.

CHOLESTATIC JAUNDICE

This type of jaundice is associated with defects in the excretion of bilirubin, the defect being present anywhere from the canalicular membrane to the level of the common bile duct draining into the duodenum. Therefore, it may be divided into intrahepatic or extrahepatic cholestasis (*see* the chapter on Cholestasis, pp. 165–75). Intrahepatic cholestatic disorders include the cholestatic phase of viral hepatitis, drug-induced cholestatic hepatitis, primary sclerosing cholangitis (PSC) and primary biliary cirrhosis (PBC). Extrahepatic cholestatic disorders are associated with obstruction to the bile flow in the extrahepatic biliary channels, and therapy usually includes endoscopic or surgical bypass of the obstructing lesion. The endoscopic and surgical aspects are discussed elsewhere (*see* pp. 46–55, 300–4); we will restrict ourselves to the medical management of these conditions. Management includes treatment of the associated symptoms of pruritus, fat-soluble vitamin deficiency and osteopenia, especially in chronic cholestatic disorders.

Treatment

Pruritus

Pruritus, which has a significant impact on the quality of life, is the most disturbing symptom in patients with cholestasis, especially those with chronic cholestatic disorders. The pharmacological agents available for the treatment of pruritus are summarized in Table I.

Ursodeoxycholic acid (UDCA) is also the drug of choice for the treatment of PBC and is the only drug that has been shown to reduce mortality in this condition.[19]

It is important to remember that cholestyramine and rifampicin act over several days and, if taken continuously, their effect is maintained; therefore, these agents should not be used on an 'as and when required' basis.

Fat-soluble vitamin deficiencies

These are common in patients with chronic cholestatic syndromes, especially PSC and PBC. Most common among these is vitamin A deficiency followed by deficiency of vitamins D and E.[20] Patients with chronic cholestasis should be screened yearly for vitamin A and D deficiencies and, if detected, these should be treated with therapeutic doses of these vitamins (Table II).

Table I. Drugs used for the management of pruritus

Ursodeoxycholic acid (UDCA)	15–30 mg/kg/day
Rifampicin	150–300 mg twice a day
Cholestyramine	4 g every 6–8 hours
Opioids (naltrexone, nalmifene)	50 mg/day

Table II. Vitamin therapy for cholestatic disorders

Vitamin A	50 000 units 2–3 times a week
Vitamin D	50 000 units 2–3 times a week
Vitamin E	100 units twice a day
Vitamin K	5 mg/day

Osteopenia

Metabolic bone disease is common in chronic cholestasis and is usually due to osteoporosis rather than osteomalacia, and is further aggravated by the use of corticosteroids in these patients.[21] This form of bone disease is very difficult to treat and various drugs, including vitamin D, bisphosphonates, oestrogen replacement therapy and calcitonin have been tried with unsatisfactory results. Ultimately, osteopenia resolves after liver transplantation.

REFERENCES

1. Berk PD, Wolkoff AW, Berlin NJ. Inborn errors of bilirubin metabolism. *Med Clin North Am* 1975;**59**:803–16.
2. Watson KJ, Gollan J. Gilbert's syndrome. *Baillieres Clin Gastroenterol* 1989;**3**:337–55.
3. Sinaasappel M, Jansen PL. The differential diagnosis of Crigler–Najjar disease, types 1 and 2, by bile pigment analysis. *Gastroenterology* 1991;**100**:783–9.
4. Sokal EM, Silve ES, Hermans D, *et al.* Orthotopic liver transplantation for Crigler–Najjar type 1 disease in six children. *Transplantation* 1995;**60**:1095–8.
5. Van der Veere CN, Sinaasappel M, McDonagh AF, *et al.* Current therapy for Crigler–Najjar syndrome type I: Report of a world registry. *Hepatology* 1996;**24**:311–15.
6. Gollan JL, Huang SN, Billing BH, *et al.* Prolonged survival in three brothers with severe type 2 Crigler–Najjar syndrome. Ultrastructural and metabolic studies. *Gastroenterology* 1975;**68**:1543–55.
7. Dubin IN. Chronic idiopathic jaundice: A review of fifty cases. *Am J Med* 1958;**24**:268–92.
8. Wolkoff AW, Wolpert E, Pascasio FN, *et al.* Rotor's syndrome: A distinct inheritable pathophysiologic entity. *Am J Med* 1976;**60**:173–8.
9. Chadha MS, Walimbe AM, Chobe LP, Arankalle VA. Comparison of etiology of sporadic, acute and fulminant viral hepatitis in hospitalized patients in Pune, India, during 1978–81 and 1994–97. *Indian J Gastroenterol* 2003;**22**:11–15.
10. Torii N, Hasegawa K, Ogawa M, Hashimoto E, Hayashi N. Effectiveness and long term outcome of lamivudine therapy for acute hepatitis B. *Hepatol Res* 2002;**24**:34.
11. Tandon BN, Nundy S (eds). *Textbook of tropical gastroenterology: Hepatobiliary diseases: Vol. 1.* Delhi: Oxford University Press; 1988.
12. Acharya SK, Dasarathy S, Tandon A, Joshi YK, Tandon BN. A preliminary open trial on interferon stimulator (SNMC) derived from *Glycyrrhiza glabra* in the treatment of subacute hepatic failure. *Indian J Med Res* 1993;**98**:69–74.
13. Maddrey WC. Alcohol-induced liver disease. *Clin Liver Dis* 2000;**4**:115–31.
14. Imperiale TF, O'Connors JB, McCullough AJ. Corticosteroids are effective in patients with severe alcoholic hepatitis. *Am J Gastroenterol* 1999;**94**:3066–8.
15. Ramond MJ, Pyonard T, Rueff B, *et al.* A randomized trial of prednisolone in patients with severe alcoholic hepatitis. *N Engl J Med* 1992;**326**:507–12.

16. Akriviadis E, Botla R, Briggs W, *et al.* Pentoxiphylline improves short-term survival in severe acute alcoholic hepatitis: A double-blind, placebo-controlled trial. *Gastroenterology* 2000;**19**:1637–48.

17. Fulton S, McCullough AJ. Treatment of alcoholic hepatitis. *Clin Liver Dis* 1998;**2**: 799–819.

18. Cabre E, Rodriguez-Iglesias P, Caballeria J, *et al.* Short and long term outcome of severe alcohol induced hepatitis treated with steroids or enteral nutrition: A multicenter randomized trial. *Hepatology* 2000;**32**:36–42.

19. Poupon RE, Lindor KD, Cauch-Dudek K, *et al.* Combined analysis of randomized controlled trials of ursodeoxycholic acid in primary biliary cirrhosis. *Gastroenterology* 1997;**113**:884–90.

20. Jorgensen RA, Lindor KD, Sartin JS, *et al.* Serum lipid and fat soluble vitamin levels in primary sclerosing cholangitis. *J Clin Gastroenterol* 1995;**20**:215–19.

21. Hay JE, Lindor KD, Wiesner RH, *et al.* The metabolic bone disease of primary sclerosing cholangitis. *Hepatology* 1991;**14**:257–61.

CHAPTER 22

Surgery in patients with jaundice

DEEPAK GOVIL

Surgery in patients with jaundice is associated with a high postoperative morbidity and mortality (8%–28%).[1] Despite considerable advances in the techniques of anaesthesia and perioperative care, the mortality rate has not changed over the past few decades. Surgery may be done in patients with jaundice in either of the following situations:

1. patients with hepatocellular jaundice requiring hepatobiliary or other surgical procedures, and
2. patients with obstructive jaundice requiring corrective or palliative surgical procedures.

SURGERY IN PATIENTS WITH HEPATOCELLULAR JAUNDICE

The factors influencing surgical risk in these patients include:

- severity of the liver disease
- urgency of the surgery (emergency *v.* elective)
- alternatives to surgery
- coexisting medical illness.

Conditions associated with an unacceptable surgical mortality and hence considered to be contraindications for elective surgery[2] include:

- acute viral hepatitis (AVH)
- acute alcoholic hepatitis
- Child class C cirrhosis of the liver[3,4]
- fulminant hepatic failure (FHF)
- severe chronic hepatitis
- severe coagulopathy (prolongation of PT >3 s despite administration of vitamin K, platelet count <50 000/cmm)

- severe extrahepatic complications
  —acute renal failure (ARF)
  —cardiomyopathy, heart failure
  —hypoxaemia.

Patients with mild-to-moderate chronic liver disease but without cirrhosis usually tolerate surgery well.[5] These conditions include:

- mild chronic hepatitis
- non-alcoholic steatohepatitis
- autoimmune hepatitis
- haemochromatosis
- Wilson disease.

Medical therapy should, however, be given to these patients prior to surgery to optimize results. The risk of surgery in patients with cirrhosis is higher and depends on the severity of the disease, in addition to the type of surgical procedure. The best predictor of risk in patients with cirrhosis is the Child–Pugh classification. The perioperative mortality rates observed in 100 patients with cirrhosis[6,7] in Child–Pugh classes A, B and C were 10%, 31% and 76%, respectively. Surgery is well tolerated by patients in Child class A, while for those in Child class B, surgery is permissible only with caution. Hepatic resection or cardiac surgery is, however, not considered for patients in Child class B.

Cardiac surgery is associated with an increased mortality and morbidity in patients with cirrhosis. The high mortality rate is usually due to postoperative infections, bleeding and progressive hepatic failure rather than cardiac dysfunction. A number of risk factors for hepatic decompensation following cardiac surgery have been identified, including the total time of cardio-pulmonary bypass, use of non-pulsatile cardiopulmonary bypass and the need for perioperative pressor support.[8] The least invasive option, e.g. angioplasty, valvuloplasty, etc. should be chosen for patients with advanced cirrhosis.

Patients with cirrhosis undergoing resection for hepatocellular carcinoma (HCC) are at an increased risk for hepatic decompensation as compared to other procedures. A substantial portion of functioning hepatic mass is removed in an already diseased liver. Though cirrhosis was earlier considered to be a contra-indication for the resection of hepatic tumours; due to improved surgical techniques, better patient selection (including earlier detection of tumours), better perioperative care and advances in the medical management of cirrhosis, the outcome has greatly improved and cirrhosis is no more considered an absolute contraindication for hepatic resection.[9]

SURGERY IN PATIENTS WITH OBSTRUCTIVE JAUNDICE

These patients are at an increased risk of developing complications such as renal failure, sepsis, coagulation disorders, delayed healing and wound infection, cholangitis and ascites.

Renal impairment

Renal failure occurs in 9% of jaundiced patients and accounts for more than one-third of deaths in them.[10] The overall mortality rate in these patients is >50%. Cholangitis and operative intervention are the two important precipitating factors for renal failure in patients with obstructive jaundice.[11,12] Following surgery, 60%–75% of patients with obstructive jaundice develop a fall in the glomerular filtration rate; of these, 30% have a substantial decrease in creatinine clearance before surgery.[13] Preoperative ARF has been found, especially in the presence of sepsis and cholangitis.[14] However, when various renal parameters were studied in detail before and after surgery for obstructive jaundice, no occult renal impairment was identified.[15]

The aetiology of ARF in the presence of obstructive jaundice is multifactorial and includes renal ischaemia, prostaglandin-mediated alterations in the renal microcirculation, myocardial depression, reduction in the intravascular volume and sepsis.

The following categories of patients are particularly at risk:

- the elderly (>60 years of age)
- decreased serum albumin level (<3 g/dl)
- poor renal function (raised serum creatinine level)
- low haematocrit value (<30%)
- leucocytosis (>10 000/cmm)
- high serum bilirubin level (>12 mg/dl)
- malignant biliary obstruction
- diabetes mellitus.

Prevention of acute postoperative renal failure

General measures

1. Early diagnosis and recognition of precipitating factors such as sepsis, pre-existing renal impairment, raised serum creatinine and low serum albumin concentrations are essential to take prompt, corrective action.
2. Renal function is assessed by the measurement of serum creatinine concentration for 2–3 consecutive days. The measurement of blood urea is not accurate as urea production is altered by liver disease and sepsis.
3. Parenteral antibiotics must be given to treat endotoxaemia.
4. Preoperative treatment with oral bile salts may prevent endotoxaemia and thus improve postoperative renal function.[16] However, firm evidence for this is lacking.
5. Prerenal deficit can be corrected by a careful assessment of fluid balance done with measurement of CVP before and 2–3 days after surgery. Adequate hydration, pre- and perioperatively, plays a pivotal role in preventing renal derangement. A serum albumin concentration <3 g/dl is associated with diminished skin turgor and generally denotes considerable volume depletion; it must be corrected before any invasive procedure is undertaken.

6. Non-steroidal anti-inflammatory drugs (NSAIDs) and other nephrotoxic drugs must be avoided. NSAIDs impair renal prostaglandin synthesis and can precipitate ARF, especially in the elderly, and hypovolaemic and hypoxic patients. NSAIDs may themselves produce acute interstitial nephritis and renal failure.

Specific measures

1. *Use of mannitol and saline:* Mannitol is a simple sugar with a molecular weight of 182. After intravenous administration, it is not metabolized but is freely filtered by the glomeruli into the tubular fluid and causes osmotic diuresis. Thus, it flushes out tubular casts and debris, and increases the renal blood flow (RBF). It appears to prevent endothelial cell swelling, which occurs during ischaemia. Thus, it prevents the 'no-flow' phenomenon.[17] Mannitol also appears to be an effective free hydroxyl radical scavenger.[18] Since mannitol causes marked natriuresis, adequate sodium supplementation is necessary with its administration. Injudicious and excessive use of mannitol may result in intravascular volume expansion, hyponatraemia and intracellular dehydration. It is advisable to give 20 g (100 ml of 20%) of mannitol 2 hours before operation and again during anaesthesia. If the urine volume falls to <50 ml/hour on two successive occasions, mannitol (20 g intravenously) is repeated.

   Loop diuretics such as frusemide and ethacrynic acid may also improve renal function. By inhibiting luminal sodium chloride transport, loop diuretics may reduce the energy requirement of the cells of the ascending limb of the loop of Henle, thus helping them to resist hypoxia.

2. *Low-dose dopamine infusion:* Dopamine at the rate of 1–2 µg/kg/min in the early stages of incipient ARF increases the RBF. This should be used when the hourly urine volume falls to <50 ml/hour on two successive occasions.[19,20]

3. Good liver perfusion should be maintained during surgery.

Management of established acute renal failure

Preoperative acute renal failure

A few patients with cholangitis, sepsis and obstructive jaundice develop ARF in the preoperative period.[12] They should be treated with fluid replacement, antibiotics and dialysis before definitive surgery. Surgery should be performed only when the renal function is stable.

Postoperative acute renal failure

Postoperative ARF is considered potentially reversible, if the patient survives the other problems. Treatment involves proper control of fluid balance and electrolytes (mainly potassium), provision of adequate calories and amino acids, and a close watch for any complications. Haemodialysis may be required in some patients.

Sepsis

Endotoxin is a lipopolysaccharide derived from Gram-negative bacteria in the gut. Endotoxins are inactivated by bile salts and Kupffer cells in healthy subjects. The presence of bile within the intestinal lumen reduces the absorption of endotoxins into the portal blood. Due to a lack of bile salts in the gut in patients with obstructive jaundice, endotoxins reach the systemic circulation and cause endotoxaemia.[21] Approximately 50% of patients with obstructive jaundice show impaired reticuloendothelial activity or decreased phagocytic activity of the Kupffer cells, thus facilitating endotoxaemia.[22]

Sepsis associated with obstructive jaundice is manifested by two distinct syndromes—cholangitis and alterations in the host defence mechanism.

Prevention of endotoxaemia

Various agents are used to prevent endotoxaemia:

1. *Oral bile salts*: Sodium taurocholate and deoxycholate act as surfactants and disrupt the endotoxin. They also decrease the absorption of endotoxins from the gut.
2. *Lactulose*: This is a non-toxic synthetic disaccharide and prevents endotoxaemia by either reducing or altering the bacterial flora in the gut.
3. *Antibiotics*: The incidence of wound infection and other septic complications is very high following biliary surgery, hence a prophylactic antibiotic is indicated.[23] In patients with obstructive jaundice due to stones, infection of the bile with *Escherichia coli* is common, whereas in those with malignant obstruction, the bile is usually sterile,[13] but wound infection is frequently caused by staphylococci. Thus, for antibiotic prophylaxis to be effective against both *E. coli* and staphylococci, a second-generation cephalosporin is preferred. Oral antibiotics are avoided because some studies have shown that the destruction of Gram-negative organisms increases the free endotoxin available for absorption.[24]

Bleeding disorders

Bleeding is an important complication in patients with jaundice undergoing surgery. It can occur because of:

1. inadequate local haemostasis or injury to the major vessels;
2. instrumentation through the liver;
3. portal hypertension; and
4. coagulopathy.

Aetiology

Jaundice-associated coagulopathy results from hepatocellular dysfunction or vitamin K deficiency. Absorption of fat-soluble vitamins is decreased in obstructive jaundice as the bile salts required for their absorption are absent in the gut. The most important among these is vitamin K, which needs to be supplemented.

Vitamin K is needed for the synthesis of Factors II, VII, IX and X by the liver. Apart from this, coagulation defects are related to biliary tract infection and endotoxaemia. Endotoxins cause intravascular coagulation by initiating the intrinsic coagulation cascade, activating platelets and releasing prostaglandins.[25]

Gastrointestinal haemorrhage is found in 3%–14% of patients with obstructive jaundice. The most common cause of bleeding is gastric erosions subsequent to an endotoxaemia-induced increase in gastric secretions.[24] Other factors that may be responsible are the presence of intragastric bile reflux and ischaemia of the gastric mucosa produced by microvascular fibrinous thrombi in the blood vessels.[26]

Prevention of coagulation disorders

1. Parenteral vitamin K and fresh frozen plasma (FFP) are administered to keep the PT within 3 s of normal. Intramuscular injection of vitamin K (10 mg daily) is given, but discontinued if there is no further response to treatment after 2–3 days.
2. Platelet transfusions are given to maintain the platelet count at a minimum of 100 000/cmm.[27] Diamino-8-D-organine vasopressin can also be given if the bleeding time is prolonged.[28] It produces a 2–4-fold increase in the plasma level of Factors VIII and vWF, presumably by their release from storage sites.
3. Fibrinogen deficiency can be treated with cryoprecipitates (1 unit/10 kg body-weight [one unit of cryptoprecipitate contains 250 mg fibrinogen]).
4. Parenteral antibiotics and H_2-receptor blockers help in preventing GI haemorrhage and stress-induced erosions caused by endotoxaemia.[23]

Antithrombin-III concentrate is useful for the prevention of disseminated intravascular coagulation (DIC)/FHF/cirrhosis with venous thrombosis/post-transplant thrombosis in children.

Delayed wound healing and wound infection

Poor nutritional status, malignancy and postoperative sepsis are responsible for delayed wound healing. Two to four per cent of jaundiced patients develop wound dehiscence.[29] Incisional hernia is found in 10%–12% of patients.[30,31] Reduced fibroblast migration[32] and lowered propyl hydroxylase levels[33] in patients with jaundice are said to be the contributing factors. No relation has been seen with the levels of plasma bilirubin.[30] It is, however, unclear if obstructive jaundice *per se* is responsible, or malnourishment and malignancy cause the delayed wound healing.

Cholangitis

Bacterial infection of the biliary tract almost always signifies biliary obstruction. Raised ductal pressure causes bacteria to proliferate and escape into the systemic circulation via the hepatic sinusoids.[34] Intravenous antibiotics, preferably second-generation cephalosporins and aminoglycosides, are administered, depending on the severity. In these patients, it is preferable to do a preoperative endoscopic sphincterotomy and biliary drainage.

Ascites

Ascites can occur due to poor nutritional status, malignancy or decompensated liver disease. Postoperative wound dehiscence and abdominal wall herniation are frequently seen in such patients. Hence, ascites should be treated aggressively before abdominal surgery. Correction of the serum protein levels helps to control ascites. Preoperative parenteral or enteral nutrition helps to build up these patients. Postoperatively, these patients need regular diuretics apart from maintenance of nutrition.

RISK FACTORS PREDICTING OUTCOME

Preoperative risk factors

Dixon *et al.*[1] reported three independent risk factors—high plasma bilirubin levels (>12 mg/dl), initial haematocrit value <30% and a malignant obstructing lesion. When all three factors were present, the mortality rate approached 60%, whereas when none was present, it was only 5%. Blamey *et al.*[16] found eight preoperative clinical and laboratory factors which were linked with postoperative mortality. These include age >60 years, malignant disease, hyperbilirubinaemia >6 mg/dl, haematocrit <30%, TLC >10 000/cmm, serum albumin <3 g/dl, serum creatinine >1.5 mg/dl and serum ALP >600 IU/L. The risk of complications was directly related to the number of positive risk factors. Blamey *et al.*[16] further showed that the serum creatinine and serum albumin levels in the week preceding surgery had independent significance in predicting mortality. Bose *et al.*[35] found the following categories of patients to be at high risk for surgery: age >60 years, associated diabetes mellitus, previous biliary tract surgery and prolonged surgery.

Role of preoperative biliary drainage

Preoperative biliary drainage can be done endoscopically through the percutaneous route or surgically. However, whether it is beneficial for the patient is still debatable. Internal drainage should be preferred over external drainage.

Controlled trials have shown that external drainage has the following problems: (i) an increased morbidity due to excessive loss of bile; (ii) a risk of sepsis; and (iii) increased cost due to prolonged hospital stay.

Internal drainage has the following advantages: (i) it avoids external biliary losses; (ii) overcomes endotoxaemia by the reintroduction of bile; and (iii) allows flexibility in the timing of surgery.

Biliary decompression leads to clinical improvement in these patients. It improves the general condition and nutritional status of the patient. It reduces the hospital stay and cost. There is a slow but distinct recovery of hepatocyte function. The function of the Kupffer cells and gut mucosal barrier, both of which are important for avoiding renal failure and sepsis, takes 4–6 weeks to recover. Preoperative biliary drainage/stenting is not routinely needed. It is a good policy to use this technique in patients with septic cholangitis, renal dysfunction, encephalopathy, coagulation defects or a combination of these factors.

Pre- and postoperative nutritional support

Nutritional support is an essential component of management and favourably affects the morbidity and mortality in jaundiced patients. The aim of nutritional support is to maintain or restore immunity, support anabolism by altering the catabolic response to injury and restoring specific hepatoceullar functions.

The nutritional risk factors for postoperative complications in hepatobiliary surgery are:[36]

1. weight loss >14% of the lean body mass over the past 6 months;
2. serum albumin levels <3. g/dl;
3. haematocrit <30%;
4. less than the 25th percentile of midarm circumference and triceps skin-fold thickness; and
5. total body potassium <85% of normal.

Of patients with obstructive jaundice, 45%–70% are malnourished as judged by weight loss >10%, albumin <3 g/dl, decreased triceps skin-fold thickness and an impaired/delayed hypersensitivity reaction.[37,38] Primary nutritional deficits in these patients are malabsorption of fat and fat-soluble vitamins. There is a loss of trace elements such as phosphate, calcium, magnesium and zinc due to salt formation with unabsorbed dietary fat.[37,38] Ascites is present in these patients due to a decrease in the serum albumin level. The metabolism of carbohydrates and proteins is rarely altered.

In patients with obstructive jaundice, biliary sepsis contributes to malnutrition by shifting protein synthesis from the anabolic to the acute phase mode. This inhibition of protein synthesis occurs due to the production of tumour necrosis factor (TNF), IL-6, eicosanoids, nitric oxide and other inflammatory mediators by endotoxin-stimulated Kupffer cells.[39] To reverse the catabolic effect of endotoxaemia, patients with biliary infection should be treated with biliary decompression for at least 4 weeks prior to a major hepatobiliary surgery to allow the hepatocytes to recover their protein synthetic activity.

Profoundly malnourished patients with cirrhosis or chronic active hepatitis and HCC usually present at an advanced stage. These patients should not undergo surgery because of the prohibitively high operative mortality.

Nutritional management

Malnourished and vitamin-deficient patients benefit from pre- and post-operative nutritional support. Routine use of parenteral nutrition in patients undergoing hepatobiliary surgery is associated with a high incidence of postoperative complications.[40]

Routes of nutritional support

- The oral route is the commonest and most physiological route.
- If the oral route fails, a soft silastic nasogastric or nasoduodenal feeding tube is used.
- If the tube fails or is unacceptable, a feeding jejunostomy or feeding gastrostomy may be done.
- If the enteral route is unavailable, total parenteral nutrition (TPN) is given.

Patients with obstructive jaundice require approximately 25–35 kcal/kg dry weight to maintain nitrogen balance. It is recommended that 25%–40% of the total calories be provided as fat. Biliary decompression should be performed before this.[41,42] Foschi *et al.*,[38] in a prospective randomized study of patients with obstructive jaundice, subjected a group of patients to biliary decompression followed by surgery, or to biliary decompression followed by 2 weeks of alimentation and then surgery. They found that patients receiving alimentation for 2 weeks had lower morbidity (17% *v.* 46%), mortality (3.5% *v.* 12.5%) and postoperative infection (14% *v.* 28%). Whenever bile flow is not established in patients with biliary obstruction, a low-fat diet supplemented with water-soluble or fat-soluble vitamins should be given. Phosphorus, calcium and magnesium are also supplemented.

In case of malignancy, each patient must be evaluated for current nutritional status. They may need up to 35 kcal/kg dry weight/day of calories, up to 2 g protein/kg dry weight/day and micronutrient supplementation. TPN-supplemented groups show reduction in the overall postoperative morbidity (55% *v.* 35%), predominantly because of fewer septic complications. They also have a lower mortality (46% less than in controls).[43]

PREOPERATIVE EVALUATION

Preoperative evaluation involves the following measures:

- Careful history-taking to identify risk factors and bring the patient to a satisfactory state of health;
- The presence of preoperative pulmonary, cardiac or hepatic disease significantly increases the incidence of postoperative morbidity and mortality. Unless contraindicated, the use of β-blockers in patients with coronary artery disease reduces the incidence of perioperative ischaemic events and myocardial infarction;
- A routine evaluation of complete blood counts (CBC), clotting factors, PT, serum electrolytes, LFT and serum creatinine helps to assess hepatic and renal functions.

Adequate preoperative hydration and strict maintenance of an intake/output chart, maintenance of fluids and electrolytes, and measures previously mentioned to prevent renal failure, endotoxaemia, bleeding disorders and GI haemorrhage should be diligently followed. Patients with cholangitis should undergo preoperative biliary drainage. The cause of ascites, if present, should be looked for and attempts made to correct nutritional deficiencies.

INTRAOPERATIVE CONSIDERATIONS

There is a 16% drop in the hepatic blood flow associated with anaesthesia and mechanical ventilation.[44] Intraperitoneal insufflation and head-up tilt result in the impairment of hepatic blood flow secondary to a decrease in the cardiac output.[40] Halothane and enflurane reduce the hepatic arterial blood flow as a result of systemic vasodilataion and negative inotropic effect. Isoflurane has a minimal effect on these and, on the contrary, increases the hepatic arterial blood flow. Therefore, isoflurane is the preferred anaesthetic agent for patients with liver disease.

Hypercarbia should be avoided in patients with liver disease because it initiates sympathetic stimulation of the splanchnic vasculature, thereby decreasing the portal blood flow. During surgery, the pCO_2 should be maintained in the range of 35–40 mmHg.[27]

Atracurium is the neuromuscular blocking agent (muscle relaxant) of choice in patients with liver disease or biliary obstruction because its metabolism does not depend on the liver or kidney.[43] The action of other muscle relaxants is prolonged in liver disease because of the reduced activity of plasma pseudocholinesterase, reduced biliary excretion and increase in the volume of distribution of muscle relaxants. For prolonged surgery such as liver transplantation, doxacurium, a long-acting, non-depolarizing muscle relaxant, is used.[45]

Fentanyl or sufentanyl are the preferred narcotic agents because their metabolism is not affected in liver disease. The metabolism of morphine and meperidine may decrease in patients with liver disease and portal hypertension due to reduced hepatic blood flow.

Among the benzodiazepine sedatives, the metabolism of diazepam and chlordiazepoxide can be prolonged in patients with liver disease. Oxazepam and lorazepam are preferred because they are eliminated by glucuronidation without hepatic metabolism.

Barbiturates may precipitate hepatic encephalopathy by binding with the gamma amino butyric acid (GABA) receptors in the brain. Therefore, these should be used with caution, although they do not greatly affect the hepatic blood flow. Chlorpromazine has a greater depressant effect on the central nervous system in patients with liver dysfunction than healthy subjects.

POSTOPERATIVE CARE

Postoperative care in patients with hepatic disease has improved considerably. Laboratory tests needed serially in the postoperative period are: haematocrit, electrolytes, serum creatinine, BUN, PT/APTT, liver enzymes and chest X-ray.

Various postoperative concerns in patients who have undergone hepato-biliary surgery include:

- *Postoperative pain*: the preferred method for its control is patient-controlled analgesia (PCA).
- *Use of narcotics*: they should be used with caution as following hepatic resection there is an unpredictable reduction in the metabolism of narcotics.
- *Coagulation factor deficiency*: this can be corrected within 48 hours of surgery by routine parenteral administration of vitamin K. If the PT is still prolonged, then fresh frozen plasma (FFP) may be needed to rapidly correct coagulation abnormalities.
- If the standard corrective measures fail, then 1-deamino-8-D-arginine vasopressin (DDAVP) at a dose of 0.3 µg/kg IV is given every 12–24 hours, depending on the severity. DDAVP increases the concentration of Factor VIII and shorterns PT.
- *Phosphorus replacement*: this is given as potassium phosphate, particularly following partial hepatic resection, to support cellular regeneration.

Early identification of risk groups and a systematic, proactive approach to treat problems in the postoperative period is very important. Melendez *et al.*[46] showed that the mortality ranged from 37% to 79% if postoperative patients with hepatobiliary disease required admission to the ICU, regardless of the diagnosis made on admission.

Other postoperative measures to prevent complications include the following:

- Maintaining the fluid balance and preventing hypoperfusion of the tissues is an important therapeutic measure in the postoperative period.
- Renal failure must be prevented by instituting appropriate measures as mentioned earlier.
- The hepatopulmonary syndrome (i.e. the triad of liver disease, increased alveolar–arterial gradient and evidence of intrapulmonary vascular resistance) can be avoided by correcting hypoxaemia at the earliest.
- Hypoglycaemia can be corrected by routine administration of dextrose solution and monitoring the blood glucose levels. Postoperative patients are prone to hypoglycaemia due to diminished glycogen reserves, increased insulin levels and impaired gluconeogenesis. Fortunately, dangerous hypoglycaemia is rare.
- Avoiding sepsis:
  —abdominal sepsis leading to significant mortality is caused by biliary manipulation and placement of a biliary stent, the presence of culture-positive bile, retained gall stones, ascites and blood loss;
  —respiratory and urinary infection must be looked for;
  —an upper abdominal incision, pleural effusion, COPD and poor pulmonary toilet may promote the development of pneumonia;
  —the wound should be inspected regularly and the central venous catheter changed routinely;
  —GI bleeding due to stress ulceration (5%) must be prevented;
  —encephalopathy must be prevented, identified and treated early. A sudden

change in the patient's mental status or onset of asterixis or flapping tremor denotes the onset of encephalopathy;

—precipitating factors such as GI bleeding, infection, drugs, diet or dehydration must be avoided.

It is always helpful to identify early deviations from the normal rather than treat organ failure. Hence, close monitoring at every stage is the key to a good outcome of surgery in jaundiced patients.

REFERENCES

1. Dixon JM, Armstrong CP, Duffy SW, Davies GC. Factors affecting morbidity and mortality after surgery for obstructive jaundice: A review of 373 patients. *Gut* 1983;**24**:845–52.
2. Friedman LS. The risk of surgery in patients with liver disease. *Hepatology* 1999;**29**:1617–23.
3. Greenwood SM, Leffler CT, Minkowitz S. The increased mortality rate of open liver biopsy in alcoholic hepatitis. *Surg Gyn Obstet* 1972;**134**:600–4.
4. Mikkelsen WP, Kern WH. The influence of acute hyaline necrosis on survival after emergency and elective portocaval shunt. *Major Prob Clin Surg* 1974;**14**:233–42.
5. Runyon BA. Surgical procedures are well tolerated by patients with asymptomatic chronic hepatitis. *J Clin Gastroenterol* 1986;**8**:542–4.
6. Garrison RN, Cryer HM, Howard DA, *et al.* Clarification of risk factors for abdominal operations in patients with hepatic cirrhosis. *Ann Surg* 1984;**199**:648–55.
7. Mansour A, Watson W, Shayani V, Pickleman J. Abdominal operations in patients with cirrhosis: Still a major surgical challenge. *Surgery* 1997;**122**:730–6.
8. Morris JJ, Helman CL, Gawey BJ, *et al.* Three patients requiring both coronary artery bypass surgery and orthotopic liver transplantation. *J Cardiothorac Vasc Anesth* 1995;**9**:322–32.
9. Grazi GL, Ercolani G, Pierangeli F, *et al.* Improved results of liver resection for hepato-cecullar carcinoma on cirrhosis give the procedure added value. *Ann Surg* 2001;**234**:71–8.
10. Fitt HA, Cameroon JL, Poltier RG. Factors affecting mortality in biliary tract surgery. *Am J Surg* 1981;**141**:66–72.
11. Bartlett W. Renal complications of biliary tract infections. *Surg Gynecol Obstet* 1953;**56**:1080–95.
12. Bismuth H, Kuntziger H, Corlette MB. Cholangitis with acute renal failure: Priorities in therapeutics. *Ann Surg* 1975;**181**:881–7.
13. McPherson GAD, Benjamin IS, Boobis AR, Brodie MJ, Hampden C, Blumgart LH. Anti-pyrine elimination as a dynamic test of hepatic functional integrity in obstructive jaundice. *Gut* 1982;**23**:734–8.
14. Dawson JL. Jaundice, septic shock and acute renal failure. *Am J Surg* 1968;**115**:516–8.
15. Govil D. Renal function in obstructive jaundice: A pre- and postoperative assessment. *J Assoc Physicians India* 1993;**41**:151–3.
16. Blamey SL, Fearon KCH, Gilmour WH, Osborne DH, Carter DC. Prediction of risk in biliary surgery. *Br J Surg* 1983;**70**:535–8.
17. Flores J, Dibona DR, Beck CH, Leaf A. The role of cell swelling in ischemic renal damage and protective effect of hypertonic solute. *J Clin Invest* 1972;**51**:118–26.
18. Pallor MS, Hoidal JR, Ferris TF. Oxygen free radical in ischemic acute renal failure in the rat. *J Clin Invest* 1984;**74**:1156–64.
19. Carcoana OV, Hines RL. Is renal dose dopamine protective or therapeutic? Yes. *Crit Care Clin* 1996;**12**:677–85.
20. Handerson IS, Beattie TJ, Kennedy AC. Dopamine hydrochloride in oliguric states. *Lancet* 1980;**2**:827–8.

21. Allison EME, Prentice CRM, Kennedy AC. Renal function and other factors in obstructive jaundice. *Br J Surg* 1979;**66**:392–7.
22. Pain JA, Cahill CJ, Bailey ME. Perioperative complications in obstructive jaundice: Therapeutic consideration. *Br J Surg* 1985;**72**:942–5.
23. Diamond T, Paiki RW. Perioperative management of obstructive jaundice. *Br J Surg* 1997;**84**:147–9.
24. Goto H, Nakamura S. Liberation of endotoxin from *Escherichia coli* by addition of antibiotics. *Jpn J Exp Med* 1980;**50**:35–43.
25. Morison DC, Ulevitch RJ. The effects of bacterial endotoxins on host mediation systems. *Am J Pathol* 1978;**93**:527–617.
26. Margaretten W, McKay DG. Thrombotic ulcerations of the gastrointestinal tract. *Arch Intern Med* 1971;**127**:250–3.
27. Maze M. Anesthesia and the liver. In: Miller RD (ed). *Anesthesia*. 4th ed. Edinburgh: Churchill Livingstone; 1994:1969–80.
28. Burroughs AK, Mathews K, Qadiri M, *et al*. Desmopressin and bleeding time in patients with cirrhosis. *Br Med J* 1985;**291**:1377–81.
29. Wattenstein BH, Giacchino JL, Pickleman JR, *et al*. Obstructive jaundice: The necessity for improved management. *Am Surg* 1981;**47**:116–20.
30. Irvin TT, Vassilakis JS, Chattopadhyay DK, Greaney MG. Abdominal wound healing in jaundiced patients. *Br J Surg* 1978;**65**:521–2.
31. Armstrong CP, Dixon JM, Duffy SW, Elton RA, Davies GC. Wound healing in obstructive jaundice. *Br J Surg* 1984;**71**:267–70.
32. Lee E. The effect of obstructive jaundice on the migration of reticuloendothelial cells and fibroblasts into early experimental granulomata. *Br J Surg* 1972;**59**:875–7.
33. Than T, McGee JO, Sokhi GS, Patrick RS, Blumgart LH. Skin prolyl hydroxylase in patients with obstructive jaundice. *Lancet* 1974;**2**:807–8.
34. Blumgart LH (ed). *Surgery of the liver and biliary tract*. New York: Churchill Livingstone; 2002.
35. Bose SM, Babu JS, Wig JD, *et al*. Relationship of bacteria and other risk factors to complications following biliary tract surgery. *Indian J Surg* 1990;**52**:579–84.
36. Halliday AW, Benjamin IS, Blumgart LH. Nutritional risk factors in major hepatobiliary surgery. *J Parenter Enteral Nutr* 1998;**12**:43–8.
37. Shronts EP. Nutritional assesment of adults with endstage hepatic failure. *Nutr Clin Pract* 1998;**3**:113–19.
38. Foschi D, Cavagna G, Callioni F, *et al*. Hyperalimentation of jaundiced patients on percutaneous transhepatic biliary drainage. *Br J Surg* 1986;**73**:716–19.
39. O'Neil S, Hunt J, Filkins J, *et al*. Obstructive jaundice in rats resulting in exaggerated hepatic production of tumor necrosis factor alpha and systemic and tissue necrosis factor-alpha levels after endotoxin. *Surgery* 1997;**122**:281–7.
40. Ecftheriadis E, Kotzampassi K, Botsios D, Tzartinoglou E, Farmakis H, Dadoukis J. Splanchnic ischemia during laparoscopic cholecystectomy. *Surg Endosc* 1996;**10**:324–6.
41. Buzby G, Mullen JL, Matthews DC, *et al*. Prognostic nutritional index in gastrointestinal surgery. *Am J Surg* 1980;**139**:160–7.
42. McCullough A, Mullen KD, Smanik EJ, *et al*. Nutritional therapy in liver disease. *Gastroenterol Clin North Am* 1989;**18**:619–42.
43. Fan S, Lo CM, Lai EC, *et al*. Perioperative nutritional support in patients undergoing hepatectomy for hepatocellular carcinoma. *N Engl J Med* 1994;**331**:1547–52.
44. Gleman S, Fowler KC, Smith KR. Liver circulation and function during isoflurane anesthesia in dogs. *Anesthesiology* 1983;**59**:A224.
45. Hunter JM. New neuromuscular blocking agents. *N Engl J Med* 1995;**332**:1691–9.
46. Melendez JA, Arslan V, Fischer M, *et al*. Peri-operative outcome of major hepatic resection under low CVP anesthesia—blood loss, blood transfusion and risk of post-operative renal dysfunction. *J Am Coll Surg* 1998;**178**:620–5.

CHAPTER 23

Nutrition in jaundice

Y.K. JOSHI, JAYA BENJAMIN

The liver is the most versatile organ of the human body. It performs various important functions such as detoxification of harmful chemicals, storage of vitamins and minerals, synthesis of proteins and clotting factors, and metabolism of nutrients.

Although malnutrition is not the cause of liver disease, except in alcoholics and starving populations, it may be a consequence of hepatic dysfunction and has important clinical implications. Hepatobiliary diseases disturb the nutrient metabolism; conversely, liver damage could result from dietary inadequacies, dietary excess, dietary contaminants or various nutritional therapies. Nutritional requirements and tolerance vary in hepatobiliary diseases.

AETIOLOGY OF MALNUTRITION IN LIVER DISEASE

In hepatobiliary diseases, multiple factors such as altered metabolism, inadequate dietary intake, increased losses, malabsorption and drugs work synergistically, leading to nutritional deficiencies. Hepatobiliary diseases also disturb the energy balance and fuel homeostasis, which may occur due to changes in the glycogen storage capacity along with reduction in the net splanchnic glucose production. As a result, fuel homeostasis is maintained by gluconeogenesis, leading to the utilization of a fat-enriched 'metabolic mixture', which results in the depletion of protein and fat stores. The liver removes 25%–50% of the ingested glucose, which is used for energy and stored as glycogen; 50%–75% enters the peripheral tissues, where it is used as a caloric source; the remaining is stored as glycogen.

Reduction in the flow of bile due to parenchymal liver disease or chronic cholestasis leads to steatorrhoea and thereby impaired absorption of fat and fat-soluble vitamins. The coexistence of certain diseases, such as coeliac disease, frequently seen with primary biliary cirrhosis or primary sclerosing cholangitis, and concurrent inflammatory bowel disease, exocrine pancreatic dysfunction and drugs may cause further malabsorption.

The liver also plays a crucial role in protein synthesis. It deaminates the amino acids and eliminates ammonia as urea. It utilizes amino acids for gluconeogenesis and is also an important site for the degradation of many proteins and hormones. In viral hepatitis and fulminant hepatic failure (FHF), protein requirement is greater due to increased gluconeogenesis, which causes depletion of the protein stores, and a reduction in plasma proteins and ureagenesis along with an elevation in blood ammonia levels.

Although the mineral turnover may not be affected in acute liver diseases, it may be affected in some chronic liver diseases and storage disorders such as Wilson disease. Similarly, in genetic haemochromatosis, increased absorption of iron causes an increased accumulation of iron in the parenchymal cells causing liver injury.

Often, dietary intake is much below that recommended in hepatobiliary diseases due to anorexia, nausea, vomiting, and protein and sodium restriction. Thus, a diminished dietary intake of both macro- and micronutrients, and prolonged fasting leads to lipolysis and gluconeogenesis of proteins, eventually causing depletion of structural and functional proteins. Complications such as sepsis and variceal bleeding contribute to malnutrition due to increased protein catabolism and massive urinary losses of amino acid and nitrogen. Ascites is also associated with increased energy expenditure leading to a negative energy balance. About 50–100 g of protein loss occurs with each paracentesis. The resting energy expenditure increases with progressive liver disease. Sepsis and alcohol metabolism further increase the energy demands.

Drugs such as lactulose and neomycin used in hepatic encephalopathy lead to nutrient malabsorption and cause mucosal damage. Neomycin interferes with lipid absorption, and cholestyramine given for pruritus binds to bile acids leading to steatorrhoea. Diuretics may also cause depletion of potassium, magnesium and zinc.

Alcoholics may have malnutrition due to poor intake and/or metabolic derangement caused by the alcohol itself or liver cell necrosis. Though studies have shown that there is no major difference in protein depletion or energy and protein malnutrition in alcoholic compared to non-alcoholic liver disease, nutrition therapy is more important in alcoholic liver disease due to specific nutrient deficiencies, e.g. of vitamins, trace elements, etc.

GOALS OF NUTRITIONAL THERAPY

The goals of nutritional therapy could be summarized as follows:

1. Provide an adequate amount of energy and protein to facilitate hepatic cell regeneration and alleviate the metabolic derangement;
2. Avoid excess production of ammonia from endogenous and exogenous protein catabolism;
3. Correct vitamin and mineral deficiencies; and
4. Avoid potential complications that may occur as a result of inappropriate

nutritional support, which include hypo- or hyperglycaemia, hypertriglyceridaemia, hepatic encephalopathy, fluid overload, electrolyte imbalance, etc.

Thus, a large number of patients with liver disease require dietary advice,
counselling and active nutritional supplements, especially in situations such
as acute and chronic hepatic failure and alcoholic hepatitis. Nutrition
supplementation may be needed lifelong in patients with chronic liver disease.
Dietary modifications and restrictions are necessary in several hepatobiliary
diseases. Some common diseases of the liver requiring dietary and nutritional
intervention are acute hepatitis due to viral infections, drugs, toxins or alcohol,
with or without encephalopathy; and chronic liver disease or cirrhosis of the
liver with or without encephalopathy.

NUTRITIONAL ASSESSMENT

Assessment of the nutritional status of patients with liver disease is important
as it enables the identification of patients at potential risk. It also helps to
document the nutritional consequences of disease progression and monitor the
outcome of nutritional intervention. Nutritional assessment helps in the timely
identification and correction of nutritional deficiencies.[1] The assessment of
nutritional status by standard indices in patients with liver disease should be
done very carefully, as the liver disease itself might lead to a false interpretation
or estimation of the parameters of nutritional status and give an incorrect picture
of the actual status.[2]

Although most of the parameters of nutritional status are affected both by
malnutrition and hepatic dysfunction, measurement of the exact contribution
of each of these factors is not feasible.[3,4] A complete nutritional assessment
comprises clinical and dietary histories, physical examination, anthropometric
measurements and selected laboratory indices. The individual components of
nutritional assessment must be interpreted with great caution to prevent
fallacious results, e.g. though immunocompetence is affected by nutrition and
determination of the immune status may be considered a marker of malnutrition,
yet certain non-nutritional factors in liver disease may influence the immune
status.[5]

Similarly, although plasma amino acids and blood urea nitrogen (BUN) are
markers of protein nutritional status, again, in patients with liver disease, a
negative nitrogen balance can be underestimated due to a decrease in urea
synthesis and increased ammonia levels. Likewise, the simplest example of
misinterpretation is that measurement of body weight may be misleading in
hepatic disease due to oedema, as it masks the underlying severe loss of muscle
mass.[6]

At present, there is no general consensus on which technique is best suited
for the assessment of nutritional status in patients, especially those with chronic
liver disease, and there is a need to develop such a technique to obtain the best
estimate of the nutritional status.[7] However, a fairly reliable assessment can be
made by the collective information gathered from combining the data obtained

from clinical, dietary, biochemical and anthropometric evaluation, provided these parameters are gathered simultaneously and on a serial basis so that the validity of the nutritional marker cannot be questioned.

NUTRITION IN ACUTE HEPATITIS

The majority of patients with acute hepatitis, whether viral or drug-induced, do not require dietary modification or nutritional intervention. GI symptoms usually subside after the preicteric phase or after drug withdrawal (in case of drug hepatitis), and patients are usually able to eat normal food. Appetite also becomes normal by this time; therefore, patients should be encouraged to eat a normal diet of their choice. Sometimes, minor GI symptoms require symptomatic treatment to enhance oral intake, which can be given along with vitamins, providing psychological satisfaction to the patients. Small, frequent meals along with adequate fluids providing 2000–2500 kcal and 80–100 g of protein should be advised to compensate for the extra need due to the catabolic process of acute illness. Contrary to earlier practice and normal belief, fat restriction is not advised as fatless diets are bulky and not palatable.

In a few patients, enteral (tube) feeding may be necessary in case of persistent anorexia and nausea accompanying severe hepatitis with a prolonged course. Several commercial preparations with adequate amounts of nutrients are available in India. In case of persistent vomiting or abdominal pain, a small group of patients may even need parenteral supplementation. Commercial preparations of amino acids, lipids and glucose providing an adequate amount of nutrients and vitamins in the desired proportions are also available. Though fluid and electrolyte imbalance is not a common feature, a few cases of severe hepatitis may need monitoring to avoid fluid retention. Thus, patients with acute hepatitis may require dietary advice in the form of minor modifications without much restriction and, occasionally, nutritional supplements with vitamins and symptomatic therapy. However, it is advisable to persuade and encourage patients to be on a normal diet.

NUTRITION IN FULMINANT HEPATIC FAILURE

Protein–calorie malnutrition is commonly seen in patients suffering from FHF and, in spite of an apparently adequate calorie and protein intake, most comatose patients exhibit obvious muscle wasting within a week. It is very difficult to determine whether any specific nutritional support may be a decisive factor in the outcome.

Hypoglycaemia is a common feature in patients with FHF because of reduced glycogen stores, decreased glycogenolysis and gluconeogenesis. Therefore, close monitoring of the blood sugar levels along with adequate replacement of dextrose is required. A constant supply of 10%–20% of glucose is beneficial; the infusion rate should be adjusted to maintain euglycaemia. Patients with FHF need about 35–50 kcal/kg body-weight/day. Lipids can safely be used parenterally to provide non-protein calories as they are calorie-dense and especially advantageous for patients with FHF suffering from volume overload or renal dysfunction.[8,9] Such patients tolerate lipid emulsions very well.

At least 40–60 g of protein should be provided to reduce protein catabolism, increase anabolism and facilitate hepatic regeneration. It could be in the form of an amino acid mixture. Branched-chain amino acid (BCAA) infusions can also be used for this purpose, either with glucose or alone.

NUTRITION IN ALCOHOLIC LIVER DISEASE

The liver is the main site of alcohol metabolism. Indeed, alcohol is also a preferred fuel. A quantity of alcohol up to 10% of the caloric intake is oxidized by cytosolic alcohol dehydrogenase (ADH) and mitochondrial aldehyde dehydrogenase (ALDH); however, an excess (>10% of the caloric intake) is toxic rather than a dietary source. It is then that the microsomal P450 oxidizing system comes into play. The sequence of events of alcoholic injury is from fatty liver to alcoholic hepatitis and finally to cirrhosis. Many factors contribute to the development of malnutrition in chronic alcoholics with liver disease.

Reduced food intake

Alcohol replaces food in the diet. One gram of alcohol provides 7.1 kcal or 29 kJ, which means 100 ml of 70% proof spirit gives 31.5 g of alcohol or 222 kcal. Maintenance energy needs are met by alcoholic calories but the person remains malnourished because of the inadequate intake of nutrients. Thus, alcohol is a source of empty calories.

Moderate alcohol intake does not suppress the appetite; rather, it may increase it, but chronic alcohol consumption has the opposite effect. Heavy alcohol intake may suppress the appetite; hence, heavy drinkers tend to eat poorly.

In most studies, the average non-alcoholic calories are well below 1000 as more than 80% of patients with alcoholic liver disease have anorexia, nausea and vomiting leading to an inevitably reduced food intake.[10] As the food intake fails to meet basal energy requirements, body stores are catabolized to provide calories for resting energy expenditure.

Malabsorption

Alcohol causes inflammation of the stomach, pancreas and intestines. Impairment of pancreatic enzyme production hampers digestion and contributes to the malabsorption of nutrients. The absorption of thiamin, folate, vitamin B_{12}, and also of sodium, water and xylose is altered. Intestinal malabsorption and impaired folate hepatic storage contribute to folate deficiency.[11] Thiamin deficiency occurs in long-term alcohol users. Deficiency of vitamin A is partly dietary and partly due to steatorrhoea.

Altered metabolism

Hypermetabolism is associated with acute alcoholism. Hypoglycaemia occurs due to an increase in plasma insulin levels and insulin resistance. Hypertriglyceridaemia and liver steatosis is a common finding. High ammonia levels, and increased aromatic and sulphur-containing amino acid levels lead to neurological deterioration and hepatic coma. Acetaldehyde can interfere with the activation of vitamins by the liver cells. Low circulating levels of 25,OH vitamin D_3 (an active form of vitamin D) with increased conversion of vitamin D to polar metabolites is seen in cirrhotic patients.[12] The serum level of vitamin B_6 (pyridoxine) is low as aldehyde acts on hepatic vitamin B_6 stores and the vitamin cannot be converted to its metabolically active form by a diseased liver.

Altered requirements/synthesis

When more than half the total calories ingested come from alcohol, there is an increase in the metabolic need for some vitamins and minerals due to greater demands for tissue repair. The resting energy expenditure is often raised by hepatic inflammation and liver enzyme induction. The requirement of the B group of vitamins is also increased to metabolize alcohol.[13] The requirement of magnesium is higher as there is increased excretion resulting in the depletion of tissue magnesium, which may be associated with hypocalcaemia.[14] Alcohol may also increase urinary losses of zinc because of reduced synthesis of zinc-binding protein.[15]

In most alcoholics, the hepatic synthesis of transferrin is reduced, resulting in a low serum transferrin level, though serum iron levels may remain normal. Poor dietary intake, vomiting, diarrhoea and secondary hyperaldosteronism in patients with ascites cause hypokalaemia. The requirement of certain amino acids such as methionine might also change in alcoholics. Cirrhosis leads to decreased serum albumin levels with reduced hepatic synthesis. An increase in the plasma levels of aromatic amino acids (AAA) is seen with a decrease in BCAA.

Vicious cycle

The malnutrition–alcohol intake relationship is a vicious cycle because malnutrition enhances the destructive effect of alcohol on the liver and also causes GI changes that lead to malabsorption, thus augmenting the poor nutritional status.

Nutritional therapy in alcoholic liver disease

Whether malnutrition is the primary injurious factor or alcohol is the primary cause of liver disease independent of nutrition has been a topic of debate for some time. Nutritional therapy does not significantly influence the vascular complications of cirrhosis or reverse established fibrosis, but aids in the recovery of parenchymal functions in acute disease.[16,17]

Both nutritional and hepatotoxic factors may actually act synergistically. Alcohol increases the requirement for nutrients; in turn, nutritional deficiency may promote the toxic effect of alcohol. Even nutritionally adequate diets may fail to protect the liver from the toxic effects of alcohol as alcohol produces metabolic derangements and histological alterations.

Suggested nutrition therapy in alcoholic liver disease is as follows: besides abstinence from alcohol and rest, the achievement of a positive nitrogen balance either by the oral, enteral or parenteral route is important. A normal or high-protein diet is recommended, provided there is no encephalopathy. Increased protein intake is necessary to enhance the functional hepatic mass.

The minimum requirement for patients with alcoholic hepatitis to become anabolic is approximately 30 kcal/kg and 1 g of protein/kg a day.[18] If not orally, then enteral or intravenous nutritional supplements must be used for this purpose. Enteral nutrition is the preferred method of providing artificial nutrition in patients with advanced cirrhosis. Feeding an enteral formula to a malnourished patient with alcoholic liver disease increases the digestibility and absorption of fat and protein. The administration of BCAA up to 55 g/day may improve the nutritional parameters. Similarly, a casein hydrolysate providing a mean protein intake of 1.5 g/kg body-weight improves encephalopathy, albumin levels and liver functions. Nasoduodenal tube-fed, casein-based food supplements improve protein intake and enhance the nitrogen balance in patients.

A marked improvement is seen in the lean body mass, and potassium, phosphorus, serum retinol-binding protein, transferrin and bilirubin levels with a high protein intake and positive nitrogen balance by partial parenteral nutrition (PPN) supplements. Patients receiving PPN showed significant improvement and longer survival compared to those on standard hospital diets.[19]

Intravenous amino acids may help by stimulating the putative hepatotrophic factors—insulin/glucagon directly into the portal vein—and help in repairing the microsomal damage caused by alcohol.[10] Amino acid therapy results in better nitrogen balance and greater resolution of fat infiltration but has no effect on the histological findings. In cirrhotics, parenteral amino acid administration leads to a reduction in serum bilirubin level and improvement in other liver function tests with increased survival. The use of polysaturated lecithin might be a promising alternative. Malnourished and sick patients with alcoholic liver disease need zinc supplementation along with thiamin and vitamin A.[20,21]

CHRONIC LIVER DISEASE

In the absence of encephalopathy

Though cirrhotics have normal energy requirements with a basal energy consumption of 25–35 kcal/kg, in associated conditions such as metabolic stress, postoperative conditions, sepsis and GI bleed, the energy requirements may be as high as 35–45 non-protein kcal/kg for energy equilibrium.[22,23] Thus, to maintain protein anabolism and avoid fatty changes, maintenance of an energy and nitrogen balance is important. Well-compensated cirrhotics are probably in nitrogen equilibrium and so have a normal protein requirement compared to malnourished cirrhotics who are in negative nitrogen balance and have an increased protein requirement.[24,25]

Proteins should not be restricted in the absence of a prior history or current evidence of protein intolerance or encephalopathy as such patients tolerate protein in amounts comparable to normal individuals. To maintain a neutral nitrogen balance, protein consumption of 0.8–1 g/kg body-weight/day is sufficient for well-compensated, non-encephalopathic cirrhotics.[26] However, protein restriction is required during episodes of overt encephalopathy.

The nutritional status of patients can be improved by standard means, simply by increasing their nutritional intake either by encouraging them to eat normal food with or without oral supplements, or by enteral nutrition using standard polymeric enteral diets.[27]

An increase in nutritional intake and decrease in mortality is seen in cirrhotics on enteral feeding compared to those on normal hospital diets. In general, fat restriction is not necessary in cirrhotics, but patients who are intolerant to fatty foods need some restriction.[28] In cholestatic liver disease and steatorrhoea or in accompanying pancreatic insufficiency, dietary fat may be reduced. In these cases, dairy fat may be better tolerated than fried food. Medium-chain triglycerides (MCT) are good for malnourished cirrhotics with steatorrhoea since MCT bypass chylomicron formation and get absorbed directly into the portal circulation. Since prolonged use might cause essential fatty acid deficiency, MCT should be supplemented with linoleic acid.[29]

In the presence of encephalopathy

Since encephalopathy is most commonly precipitated by an acute GI bleed, septicaemia or electrolyte disturbance, efforts are directed towards treating these factors along with nutritional support designed to maintain homeostasis during liver failure and recovery.[30]

Whether nutritional support affects the outcome or only nutritional status or both remains an intriguing question for hepatologists. Various therapeutic modalities for encephalopathy have met with controversy over the years. As shown by kinetic studies, plasma amino acids are contributed mainly by protein breakdown within the body (endogenous rather than dietary protein); thus, instead of protein-free diets, some protein must be given to replace oxidative losses.

The treatment of hepatic encephalopathy is based on preventing the absorption of gut-derived toxins, mainly ammonia.[1] During the 1950s and 1960s, nitrogenous substances, including dietary protein, were thought to be the cause of the neuropsychiatric abnormalities associated with chronic liver disease, and withdrawing dietary protein for prolonged periods was widely advocated. Nearly two decades back, concern was expressed about the practice of restricting protein in cirrhotics mainly because of three factors: (i) most of these patients

(30%–70%) are malnourished; (ii) protein requirements are actually increased in cirrhotics; and (iii) there is evidence that patients with hepatic encephalopathy can tolerate high-protein diets and benefit from them.[31] In fact, a low-protein intake has been shown to be independently associated with worsening of hepatic encephalopthy.[1]

The European Association for Parenteral and Enteral Nutrition (ESPEN) consensus group recommends protein intake of 1–1.5 g/kg body-weight for cirrhotics depending on their degree of decompensation; however, protein restriction is avoided in patients with hepatic encephalopathy though, in some patients, a transient restriction to 0.5 g/kg body-weight may be necessary and, in rare cases of protein intolerance, daily protein restriction may be required. Additional nitrogen should be provided in the form of amino acid supplements.[32] Protein intolerance can also be dealt with by a standard protein formula of BCAA, casein-based diets and vegetable protein diets. A distributed meal pattern of 4–7 small meals throughout the waking hours along with a late-night snack of complex carbohydrates is recommended for optimum fuel utilization and nitrogen economy, thereby avoiding protein loading. Tolerance to dietary protein depends on its source. Dairy protein is tolerated better than protein from a mixed source and vegetable protein is better tolerated than meat protein, though 50 g of vegetable proteins are considered bulky and produce early satiety, abdominal distension, flatulence and diarrhoea.[1]

Branched-chain amino acids

The plasma amino acid profile changes, particularly in flux and oxidation. A higher concentration of AAA accumulate in the plasma; consequently, the exclusion of AAA or protein from the diet would cause negative nitrogen balance. BCAA (leucine, valine and isoleucine) are beneficial for malnourished patients with liver disease as BCAA, especially leucine, decreases muscle protein breakdown through the formation of ketoisocaproate. BCAA increase the synthesis of hepatic and muscle protein, and also serve as an energy source for muscle tissue. The use of BCAA results in marked improvement in the nitrogen balance, fat stores and anthropometric parameters.[33] BCAA are anticatabolic, thus promoting positive nitrogen balance and improving nutritional status in those with neurological dysfunction.[34] BCAA should be used only for patients with demonstrated intolerance to protein or those who have suboptimal protein intake for long periods, as patients with cirrhosis and malnutrition can be treated with standard protein instead of BCAA.[35,36] On the other hand, studies suggest that an increase in the dose of BCAA does not consistently increase protein synthesis or decrease degradation; but the situation may be different in severely malnourished or decompensated cirrhotics with hypercatabolic complications.[2]

Standard protein and amino acid solution

Orally administered protein from mixed sources is recommended for cirrhotics but in patients with encephalopathy, anorexia and ascites, the enteral route, bypassing the mouth and oesophagus, may be used. The osmolarity of the feeding formula is important. Feeding should be started at a low rate of 20–40 ml/hour supplying 20–30 g of protein/24 hours. Subsequently, the protein intake is increased successively by 10–20 g with careful monitoring of hepatic encephalopathy.[37] In fact, in patients at risk of encephalopathy, a central or peripheral venous infusion is preferable to the enteral route.

Casein-based diets

The exact mechanism of action of casein-based diets in chronic hepatic encephalopathy is not clear. Casein-based diets have a low ammoniagenic property and they are tolerated in a fashion similar to BCAA. Casein is a high-quality protein providing adequate amounts of essential amino acids (EAA). It has 22% of BCAA and a favourable ratio of BCAA:AAA, i.e. 2:1, and low methionine content. Casein-based, high-caloric supplements with protein equivalent to 143 g are well tolerated by patients with low-grade chronic encephalopathy.[37,38] Casein-based diets are especially advantageous for patients requiring fluid restriction and those with some degree of intestinal malabsorption.

Vegetable proteins

Vegetable protein might be useful for patients with encephalopathy as it has a low methionine content and rapid transit time, but diets based solely on vegetable protein become impractical because of their large volume and unpalatability.[39]

Salt and fluid

Chronic and subacute liver diseases manifest as ascites and peripheral oedema. Dietary sodium restriction is the key element since the total amount of sodium retained reflects the balance between dietary sodium intake, and urinary and non-urinary sodium losses.[40]

A rigid restriction of sodium to 10–20 mEq/day will control ascites even in patients with little or no sodium excretion. If diuretics are used, then a daily restriction of 60–80 mEq should not be followed on a long-term basis, as such a diet is unpalatable.

CHOLESTASIS

The severity of cholestasis depends on the site and degree of obstruction in the biliary system. In prolonged obstruction, steatorrhoea and fat-soluble vitamin deficiency may occur. In conditions such as sclerosing cholangitis, biliary atresia and primary or secondary biliary cirrhosis, dietary advice should be given to patients. Fat intake should be reduced, though not completely restricted; preferably, it should be given in the form of MCT. Supplements of fat-soluble vitamins should be provided on an empirical basis to all jaundiced patients. In case of inability to provide oral supplements, these vitamins should be given parenterally. In a nutshell, patients with obstructive jaundice should be provided a high-protein, high-energy, low-fat diet, preferably in the form of MCT, along with vitamins and minerals.

CONCLUSION

The liver plays a central role in metabolism. Hepatobiliary diseases disturb liver function leading to malnutrition. Inadequate intake further enhances liver damage. Hence, in diseases of the liver, dietary or nutritional management plays an important role. It is advisable to monitor the nutritional status of all patients with liver disease, especially those with chronic liver disease, and a modified diet with specific nutritional supplements should be provided to these patients. In patients with alcoholic hepatitis, FHF and decompensated chronic liver disease, nutritional support is an essential part of the treatment.

REFERENCES

1. Morgan MY. Nutritional aspect of liver and biliary disease. In: Bircher J, Benhamou JP, McIntyre N, Rizzetto M, Rodes J (eds). *Oxford textbook of clinical hepatology. Vol. 2.* 2nd ed. New York: Oxford University Press; 1999:1923–81.
2. Munoz SJ. Nutritional therapies in liver disease. *Semin Liver Dis* 1991;**4**:278–88.
3. Butterworth CE Jr, Weinsier RL. Malnutrition in hospital patients: Assessment and treatment. Goodhart RS, Shils ME (eds). In: *Modern nutrition in health and disease.* Philadelphia: Lea & Febiger; 1978:667–84.
4. Jelliffe DB. *The assessment of the nutritional status of the community.* Geneva: World Health Organization; 1966. WHO Monograph 53.
5. Dominioni L, Dionigi R. Immunological function and nutritional assessment. *J Parenter Enteral Nutr* 1987;**11**:70S–72S.
6. Shenkin A. Assessment of nutritional status: The biochemical approach and its problems in liver disease. *J Hum Nutr* 1979;**33**:341–9.
7. Merli M, Romiti A, Riggio O, Capocaccia R. Optimal nutritional indexes in chronic liver disease. *J Parenter Enteral Nutr* 1987; **11** (Suppl):S126–S129.
8. Forbes A, Wicks C, Marshall W, *et al.* Nutritional support in fulminant hepatic failure: The safety of lipid solutions. *Gut* 1987;**28**:1347–8.
9. Forbes A, Wicks C. Fulminant hepatic failure—nutrition and fat clearance. *Recent Advan Nutr* 1990;**1**:67–9.
10. Achord JL. Review of alcoholic hepatitis and its treatment. *Am J Gastroenterol* 1993;**88**:1822–31.
11. Herbert V. Correlation of folate deficiency with alcoholism and associated macrocytosis, anemia, and liver disease. *Ann Intern Med* 1963;**58**:977–88.
12. Hepner G. Abnormal vitamin D metabolism in patients with cirrhosis. *Am J Dig Dis* 1976;**21**:527–32.
13. Leevy CM, Thompson A, Baker H. Vitamins and liver injury. *Am J Clin Nutr* 1970;**23**:493–9.
14. Elin RJ. Magnesium metabolism in health and disease. *Dis Mon* 1988;**4**:161–218.
15. Weismann K. Zinc supplementation in alcoholic cirrhosis. *Acta Med Scand* 1979;**205**:361–6.
16. Sherlock S. Nutrition: The changing scene. *Lancet* 1984;**1**:436–8.
17. Achord J. Malnutrition and the role of nutritional support in alcoholic liver disease. *Am J Gastroenterol* 1987;**82**:1–4.

18. Morgan TR. Treatment of alcoholic hepatitis. *Semin Liver Dis* 1993;**4**:384–94.

19. Nasarallah SM, Galambos JJ. Amino acid therapy of alcoholic hepatits. *Lancet* 1980;**2**:1276.

20. McClain CJ, Sul C. Zinc deficiency in the alcoholic: A review. *Alcohol Clin Exp Res* 1983;**64**:527–35.

21. Hoyumpa AM Jr. Alcohol and thiamin metabolism. *Alcohol Clin Exp Res* 1983;**7**:11–14.

22. Shronts EP. Nutritional assessment of adults with end stage hepatic failure. *Nutr Clin Pract* 1988;**3**:113–19.

23. Qwen OE, Trapp VE, Richard A, *et al*. Nature and quantity of fuel compound in patients with alcoholic cirrhosis. *J Clin Invest* 1983;**72**:1821–32.

24. Mullen KD, Denne SC, McCullough AJ, *et al*. Leucine metabolism in stable cirrhosis. *Hepatology* 1986;**6**:622–30.

25. O' Keefe SJD, Abraham R, Davis M, Williams R. Protein turnover in acute and chronic liver disease. *Acta Chir Scand* 1980;**507** (Suppl):91–101.

26. Weber FL, Bagby BS, Licate L, Kelser SG. Effect of branched chain amino acid on nitrogen metabolism in patients with cirrhosis. *Hepatology* 1990;**11**:942–50.

27. Silk DB, O'Keefe SJ, Wicks C. Nutritional support in liver disease. *Gut* 1991; (Suppl):S29–S33.

28. Morgan MY. Enteral nutrition in liver disease. *Acta Chir Scand* 1981;**10** (Suppl):81–91.

29. Greenberg NJ, Skillman TG. Medium chain triglycerides. Physiologic considerations and clinical implications. *N Engl J Med* 1969;**280**:1045–58.

30. George L, Blackburn GL, Stephen J, O' Keefe D. Nutrition in liver failure [Editorial]. *Gastroenterology* 1989;**97**:1049–51.

31. Mendenhall CL, Tosch T, Weesner RE, *et al*. VA Cooperative study on alcoholic hepatitis II: Prognostic significance of protein–calorie malnutrition. *Am J Clin Nutr* 1986;**43**:213–18.

32. Plauth M, Merli M, Kondrup J, Weimann A, Ferenci P, Muller MJ. ESPEN guidelines for nutrition in liver disease and transplantation. *Clin Nutr* 1997;**16**:43–55.

33. Marchesini G, Dioguardi FS, Bianchi GP, *et al*. Long term oral branched chain amino acid treatment in chronic hepatic encephalopathy. A randomized, double blind, casein controlled trial. *J Hepatol* 1990;**11**:92–101.

34. Shanbhogue RLK, Bristrian BR, Lakshman K, *et al*. Whole body leucine, phenylalanine, and tyrosine kinetics in end stage liver disease before and after hepatic transplantation. *Metabolism* 1987;**36**:1047–53.

35. Morgan MY. Branched chain amino acids in the management of chronic liver disease: Facts and fantasies. *J Hepatol* 1990;**11**:133–41.

36. McCullough AJ, Muller KD, Tavill AS. Branched chain amino acid as nutritional therapy in liver disease: Dearth or surfeit? *Hepatology* 1983;**3**:269–71.

37. Smith J, Horowitz J, Henderson JM, Heymsfield S. Enteral hyperalimentation in undernourished patients with cirrhosis and ascites. *Am J Clin Nutr* 1982;**35**:56–72.

38. Hambraeus L. Importance of milk proteins in human nutrition: Physiological aspects. In: Galestool TE, Tinberger BJ, Wageninger P (eds). *Milk Proteins, 84*. Proceedings of the international congress on milk protein. Luxembourg, 1985.

39. Weber FL, Minco D, Fresard KM, Banwell JG. Effects of vegetable diets on nitrogen metabolism in cirrhotic subjects. *Gastroenterology* 1985;**85**:538–44.

40. Runyon BA. Treatment of patients with cirrhosis and ascites. *Semin Liver Dis* 1997;**17**:249–60.

Index

The letters 'b', 'f' and 't' after the numbers indicate boxes, figures and tables, respectively.